Hair Replacement Surgery

Springer
Berlin
Heidelberg
New York
Barcelona
Budapest
Hong Kong
London
Milan
Paris
Santa Clara
Singapore
Tokyo

P. Bouhanna J.-C. Dardour

Hair Replacement Surgery

Textbook and Atlas

Translated by D. le Vay

With 310 Figures, Some in Colour, and 18 Tables

Springer

Dr. Pierre Bouhanna
14, rue Théodore de Banville
75017 Paris
France

Dr. Jean-Claude Dardour
146, rue de Longchamps
75116 Paris
France

Translator:
Dr. David le Vay
6 Garstons
Burwash, East Sussex TN19 7EZ
England

ISBN 3-540-59030-7 Springer-Verlag Berlin Heidelberg New York

Library of Congress Cataloging-in-Publication Data. Bouhanna, P. (Pierre), 1947- [Chirurgie de la calvitie. English] Hair replacement surgery: textbook and atlas/P. Bouhanna, J.-C. Dardour. p. cm. Includes bibliographical references and index. ISBN 3-540-59030-7 (hardcover) 1. Hair - Transplantation. 2. Scalp - Surgery. 3. Baldness - Surgery. I. Bouhanna, P. (Pierre), 1947- . II. Dardour, J.C. III. Title, [DNLM: 1. Alopecia - surgery. 2. Alopecia - atlases. 3. Scalp - surgery. 4. Scalp - atlases. 5. Hair - physiology. 6. Hair - atlases. WR 460 8759c 1996a] RD121.5.86813 1996 617.4'779-dc20 DNLM/DLC for Library of Congress 96-31817

Cover design: Springer-Verlag, E. Kirchner

Typesetting: Thomson Press (India) Ltd., New Delhi

SPIN: 10497348 23/3132/SPS - 5 4 3 2 1 0 - Printed on acid-free paper

Contents

Introduction

The subject we deal with here is male baldness, often still termed androgenic or androgenetic baldness. Very important research studies have shown that practically 98% of men who are losing or who have lost their hair have at some time or other taken steps to try to arrest this process. In other words, only those who are not affected by baldness are indifferent to it. And it is surprising how many preventive consultations are sought by people whose hair is normal, but who are simply afraid that the day may come when they will lose it.

It is precisely because the ideal procedure, preventive as well as curative, does not yet exist that so many treatments have been suggested. The physician or surgeon desirous of treating baldness must therefore be acquainted with and practice all these techniques.

Male baldness is in fact not a single entity, but consists of numerous types. Each calls for its specific treatment, and the aim of a good classification should be to take account of the greatest number of factors, or at least the more important ones, as simply as possible.

The surgeon's own experience will fill in any gaps, in the knowledge that ultimately it is as important to treat the scalp as what is beneath it: the brain.

Anatomy

Hair

Embryology

The embryological origin of the hair is twofold:

- Ectodermal: the hair itself and the pilo-sebaceous follicle
- Mesodermal: the dermal papilla

The hair appears in the third month of fetal life by invagination of the basal germinal layer of the epidermis. A small bud progressively embeds itself in the mesenchyma, and the lower end of this progressive elongation becomes depressed and hollowed out to form a compartment colonised by mesenchymal cells, the future dermal papilla (Fig. 1).

Two swellings develop in these pilo-sebaceous rudiments: one superior, giving rise to the sebaceous gland, functional and secreting lipid droplets from the 17th week, the other below the bulb at which the mesenchymally derived arrector muscle of the hair is attached.

The synthesis of melanin pigment begins around the fourth month after the formation of pigment cells (melanocytes) derived from the neural crest. The origin of the lines of implantation of the scalp hair constitutes the "crown", whose centre is situated at the top of the vertex; the curving lines of hair distribution diverge progressively as they depart from the centre of the crown (Fig. 2a,b). Thus formed, the hair serves as a model for subsequent hair cycles. The first cycle occurs from the 22nd week of fetal life, and subsequent hair cycles follow throughout life.

Macroscopy

The different aspects of the hair are genetically determined and vary widely from one individual to another, and with race and sex, and even in the same individual depending on the region of the scalp and his or her age. Thus, in man the hair assumes four aspects in succession: at first, the unpigmented intrauterine lanugo, then the down of the infant lacking a medulla, then the thicker and pigmented intermediate hair and finally the terminal hair that appears at puberty. The hair

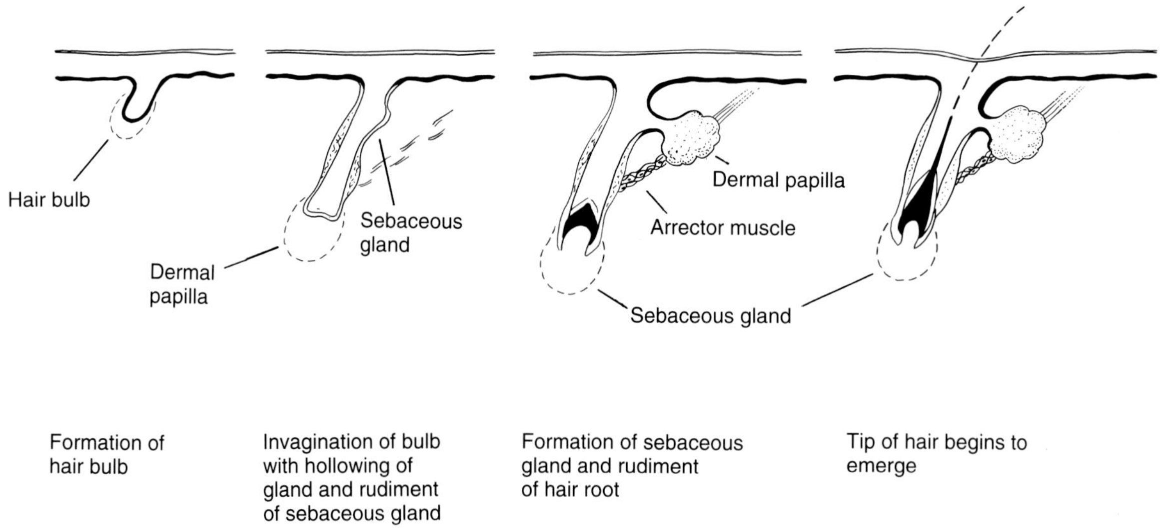

Fig. 1. Foetal development of the hair bulb

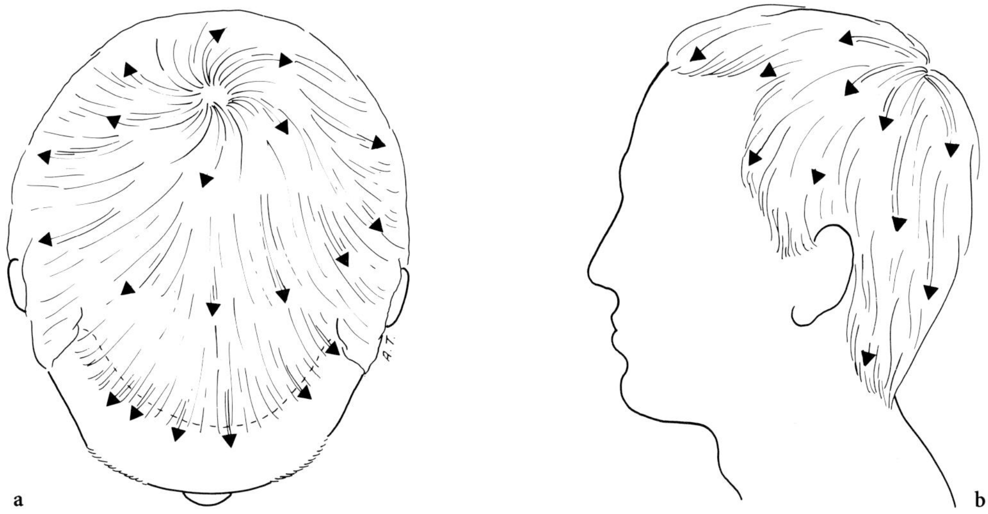

Fig. 2a,b. Direction of emergence of the hairs

has physical properties which determine the following:

Visual and Textural Characteristics

Colour

Colour is classified into ten shades, from black to very light blond. Red hair is just a subdivision of chestnut shades.

Shape

Four types of hair may be routinely distinguished:

- Stiff
- Ringleted, wavy
- Frizzy
- Crinkly

The shape of the hair stem corresponds to the shape of its cross-section:

- Stiff hair has a round section.
- Wavy hair has an oval section.
- Frizzy hair is flattened in section.

Shape and colour are determined by heredity and ethnic origin:

- Shades and varieties are numerous in the white races.
- Asiatics usually have markedly pigmented and stiff hair.
- Negroid populations have dark, crinkly hair.

We have sometimes observed a transient modification of the stems of grafted hairs, which become frizzy.

Thickness

Thickness varies from 50 to 90 µm (in white races); the hair is rather thicker in black people and may reach 120 µm in Asiatics. The hair is usually finer in women.

Texture

The hair stem is normally smooth and soft, but certain external insults may make it rough and raspy.

Greasiness

The hair is usually shiny, neither too greasy nor too dry. It may become dry and often lacklustre after various insults. Excessive seborrhoea can make it too greasy, shiny and sticky and less bouffant.

Tonicity

Normal hair should have a certain degree of tonicity and not fall back limply after lifting a lock; only suitable shampoo allows maintenance of this tonicity.

Laxity

Usually supple and more or less "lively", the hair may become brittle and very fragile, due to congenital anomalies or to certain external insults.

Mechanical Properties

The mechanical properties of hair are essentially its resistance and its elasticity.

Resistance and Firmness

Normally, the hair should resist traction until its avulsion from the scalp (rupture load), which takes place between 60 and 90 g for normal European hair of 60–90 μm diameter, 100–110 g for Asiatic hair and 40–60 g for Negro hair.

Elasticity

Elasticity has been studied by measuring the stretching of hair depending on the load applied. The hair can elongate by up to 30% before undergoing irreversible changes in texture; this stretching is considerably increased when it is damp.

Quantitative Data

Density

The density of hair per square centimetre varies with age (considerable in the newborn, less after 50 years) and with the regions of the scalp. On average, in the adult, density ranges from 200 to 400 hairs/cm^2, but this density may decrease enormously in androgenetic alopecia.

A cylindrical graft of 5 mm in diameter, i.e. 19.6 mm^2, may thus consist theoretically of 20–80 hairs, whereas a graft of 4 mm (12.56 mm^2) will have 15–50 hairs. In practice, we have counted between eight and 25 hairs on average on a graft of 4 mm in diameter (Photos 1, 2).

One to three hairs may naturally emerge from a single orifice (uni-, bi- or trigeminal); this is a genetically transmitted characteristic.

Total Number of Hairs

In a full head of hair there are 100–150000 hairs over a total surface area of 600–700 cm^2.

Implantation

The hairs are implanted obliquely in the scalp. The direction of implantation varies with the region:

- Downward in the occipital region.
- Forward in the frontal and tonsural regions.
- Downward and slightly forward in the parietal regions.
- At the vertex there is a point (sometimes two symmetric points) where the hairs are arranged in a radiating and rather spiral manner.

The direction of implantation should be constantly observed in the surgical treatment of baldness (Fig. 2).

Interaction of All These Factors

The apparent clinical density depends on the number of hairs per square centimetre and their thickness. The covering power of the hair is very variable:

- Dry hair is more bouffant than damp or greasy hair.
- Wavy hair has better covering power than stiff or curly hair, but is unattractive if too long. On the

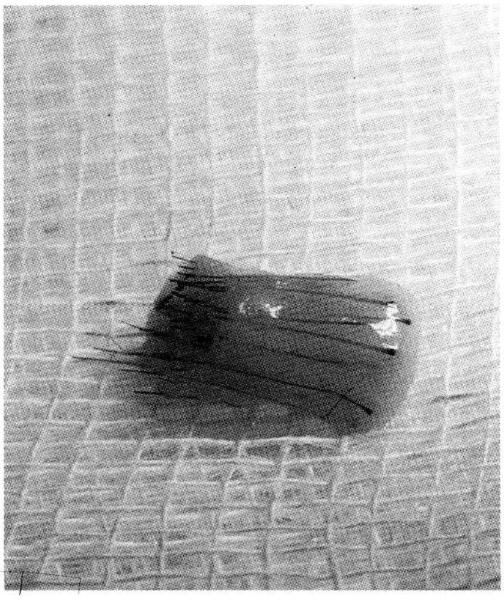

Photo 1. A graft 4 mm in diameter may include between eight and 25 hairs. Note that one to three hairs may emerge at a single orifice

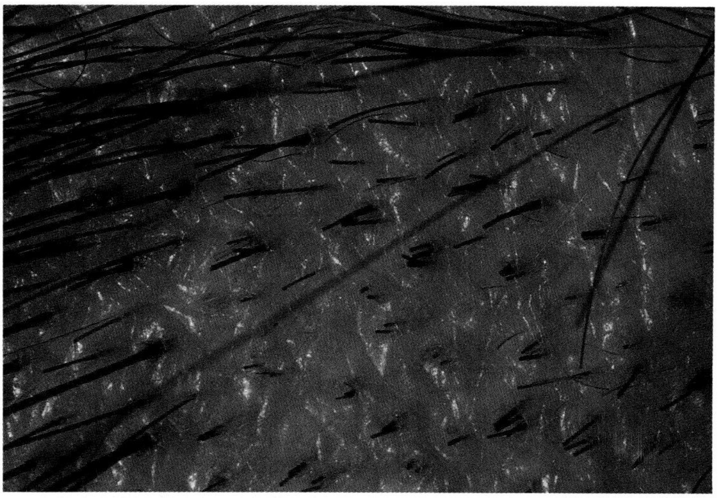

Photo 2. Emergence of one to three hairs per skin orifice

other hand, stiff hair has good covering power when very long, provided it is styled.
- The crinkly hair of Blacks has excellent covering power in situ but not at a distance. A few grafts suffice to give it an agreeable appearance.
- Dark hair has better covering power than fair hair, but is less tolerant of lack of uniformity. This is why grafts give a "doll's hair" or "leek row" aspect in dark-haired persons, whereas the effect is more blurred in blond or greying individuals and gives them an acceptable appearance.

Optical Microscopy

The hair is divided into two parts: the stalk and the root.

Shaft

The shaft is the part of the hair visible at the scalp surface and is free and mobile. Its length varies (and may reach over a meter) and its diameter varies from 60 to 100 μm. The shaft consists of three concentric layers: cuticle, cortex and medulla:

- The cuticle, totally keratinised, consists of square, flattened cells, imbricated in scales like roof-tiles. They have no nuclei or pigment and their free edge faces upward; this layer is very important in protection and appearance.
- The cortex is the most important part of the hair shaft. It is formed of completely keratinised, elongated cells containing pigment (as melanin granules). It therefore forms the central part of the shaft and is largely responsible for its mechanical properties.
- The medulla is the central column, sometimes discontinuous, composed of non-nucleated and loosely interconnected cells. It is weakly pigmented.

Thus the structures of the shaft amount to the juxtaposition of completely keratinised cells cemented by amorphous material.

Root

The root (Fig. 3, Photo 3), also called the bulb or follicle, is the fixed part of the hair, implanted obliquely in the scalp, with its lower pole swollen like a bulb and hollowed into a papilla, where the nutrient elements of the hair arrive. It is surrounded by a sort of sac (hair follicle), itself formed of two epithelial sheaths (internal and external); one or more sebaceous glands, as well as an erector muscle of the hair, are appended to the follicle, forming a true pilosebacous entity.

Transverse and longitudinal sections of the hair follicle under optical microscopy (Photo 4a,b) reveal, from the periphery towards the centre, the vitreous membrane, the sebaceous glands and the arrector muscle of the hair.

The vitreous membrane, a fibrous sac made of dense connective tissue, surrounds the external epithelial sheath, consisting of glycogen-rich cells, and the internal epithelial sheath, formed of two cell layers, both rich in trichyalin:

- The unicellular sheath of Henle
- The stratified sheath of Huxley

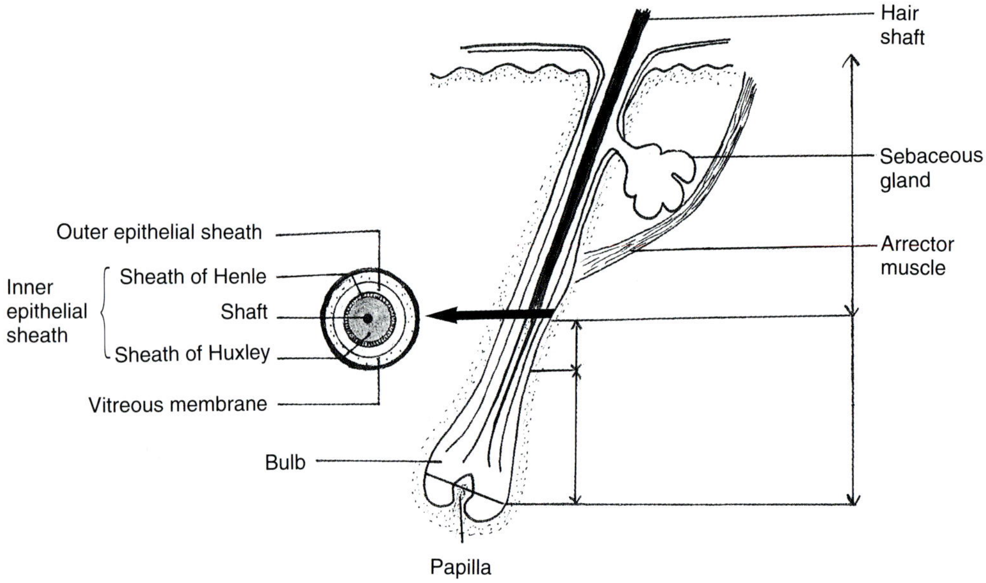

Fig. 3. Longitudinal and transverse sections of a hair

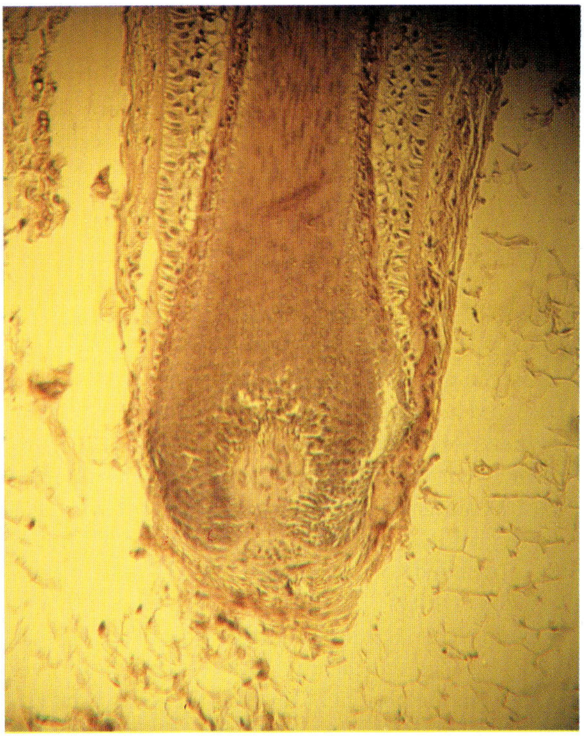

Photo 3. Section of root

These structures envelop the shaft, which was described above.

In longitudinal section, the base of the bulb near the dermal papilla constitutes the epidermal matrix. It is filled with very active germinal or matrix cells arranged around the dermal axis formed by the papilla. These cells become keratinised and progressively lose their nuclei to become the cortical cells of the hair shaft, whereas the melanocytes are interposed among the matrix cells. One or more sebaceous glands and the erector muscle of the hair are appended to the hair follicle.

The sebaceous glands are acinous glands of the simple alveolar holocrine type that are seven to eight

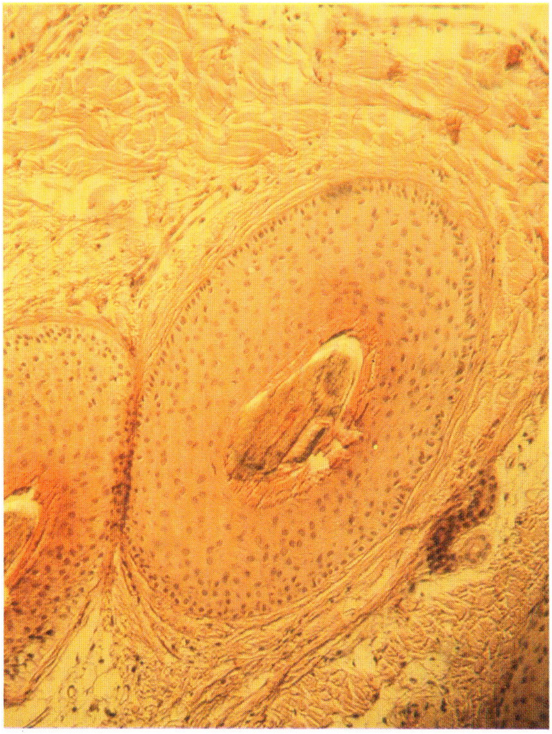
a

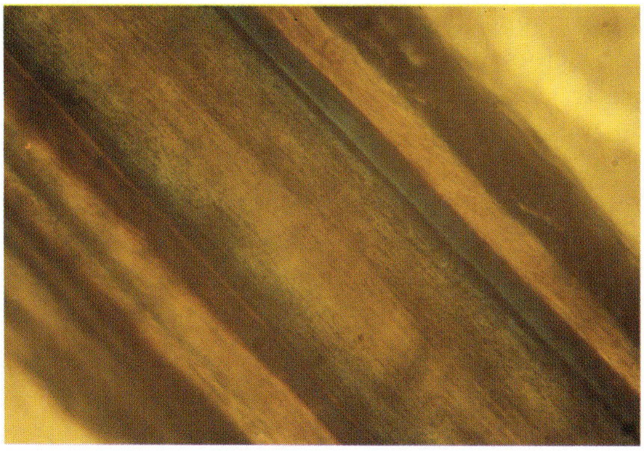
b

Photo 4. a Transverse section and **b** longitudinal section of hair follicle

times as numerous on the scalp (700/cm^2) than on the rest of the body. The dimensions of the glands are inversely proportional to the diameter of the hair.

The arrector muscle of the hair is situated in the obtuse angle between the hair and the dermis. It is formed of smooth muscle fibres, inserted deeply on the fibrous sac and superficially at the dermal papilla. It is innervated by sympathetic fibres.

Electron Microscopy

The ultrastructure of keratinised hair is as follows:

Structure of Cuticle

Human hair is surrounded by seven to ten layers of cuticular cells imbricated like the tiles of a roof. Each cuticular cell (whose external membrane is 5–25 μm thick) consists of lamellar components organised in three principal layers:

- Layer A, rich in cystine (40 μm thick)
- The exocuticle (0.2 μm)
- The endocuticle (0.1 μm)

The junction between the two last layers is often irregular.

Structure of Cortex

Two types of cortical cells can be distinguished:

- The cells of the paracortex, which have a very dense macrofibrillary content
- The cells of the orthocortex, whose fibrils are less dense and arranged like a fingerprint

The cortical cells are very coherent, fusiform and orientated along the hair axis; they are 3–6 μm wide and 100 μm in length. They contain nuclear remnants of stellate aspect in transverse section ("muscle ghosts"), surrounded by densely packed macrofibrils, each a cylinder of 0.10–0.40 μm in diameter and of variable length, but often the entire length of the cell. Between the macrofibrils there is a variable amount of intermacrofibrillary matrix and melanin granules. The macrofibrils consist of packed microfibrils (7 μm in diameter) arranged in a spiral and embedded in an intermicrofibrillary matrix; the microfibrils themselves consist of protofibrils (0.2 μm in diameter), formed of two or three polypeptide chains in an alpha helix.

Medulla

Medulla is found only in the terminal part of the hair and may be continuous, discontinuous or even absent. The medullary cells have lost their nuclei and organelles; they consist of large vesicles, granules and proteinic filaments. These cells have both intra- and extracellular air spaces.

Histological Changes in Male Baldness

Initially, the hair follicle shows collagen degeneration around the vessels; then the follicle becomes progressively smaller, while the proportion of quiescent follicles increases. The atrophic follicles become more superficial in the subcutaneous fat, far from their original position. At the same time, the diameter of the hairs decreases from 0.08 mm to around 0.005 mm. However, electron microscopy does not show any change in the ultrastructure of the hair sheath at this stage.

The degree of atrophy varies from one hair to another and there is no obvious modification in the sebaceous or sweat glands, nor any signs of inflammation. The erector muscles atrophy, but to a much lesser degree than the follicle. It may be concluded that, in baldness, the hair follicles are not dead but simply increasingly atrophic. It is perhaps not illusory to conceive the possible discovery of a substance which would allow the bulb to regain its initial shape and function. In his thesis, Bouhanna has reported the "stimulating" effect of postoperative phenomena on the growth and pigmentation of the bulb.

Chemical Composition

Keratins

The hair essentially consists of a fibrous protein of high molecular weight, keratin (Fig. 4), which is characterised by the following:

- Its strictly intracellular site (mainly in the cortical cells)
- Its insolubility and resistance to proteolytic enzymes
- Its structure, consisting of polypeptide chains containing 18 amino acids, of which the most important are tyrosine and especially cystine (15%–16%); it is rich in sulphur, but cystine is found only in minimal amounts. These chains are parallel, very elongated and orientated in the axis of the hair shaft.

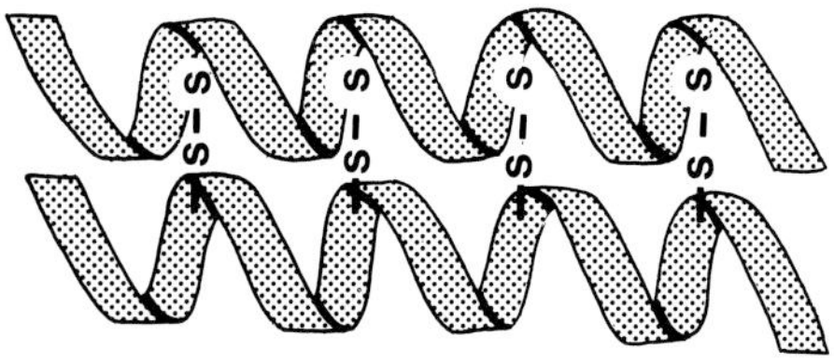

Fig. 4. Structure of keratins: polypeptide chains with disulphur bonds

X-ray diffraction methods have shown, in the unstretched human hair, an organisation of the polypeptide chains stabilised in an alpha helix (diameter, 9.8 Å) by hydrogen bonds. The cohesion between adjacent chains is essentially maintained by disulphur bonds (-S-S-) between the cystine residues, derived from the combination of two cysteine molecules (SH groups) during keratinisation, and by an oxidation – reduction reaction. However, this cohesion is also ensured by more labile linkages: hydrogen bonds, saline bonds (electrovalences), Van der Waal forces (hydrophobe linkages); rupture of these linkages, especially of the covalent disulphur linkages (largely responsible for the cohesion of keratin) by different external agents may lead to instability of the molecular structure.

Biochemical analysis of the cortex makes it possible to specify its composition, which comprises 40% of fibrillary protein (in alpha helix), poor in sulphur. The amorphous matricial substance is also joined to the organised fibrillary structures by strong disulphur bonds (Fig. 4).

Within the hair itself several structural keratins seem to exist whose composition is not constant, as they are subject to modification by individual genetic factors, diet and various toxic agents. Finally, chemical analyses have shown the presence of traces of metals (Ca, Cd, Cr, Cu, Hg, Zn, Pb, Fe, As and Se) in the form of cations, most of which derive from the environment and are integrated in the hair fibres by linkage with the lateral chains of the proteins.

All previous studies have shown that there is no alteration in the chemical composition of the hair in cases of baldness.

Natural Colouration of Hair

Hair colour is genetically determined by a pigment, the melanin manufactured by the melanocytes. These are essentially active in the anagenic phase of the hair cycle. They exist in the upper part of the bulb in the form of granules or melanosomes, which are then transferred into the cortical cells of the shaft. The granules are distributed throughout the cortex, but with a greater peripheral concentration in the paracortex.

The pigmentation of the hair is due to two types of melanin:

- Eumelanin, contained in the large melanosomes shaped like rice grains, which gives the darker hues

- Pheomelanin, contained in small ellipsoidal or spherical melanosomes, responsible for light colours

The two pigments often co-exist and their relative proportions determine the immense variety of natural shades of the hair, the colour of which also depends on the quality, localisation and especially the distribution of the pigment granules.

Melanin is a polymer of high molecular weight, insoluble in water and in most other solvents. It is of weak chemical reactivity and can only be broken down by intense oxidation reactions or by very concentrated alkaline solutions (the active agents of bleaches). Eumelanin is formed biochemically by the polymerisation of dopaquinone, itself derived from the conversion of tyrosine into dopa and then into dopaquinone by means of tyrosinase.

Dopaquinone may be combined with cysteine to give cysteinyldopa, which polymerises into pheomelanin. Recent discoveries have shown possible interference between these routes of synthesis, due to the possible formation of a co-polymer derived from the two melanins and suggesting the existence of several varieties of melanin.

Action of External Agents

Water

Keratin has a special affinity for water, absorption of which can lead to rapid swelling of the hair due to porosity by up to 30%–40% of its dry weight. as it penetrates into the fibres, the water molecules relax their cohesion and act on the linkages between the chains – the saline bonds and especially the hydrogen bonds – inserting themselves between the polypeptide chains, which is how damp hair loses its waviness. If it is dried while this stretching is maintained, it keeps the fold imparted to it, but only temporarily until the next time it becomes wet.

Permanent Waving

Permanent waving is based on rupture of the disulphur bonds by the action of a caustic agent such as soda or reducing agents. Recent findings seem to indicate that this action takes place mainly at the level of the disulphur bonds between the amorphous substance and the organised fibrillary structures, thus destabilising the whole hair; then, when moulded on the roller, a different restructuring of these linkages takes place. The hair, thus chemically altered and then rearranged, retains its new shape even after several shampooings.

Sun

In the presence of oxygen and in high-dosage, ultraviolet light acts essentially by oxidant hydrolysis, further augmented by the ambient humidity, not only on the colour, having a lightening effect, but also on the structure of the keratin, weakening the disulphur bonds, the hair becoming brittle, lacklustre and rough. The same effects can also result from various traumatic or chemical insults, such as oxidative dyes and incautious permanent waving.

Temperature

The hair is resistant to heat up to 145°C.

Special Features of Hair

Static Electrical Phenomena

The hair is tricho-electric, i.e. it becomes charged with static electricity by friction. This charge is negative, the keratin having an anionic tendency due to the presence of acid-base poles. This explains the possibilities of fixation of microbes, pollutants etc., as well as the possible repulsion of the hairs between themselves, with resulting difficulties in styling.

Dry Hair, Greasy Hair

As will be seen later, the variable degree of greasiness of the hair is due essentially to the fluidity of the sebum (and partly to its rate of excretion onto the scalp).Conversely, hair insufficiently lubricated with sebum becomes sensitive to every trauma and will become brittle and rough.

Split Ends (Trichoptylosis)

While the main portion of the shaft is protected by a cuticle (seven to ten cell layers), at the tip this is progressively diminished to one to two layers, rendering it more fragile, especially after incautious handling (brushing, some forms of waving, etc.), leading to splitting of the fibres into two (trichoptylosis) or even more branches (trichoclasia, "split ends").

Seborrhoea and Dandruff

In the normal state, in the epidermis of the scalp, the phenomena of cellular renewal and of desquamation of the cells of the superficial horny and normally keratinised layer (corneocytes) lead to separation of the cells and their elimination, usually invisible to the naked eye. Dysfunction arises from increased production of the basal cells, and thus of epithelial turnover, and an acceleration of these desquamation phemonena. Thus, the more superficial cells no longer have time to separate (remaining joined by their desmosomes), nor to keratinise, because of the over-rapid migration of the cells to the surface. Thus dandruff consists essentially of cell agglomerates, often still nucleated (in parakeratosis). There is a distinction between pityriasis simplex (often due to dryness of the scalp and with more or less seasonal exacerbations) and its coexistence with excessive seborrhoea, which makes the greasy scales stick together (steatoid pityriasis).

The exact cause is obscure. The role of saprophytic microbial flora (particularly pityrosporum ovale) and of general factors (e.g. nervous, digestive) is debatable. It should be noted that the most effective anti-dandruff treatments are keratolytics and may lead to elimination of the horny layers. These have a role in reabsorption of the sebum, which may account for the accelerated relubrication of the hair after such treatments.

Seborrhoea is due to hypersecretion of the sebaceous glands. In the normal state, the sebum (which contains 92%–100% of lipids, a mix of squalene, triglycerides and waxes) has a beneficial action on the hair, making it glossy and soft by providing a protective coating with a bacteriostatic role. After its excretion, the sebum migrates onto the hair and impregnates the superficial horny cells, and this passage is accelerated by brushes, combs or the fingers passing through the hair.Thus, the rheological properties of the sebum are very important in lubrication of the hair, producing a greasier appearance when more fluid.

The determination of sebaceous hypersecretion itself is essentially hormonal and probably genetically programmed. Certain pilo-sebaceous receptors have a greater aptitude for ensuring the local metabolism of androgens (role of 5-alpha-reductase), dihydrotestosterone stimulating directly the biosynthesis of the lipid sebaceous material. The role of the nervous system and other factors is not clearly demonstrable. Some authors have suggested a possible regulation of secretion by a feedback mechanism. Finally, as we have seen, the horny layers may have an action on the reabsorption of sebum at the surface of the scalp.

As regards the consequences of very frequent shampooing on seborrhoea, it has been definitely shown that even after daily shampooing there is no change in the rate of excretion of sebum; on the contrary, the kinetics of relubrication of the hair varies with the type of shampoo and the treatment applied, as the sebum may then undergo certain modifications of its rheologic properties (more fluidity etc.).

Scalp

Microscopy (Photo 5)

Histological Section

A histological section of the skin of the scalp reveals the following:

- The epidermis (0.1 mm thick) – this is a keratinised malpighian epithelium and therefore consists of several successive layers (from the outside in-

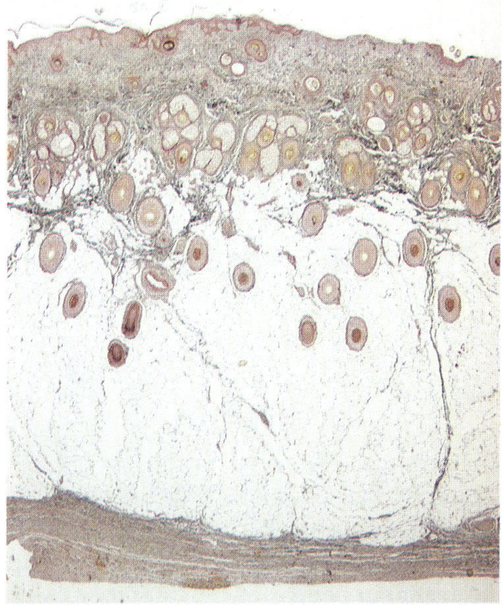

Photo 5. Histological section of scalp. The hair bulbs are located at a mean depth of 3.5 mm

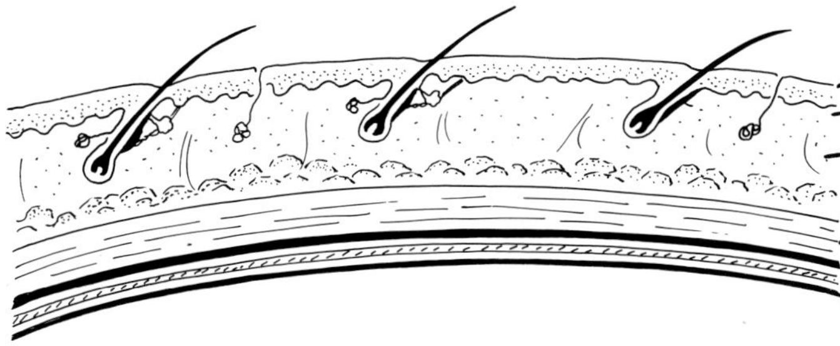

Fig. 5. The different planes of the scalp

wards: granular layer, filamentous layer, basal layer).

- The dermis – this is separated from the epidermis by a variably thick basal membrane. It contains dermal cells (fibroblasts, histiocytes), a framework of fibres (collagen, elastic, reticular fibres), itself coated by basic substance. It comprises two successive layers, the superficial or papillary dermis (0.2 mm) and the reticular dermis (1.1 mm).

The dermis is traversed by multiple blood-vessels. Ascending branches traverse the superficial fascia, only a few branches leading to the hypodermis, and join the subdermal plexus, which then reaches the very rich subpapillary or subdermal plexus, from which collateral branches emerge for the pilo-sebaceous systems and the terminal arterioles [2].

The Different Layers (Fig. 5)

In addition to the skin, which is described above, the following layers are present (from the inside outwards):

- The periosteum, a thin membrane which covers the entire outer table of the cranium up to the lines of attachment of the muscles. It is embedded and firmly fixed at the sutures, which makes its excision difficult at this site, whereas over the rest of this area it is easy to strip despite its thinness and fragility.
- The space of Merkel, a zone made up of loose and relatively avascular connective tissue; this is a very strippable zone, clearly demarcated from the second layer.
- The supraperiosteal layer, a quite thin but resistant layer, easily stripped, which appears to be closely joined with the periosteum itself at the lateral aspects of the cranium, continuing jointly with it on the aponeurosis of the temporal muscle at the superior curved temporal line. On the other hand, the superficial aspect of this layer is firmly attached to the third and overlying layer.
- The subepicranial layer, attached to the superficial aspect of the supraperiosteal layer by very dense and tenacious fibrous tracts, giving a fleecy aspect and rasping on dissection. The subepicranial layer is well marked and quite firm, but even macroscopically the orientation of its constituent fibres differs from that of the supraperiosteal layer.
- Above this layer, there is a component of spiderweb texture, the epicranial aponeurosis itself. Its thinnness and fragility, the structure of its weave made of interlacing fibres in a single layer and its great adherence to the overlying layers render its dissection awkward. Its deep aspect appears shaggy with a fine down, a residue of the tracts of the space of Merkel. Its superficial aspect is joined with the overlying layer, especially at the mid-line and up to 3 cm on either side of it.
- The supra-epicranial layer, like the subepicranial layer, is easily identified, though more difficult to dissect, especially when approaching the mid-line. Its aspect corresponds entirely to that described for the subepicranial layer, but it seems to stop at a convex margin at the periphery of the cranial vault. There, in the manner of an intermediate tendon, the fronto-occipital muscles and the superior and anterior auricular muscles attach. This aspect is reinforced when the dissection is continued towards the muscles, particularly at the two frontal muscles, which are separated at the mid-line; it then seems to divide into small, closely packed strips of at most 0.5 cm in width. The classical authors always described the epicranial aponeurosis and the supra-epicranial layer as a single structure, the galea aponeurotica, giving attachments to the "cutaneous muscles of the scalp", whereas in fact the epicranial aponeurosis appears in dissec-

tions as a thin layer divided between one part that covers the cranium and another belonging to the scalp proper.
- Above the supra-epicranial layer there is a thick, dense superficial fascia, whose deep aspect can be very easily separated from the supra-epicranial layer, but whose superficial aspect is much less readily detached from the overlying dermis. It is this fascia which sends fibrous septa vertically and very deeply into the hypodermis, which divide this fatty layer into small separate compartments.
- Above these six layers is the variably thick hypodermis (2.5–4.5 mm) with the subcutaneous fatty tissue, lobulated by strands of connective elastic tissue.

Implantation of Hair Follicles

In the scalp the hair follicle is within the hypodermis. Whatever the zone (temporal, parietal etc.), the bulb is always an average of 3.5 mm from the surface (Photo 5) and in the hypodermis [13]. However, there are major variations with age, sex and ethnicity.

Scalp Vessels

The scalp vessels have no tendency to contractility and spontaneous haemostasis for the following reasons [15]:

- In the subdermal plexuses the arteries are always gaping because of their strong adherence to the surrounding connective tissue.
- At the galea, the vessels travel in a fascio-aponeurotic double-layered compartment between the superficial fascia and supra-epicranial layer and adhere to it, forming kinds of sinuses which do not stretch and hardly contract when cut.
- Finally, it should be noted that, in the elderly, the vessel walls are often thickened, especially in the capillaries and postcapillary venules [1, 7, 9].

Glands

Glands are mainly sebaceous and attached to the hair follicle, into which they empty their lipid (holocrine) excretions; there are one or more per follicle, situated in the middle dermis, and they have a racemose arrangement. The sweat (exocrine) glands are tubed glands with an excretory duct. They predominate mainly at the forehead.

Variations

With Age. The hypodermis is thicker than in the young, and vascularisation, especially terminal, decreases after the age of 60. This implies very great caution in the shaping of flaps.

With Race. The pilo-sebaceous follicles are curved and superficial in the scalp in black races. In contrast, they are straight and deep in Asiatics. This factor must be considered in the taking of grafts.

Macroscopy [23, 27, 30, 31]

Topography

Boundaries

The scalp is an anatomic entity covering the top of the skull and is defined by the presence of hair (currently, or formerly in the case of baldness). It is bounded in front by the frontal region, laterally by the auricular and mastoid region and behind by the smooth lower part of the nape of the neck.

Relations

Superficial Relations. At the front, the frontal region is bounded by the frontal and temporal lines of hair implantation. These two lines are convex at the front join to follow a concave line of variable depth called the fronto-temporal recession. The temporal line is variably sited and often tends to recede as baldness increases. The frontal line forms an acute angle with the frontal plane which tends to increase with baldness, thus adding to the depth of the fronto-temporal recession.

In women and children, the frontal and temporal lines are sometimes continuous without any recession, and this may constitute a secondary sex characteristic (Photos 6–9). In cases of frontal baldness, the frontal muscle and therefore the zone of superior forehead mobility defines its boundary with the scalp.

As will be seen, in our classification we have termed the anterior frontal line *f*, the temporal line *t* and the deepest point of the recession *G*. During the

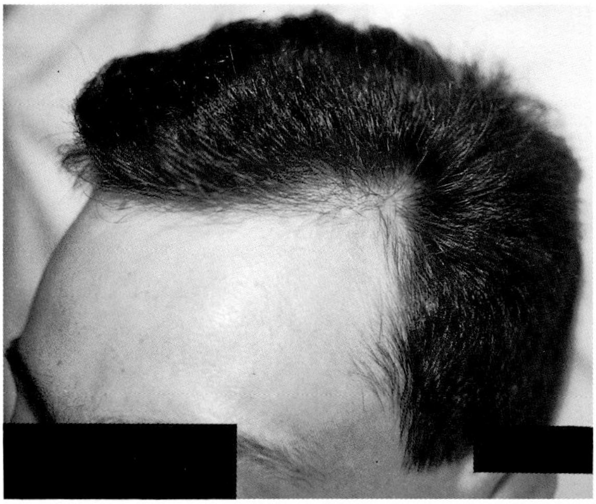

Photo 6. Harmonious fronto-temporal line of implantation in man with deep fronto-temporal recession

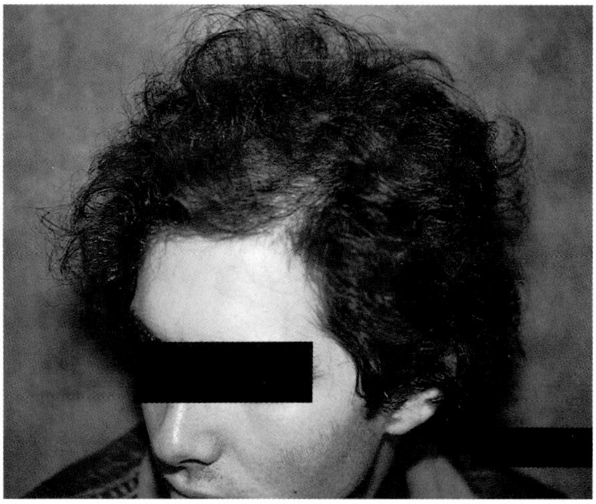

Photo 7. Absence of fronto-temporal recession in young boys, often of Latin American origin

a

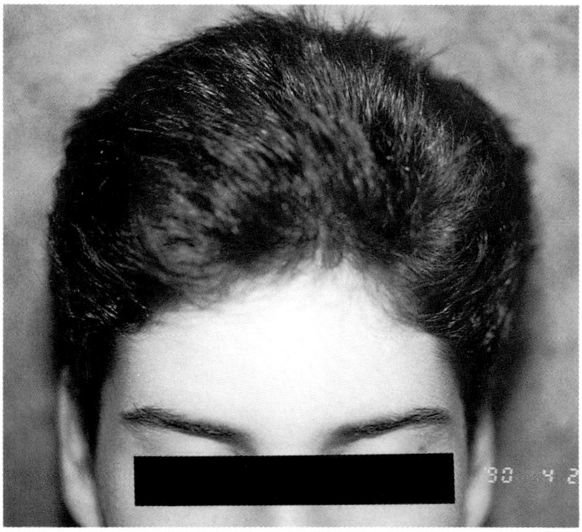

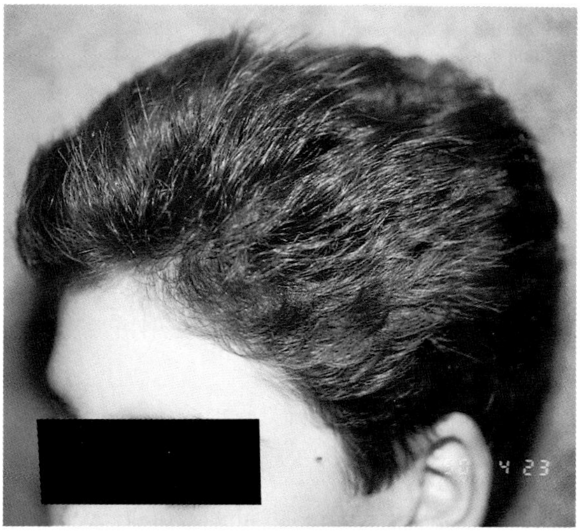

b

Photo 8a,b. Anterior line in male child

a

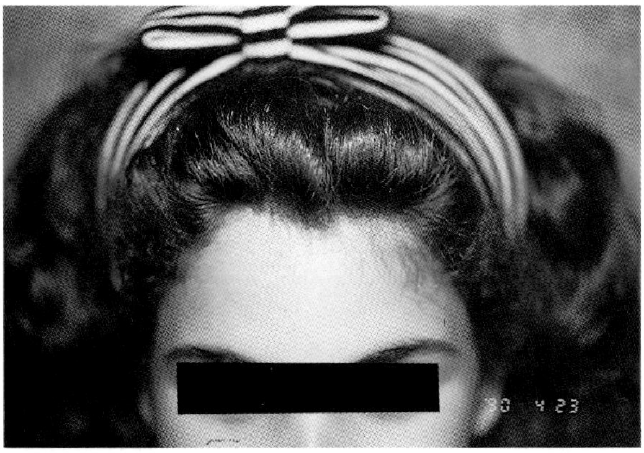

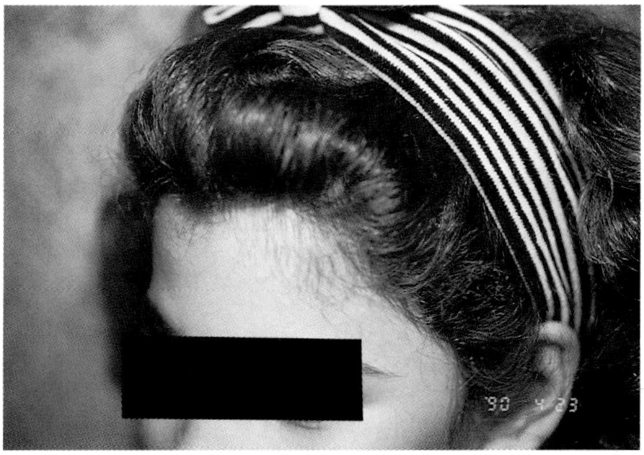

b

Photo 9a,b. Anterior line in female child

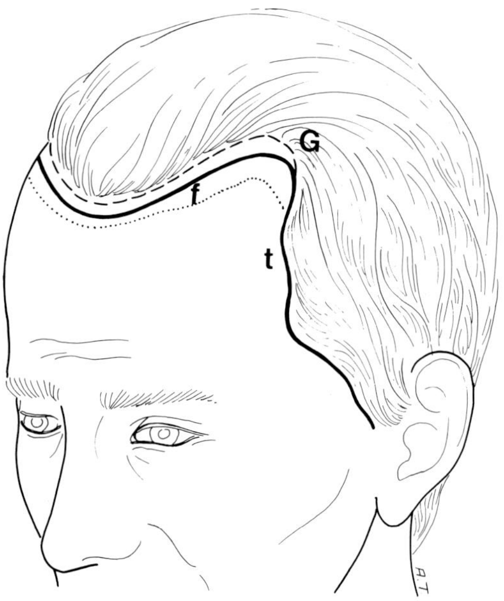

Fig. 6. Position of *f* and *t* defining frontal line

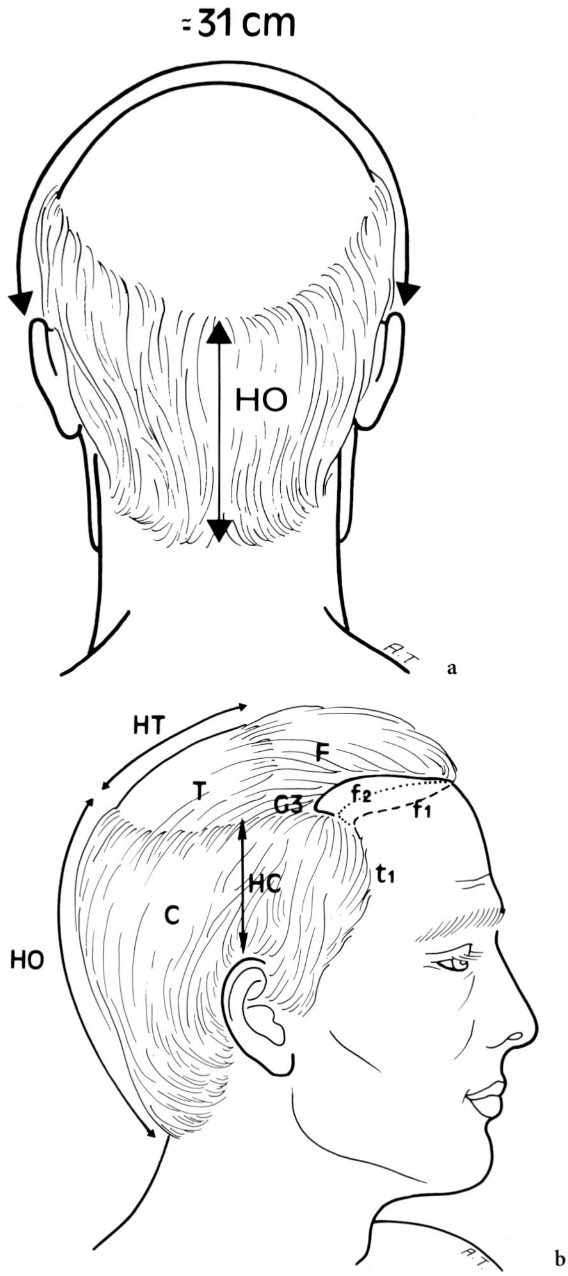

Fig. 7. a Posterior view: definition of bi-auricular distance and of OH (occipital height). **b** Regions and measurements

course of the alopecia process, these two lines do not necessarily recede in a symmetric manner (Fig. 6).

Laterally, from the back forwards, the skin is smooth and fine at the mastoid and supra-auricular areas and then there is a rectangular pre-auricular hairy zone or sideburn, which is covered with hair or beard of a different nature in different individuals. Therefore, it should not be used a donor area for grafts or flaps. At the back, the posterior cervical region has an ill-defined boundary with the scalp, whose hair often assumes a downy aspect.

Deep Relations. The scalp is separated from the cranial vault by an easily stripped and virtually avascular space situated beneath the galea – the space of Merkel.

Regions

The area of the scalp may be separated into several regions: frontal, parieto-temporal or crown, vertical and occipital.

Description [3]

Shape

The scalp is roughly the half of a sphere, following the shape of the cranium to which it is attached. However, the latter varies widely between different individuals: in dolichocephalics the cranium is very elongated, whereas in brachycephalics it is flattened. The shape of the frontal lines (*f*) and temporal lines (*t*) was defined in the previous paragraph.

Dimensions (Fig. 7)

The area is estimated to be 600–700 cm^2 in the adult. The length of the bi-auricular line (in a frontal plane from one ear to the other) is 30–32 cm. The length of the scalp from forehead to nape is 32–34 cm. The perimeter measured from one temporal line to the other is about 40 cm.

Total Thickness

Total thickness varies in between 5.7 and 6.4 mm, varying with the region, thicker at the nape and decreasing in front and at the sides; the scalp skin is the thickest of the whole body [13].

Elasticity

Table 1. Age distribution of degrees of baldness, scalp thickness and elasticity

		≤ 25 years		25–45 years		≥ 45 years		Total
		(n)	(%)	(n)	(%)	(n)	(%)	
Baldness	I	13	40	17	15	1	11	31
	II	17	50	44	39	3	30	64
	III	3	10	51	46	7	59	61
Elasticity	I	3	10	25	22	3	30	31
	II	25	75	696	62	7	59	101
	III	5	15	18	16	1	11	24
Thickness	I	0	0	3	3	3	30	6
	II	26	80	82	73	7	59	115
	III	7	20	27	24	1	11	35
Total		33	21	112	72	11	7	156

The scalp has only weak elasticity, due essentially to its adhesion to the galea (epicranial aponeurosis), which is itself barely stretchable. However, it can be gradually stretched and such elongation takes the form of an exponential curve.

We may distinguish zones of greater laxity: the temporal zones and especially at the back of the neck below the external occipital protuberance. The laxity of these peripheral zones, their particular shape, as well as the existence of more adherent zones, contribute to an elasticity which is even less in the longitudinal (front to back) direction than in the transverse direction (top to bottom). The maximum breadth of a flap for a very elastic scalp may be 5 cm in the Juri type of horizontal flap and only 4 cm with vertical types of flaps (Nataf or Dardour).

Age Variations

While the degree of baldness certainly increases with age, there does not seem to be a very marked correlation between age and the elasticity or thickness of the scalp. Before 25 years and after 45 years, the proportion of patients with very poor elasticity of the scalp is stable, between 11% and 16%. It may well be that there is a greater percentage of patients with excellent elasticity after the age of 45 (30%) than before 25 years (10%). The same can be said about the thickness of the scalp, which seems to increase with age (Table 1).

Stripping

While classically subgaleal stripping of the scalp is relatively easy, there is a zone where stripping is more difficult: the occipital region; at the nape of the neck, below the external occipital protuberance, the skin is firmly attached by numerous fibrous septa to the fascia of the superficial occipital, trapezius and sternocleidomastoid muscles. This region is rich in neurovascular perforants.

Galea

The galea (or epicranium) [5, 19] is a fibro-aponeurotic layer formed of several sublayers [20]: superficial fascia, supra-epicranial layer, epicranial aponeurosis, subepicranial layer, supraperiosteal layer (Fig. 5). It is continuous at the front with the frontal muscle and laterally with the auricular muscles, thus forming an actual digastric muscle system. It may be regarded as the cranial equivalent of the superficial facial musculo-aponeurotic system (SMAS) [10]. It is 1.5 mm thick. Finally, we have noted the numerous adhesions between skin and galea, responsible for the lack of scalp extensibility.

The galea is also richly vascularised, acting as a vessel-carrying layer; the plane of passage of the vessels is between the supra-epicranial layer and the superficial fascia (Fig. 8).

Vascularisation

Static Vascularisation

A particular feature of the scalp circulation is the great wealth and the extent of the anastomoses between the different systems. The arterial anatomy is well known, but that of the venous plexus is less well systematised.

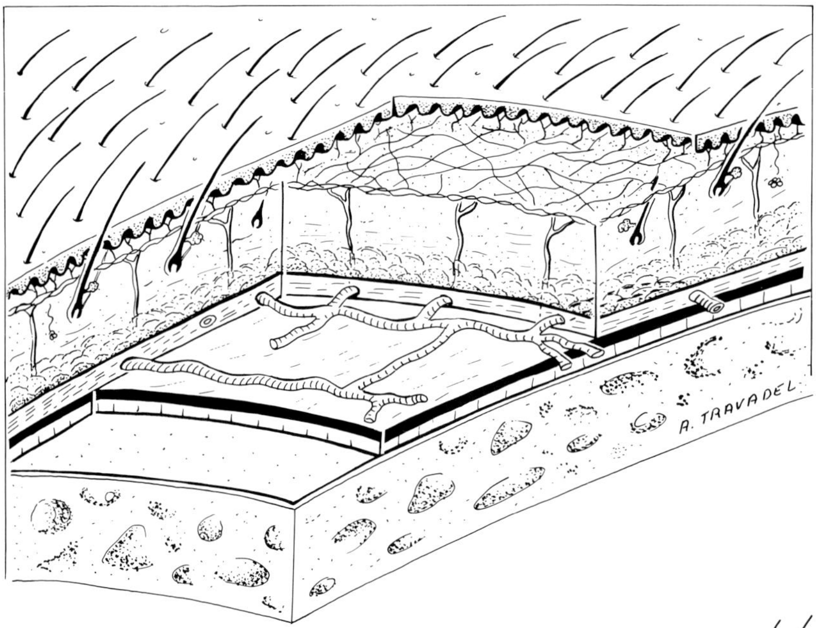

a

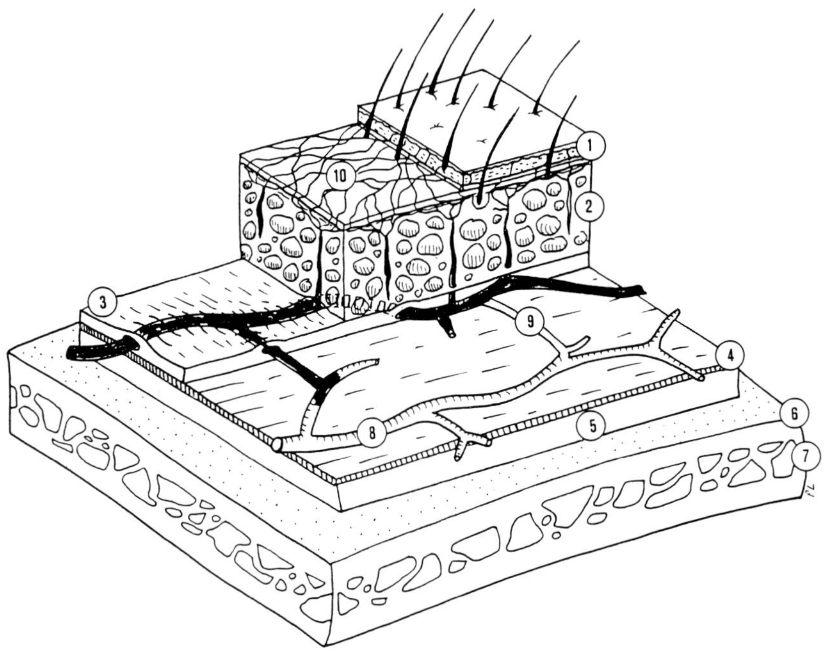

1 Skin
2 Subcutaneous tissue
3 Superficial fascia
4 Galea
5 Space of Merkel
6 Periosteum
7 Diploë
8 Superficial temporal artery
9 Intra-aponeurotic anastomosis
b 10 Subdermal anastomosis

Fig. 8a,b. Relations of arterial plexus and galea

Arterial Vascularisation

Arterial vascularisation [2, 8, 11, 25, 26, 28, 29] (Fig. 9) is essentially ensured by three branches of the external carotid:

a) The superficial temporal artery [12, 14]. This is the main artery and effects the major part of the supply of the scalp (reimplantation of the scalp is possible on a single temporal artery). The superficial temporal artery appears in the supra-aponeurotic plane very low down at the level of the zygomatic arch, thus allowing very low stripping of the scalp without vascular damage. The point of emergence of its superficial subcutaneous segment in the subcutaneous areolar tissue is at 4–5 mm in front of the upper border of the external

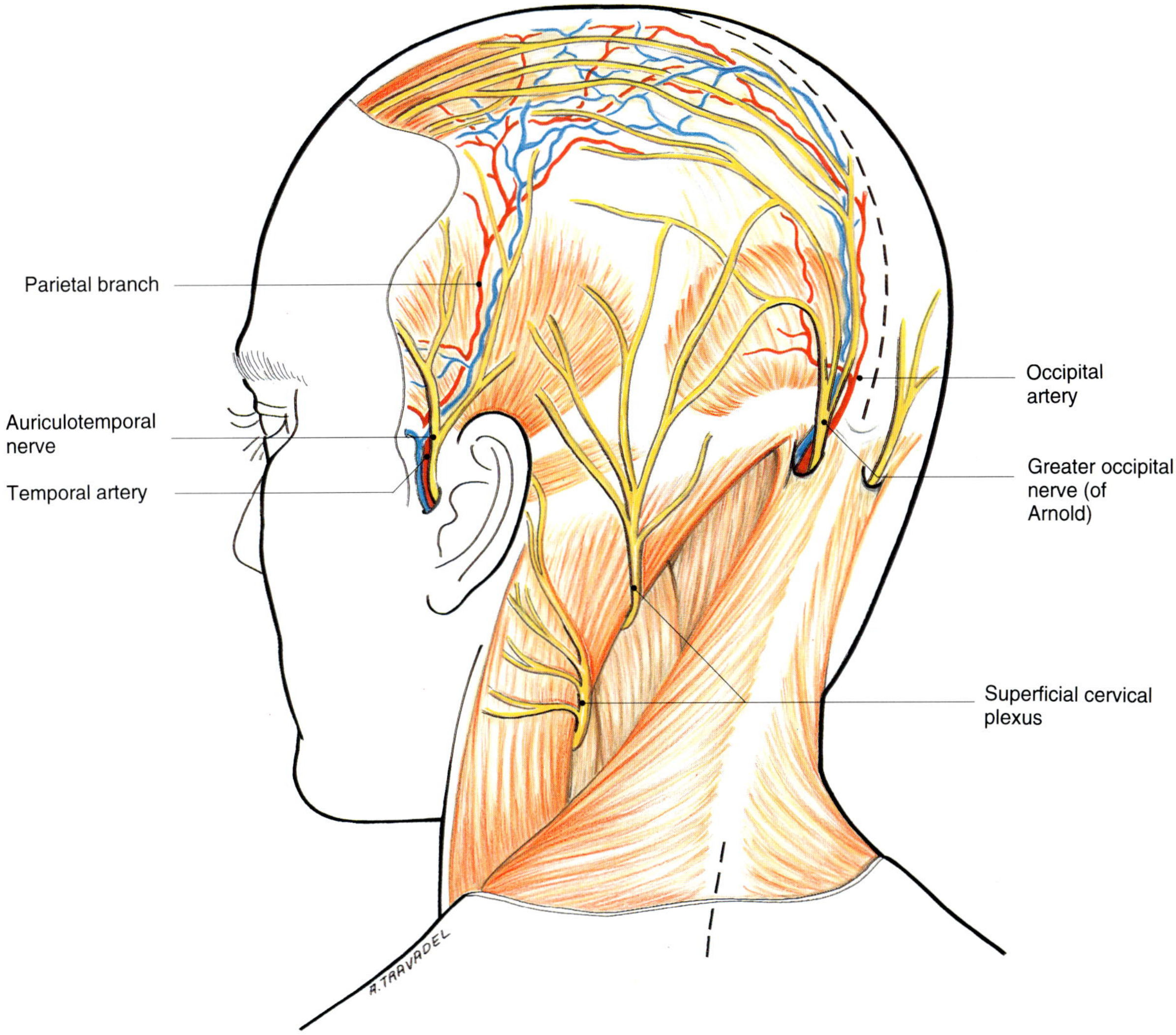

Fig. 9. Arteries and nerves of scalp

auditory meatus on a line joining the upper border of the meatus to the middle part of the upper border of the orbit; this portion has a winding course and ends at a variable level by dividing into two terminal branches:

- Anterior (temporo-frontal) branch
- Posterior (temporo-parietal) branch

None of the collateral branches of the superficial temporal artery are involved in the supply of the scalp. This does not apply to the terminal branches, which ensure vascularisation of a great part of the scalp:

- The temporo-frontal branch, which passes obliquely forward in relation to the trunk of the superficial temporal artery and is often sinuous. It forms a curve with a postero-superior concavity passing 2 cm behind the external orbital margin. It gives off numerous collaterals on its posterior aspect and ends in a branch which seems to continue it posteriorly, a lateral superciliary artery, anastomotic branches with the palpebral circle and, finally, in ascending branches to the scalp which cross the mid-line to anastomose with their homologues from the opposite side. Its calibre is of the order of 1.4 mm.
- The parietal branch, which ascends more or less vertically, seeming to continue the course of the superficial temporal artery. Its calibre is of the order of 1.2 mm. Its collaterals supply the scalp in an arborescent manner. It terminates beyond the mid-line by anastomosis with the branches

of the occipital and posterior auricular arteries and with those of its homologue of the opposite side. The location of the parietal branch is virtually constant. It is found in continuity with the trunk of the artery in a strip 2 cm wide, axised on the external auditory meatus and parallel to a frontal plane. It is initially close to the anterior limit of this strip and then ascends with a slight posterior concavity and reaches the posterior limit.

The calibre of these vessels exceeds 1 mm and therefore allows microanastomosis in the transplant context, using the temporal region as the donor or receptor zone. The available length of pedicle is variable: 10 cm for the parietal branch, varying from 4 to 13 cm; 11 cm for the frontal branch (7–13 cm). To this length that of the tissue island may be added, some 6 × 3 cm. The depth of the artery in the subcutaneous areolar tissue is practically constant at 5 mm from the surface. It is only at 2–3 cm from the mid-line that it approaches the dermis.

Anastomoses. The anastomotic plexus is extraordinarily abundant. Left–right anastomoses are constant in the scalp. The superficial temporal artery gives off ascending vertical branches at its superior aspect, so that there is a double anastomotic plexus: the subdermal plexus and the wide intra-aponeurotic anastomosis. This explains how, in extensive flaps, a contralateral zone can be employed, the arterial plexus supplying receptor channels. The antero-posterior anastomoses between the superficial temporal, posterior auricular and occipital arteries permit major scalp plasties. The anastomoses between both superficial temporal arteries permit transverse flaps, particularly the bipedicled scalp flap.

b) The occipital artery. This arises from the posterior aspect of the external carotid. It can be divided into three parts:
   - Oblique ascending posterior and deep in the parotid region
   - Horizontal under the muscles of the back of the neck
   - Finally, it bends to become vertical and superficially subcutaneous, after having perforated the trapezius. This part measures 3 cm on average and it ends in two branches, lateral and medial.

   The point of subcutaneous emergence is constant and easy to locate by following the curved superior occipital line to 3.5 or 4 cm from the mid-line. At this level it is accompanied by the occipital nerve (of Arnold). Any stripping of the scalp which transgresses this lower limit risks damaging the occipital artery, so that its location is important when designing occipital flaps.

   Its calibre is on average 1.6 mm in the third part. It anastomoses with the posterior auricular artery by its lateral branch and with the terminal medial branches of its opposite homologue across the mid-line.

c) Posterior auricular artery. This is a branch of the external carotid and travels obliquely upwards and backward. It passes toward the tip of the mastoid process and then toward the auriculo-mastoid groove, where it terminates by bifurcating into an anterior auricular branch and a posterior mastoid branch. It has a small calibre and supplies a minor territory above and behind the ear.

Accessory Vascularisation

Vascularisation occurs much more accessorily, and for the frontal territory mainly, by two branches of the internal carotid: the medial frontal or supratrochlear artery and the lateral frontal or supraorbital artery, both branches of the ophthalmic artery.

Anastomoses [21]. These are very numerous between the different branches and occur not only between the branches of the homolateral pedicles, but also, after crossing the mid-line, between each side (the latter decreasing after the age of 60). The vascularisation of the scalp is essentially ensured by a rich subdermal anastomotic plexus fed by ascending branches derived from the wide-channel plexus mentioned above and carried by the galea. Apart from the inferior nuchal region, there is no supply from perforating vessels. Thus, apart from this zone, flaps may be autonomised by simple incision without subcutaneous stripping.

Veins

The arrangement of the veins is more variable. Essentially, they follow the course of the arteries, but there are also major variants, especially at the fronto-temporal region, where the venous system is often scanty. Drainage occurs essentially towards the jugular vein at the front, the external jugular vein laterally and the vertebral vein behind. In addition, a small part of the scalp (mainly parietal) drains into the intracranial system via emissary veins perforating the cranium.

Dynamic Vascularisation

The terminal branches have a particular course and are tethered in a special way to the scalp planes. This they approach by passing beneath the cutaneous muscles to travel between the supra-epicranial layer and the superficial fascia. At this level the latter, just as it has given off connective tissue septa to the hypodermis, sends arches of connective tissue fibres, transforming the space between its deep aspect and the superficial layer of the supra-epicranial aponeurosis into tunnels in which the arteries travel without friction. Throughout their course, and especially at their upper aspect, these terminal branches give off branches which traverse the superficial fascia to reach the hypodermis, forming the "chandeliers" described by Cormia [7]. These branches are destined either for the baskets surrounding the hair follicles, sebaceous and sweat glands, or for the dermal papilla.

The separation of the arterial branches by the aponeurotic layer in relation to the subjacent plane explains the almost bloodless stripping of the scalp. Unlike the face, where flaps may be of varying thickness, the scalp imposes flaps of uniform thickness.

The abundance of anastomoses in the scalp explains why:

- There is a system of compensation such that failure of one branch is compensated for by an adjacent branch.
- It is possible to construct very large and extensive vascular flaps (since the superficial temporal vessels by themselves serve to ensure virtually the entire supply of the scalp) and on homo- or contralateral sides (since the anastomoses then serve as passive channels).
- Flaps based solely on the rich subdermal plexus and not including a major pedicle may be much longer than they are wide (5:1 or even 6:1).

Finally, it should be noted that at the pilo-sebaceous follicle the vascularisation is more considerable when hair growth is more active and becomes more sparse when the hair enters a quiescent phase.

The flow in the subcutaneous plexus is strongly influenced by the vasoconstriction created by local injection of adrenaline, provided the injection is made into a layer superficial to the galea. Scalp incisions then cease to be very haemorrhagic.

In smokers, there is also a marked decrease in blood-flow, as proved by the greater vulnerability of flaps. This decrease is probably due to a chronic factor of vascular damage, but also to a factor of acute vasoconstriction appearing after every cigarette and lasting about 20 min. Other factors such as stress, which excites adrenaline discharge, very probably play a part in the blood-flow of the scalp.

Innervation [22–31] (Fig. 9)

Motor innervation is through the branches of the facial nerve distributed to the frontal and occipital muscles. Sensory innervation is effected by branches of the trigeminal at the front and of the superficial cervical plexus at the back.

Frontal Nerve

The frontal nerve is given off from the ophthalmic nerve, itself a branch of the maxillary nerve. It divides a little behind the upper orbital margin into two branches: the lateral frontal or supraorbital nerve, which passes into the supraorbital notch (it is at this site that injections are given to obtain regional anaesthesia) and the medial frontal nerve, medial to the foregoing. These branches provide sensory innervation of the forehead and the entire antero-lateral part of the scalp as far as the vertex.

Auriculotemporal Nerve

The auriculotemporal nerve issues from the mandibular nerve and travels with the superficial temporal vessels through the retrocondylar buttonhole of Juvara. It then skirts the origin of the zygomatic arch and perforates the supra-aponeurotic layer before being distributed to the skin of the temporal region.

Superficial Branches of the Cervical Plexus

The superficial branches of the cervical plexus emerge from C2 (greater occipital nerve of Arnold) and C3 and innervate the skin of the posterior aspect of the skull and neck. After emerging at the posterior border of the sternocleidomastoid muscle, these nerves travel on its deep aspect and then perforate the galea at the curved occipital line together with the occipital artery to become superficial (it is here that injections for regional block are given, 3 cm from the mid-line). Thus they are normally sacrificed at this level in inferior stripping of this region, but careful dissection may preserve them and prevent their stretching after freeing.

References

1. Ainsworth RW, Gresham GA, Balmforth GV (1961) Pathological changes in temporal arteries removed from unselected cadavers. J Clin Pathol 14: 115–119
2. Bellocq P (1925) Étude anatomique des artères de la peau chez l'homme. Strasbourg Med 2: 63
3. Bourgery JM (1844) Traité complet de l'anatomie chez l'homme, anatomie descriptive et physiologique, vol 3. Delaunay, Paris
4. Bouhanna P (1980) Anatomie et physiologie du cuir chevelu. Bull Soc Med Paris 8(5): 132–135
5. Chayen D, Hillel (1974) Anatomical observations on the subgaleotic fascia of the scalp. Acta Anat (Basel) 87: 427–432
6. Converse JM (1964) Reconstructive plastic surgery, vol 3. Saunders, Philadelphia, pp 1087–1088, 1340
7. Cormia FE (1961) Circulatory changes in alopecia. Arch Dermatol 84: 493
8. Cormia FE (1963) Vasculature of normal scalp. Arch Dermatol 88(6): 692–701
9. Corso PF (1961) Variation in head circulation. Plast Reconstr Surg 27(2): 160
10. Couly G, Hureau J, Vaillant JM (1975) Fascia superficialis céphalique. Ann Chir Plast 20(2): 171–182
11. Crepy (1967) Anatomie cervico-faciale. Masson, Paris
12. D'All Acqua V (1906) Artère temporale superficielle chez l'homme. Acta Ital Biol 36
13. Dardour JC, Noury-Duperrat G, Dufourmentel C (1977) Le cuir chevelu, zone donneuse de greffes minces. Ann Chir Plast 22 (3): 169–175
14. Eustathianos N (1932) Étude anatomique sur les artères temporales uperficielles. Ann Anat Path 9: 678–684
15. Irague M (1971) Les artères du cuir chevelu; disposition des artères dans l'épaisseur du cuir chevelu. C R Assist Anat: 177–180
16. Kazanjian WH, Converse JM (1974) Reconstructive plastic surgery, vol 1. Saunders, Philadelphia, pp 585–586
17. Larmanaud H (1882) Des téguments du crâne, recherches d'anatomie et de pathologie. Thesis, Lyon
18. Lebeau J, Antoine P, Raphael B (1986) Introduction angéologique à la chirurgie du scalp. Ann Chir Plast 30(4): 321–324
19. Libersa C, Laude M (1961) À propos de l'aponévrose épicrânienne (galéa aponévroticocupitis). Arch Anat Cytol Pathol 12: 149–152
20. Marie M (1967) Cuir chevelu: études anatomiques et anatomo-radiologiques – incidences cliniques. Thesis, Paris
21. May NDS (1967) Arterial anastomoses in the head and neck of sheep. J Anat 101: 381–387
22. Montagna W, Ellis RA (1958) The vascularity and innervation of human hair follicles. In: Montagna W, Ellis RA (eds) Biology of hair growth 10: 219–226
23. Paturet P (1958) Traité d'anatomie humaine, III, 1. Masson, Paris, p 285
24. Poirier P, Charpy A (1902) Traité d'anatomie humaine, III. Masson, Paris, pp 690–691
25. Ricbourg B (1974) Artères et veines cutanées de la face et du cuir chevelu. Thesis, Paris
26. Ricbourg B, Mitz V, Lassau JP (1975) Étude anatonique et déductions pratiques. Ann Chir Plast 20(2): 197–213
27. Rouvière H (1970) Anatomie humaine, 10th edn. Masson, Paris
28. Salmon M (1936) Artères de la peau. Masson, Paris, pp 114–116
29. Salmon M (1936) Artères des muscles de la tête et du cou. Masson, Paris, p 75
30. Spalteholtz W (1970) Hand Atlas der Anatomie des Menschen. Hirzel, Heipzig
31. Testut-Latarjet (1948) Traité d'anatomie humaine, II. Masson, Paris, pp 233–236

Biology and Physiology of Hair Growth

Adults

Growth of Hair: The Hair Cycle (Fig. 1, Photo 1a–c)

Hair growth is effected by multiplication of the generative cells of the root, the mitotic activity of which varies from one cycle to another. The average growth of the scalp hair, which is faster than that of hair elsewhere, is from 0.35 to 0.45 mm/24 h, i.e. over 1 cm a month. This growth varies with sex (it is faster in women) and with the scalp region (growth is faster at the vertex than at the temples). Again, it seems to be subject to seasonal rhythms, being greater in winter than in summer and more marked during the day than at night.

Moreover, the hair renews itself throughout life. Each hair is in effect the permanent site of cyclical activity independent of that of other hairs: the so-called mosaic activity.

Anagenic Phase

The anagenic phase lasts for 2–6 years (mean, 3 years) and is the phase of active growth. There is an early anagenic phase, characterised by intense mitotic activity starting quite suddenly in a group of cells situated below the former bulb (previously the follicle, now in telogenic phase, see below); these cells multiply and arrive at the papilla and surround it to form a new bulb.

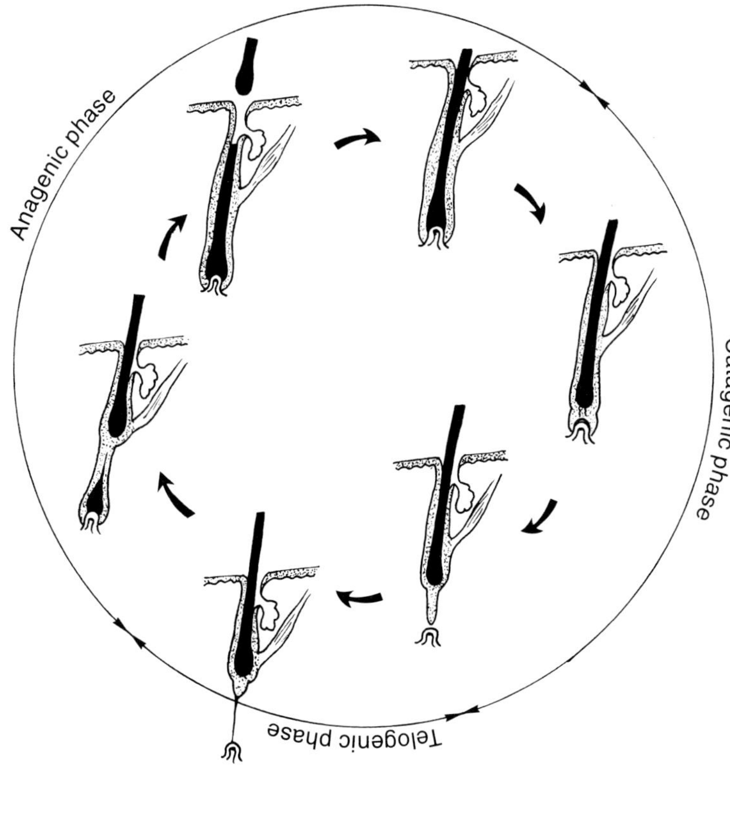

Fig. 1. Hair cycle

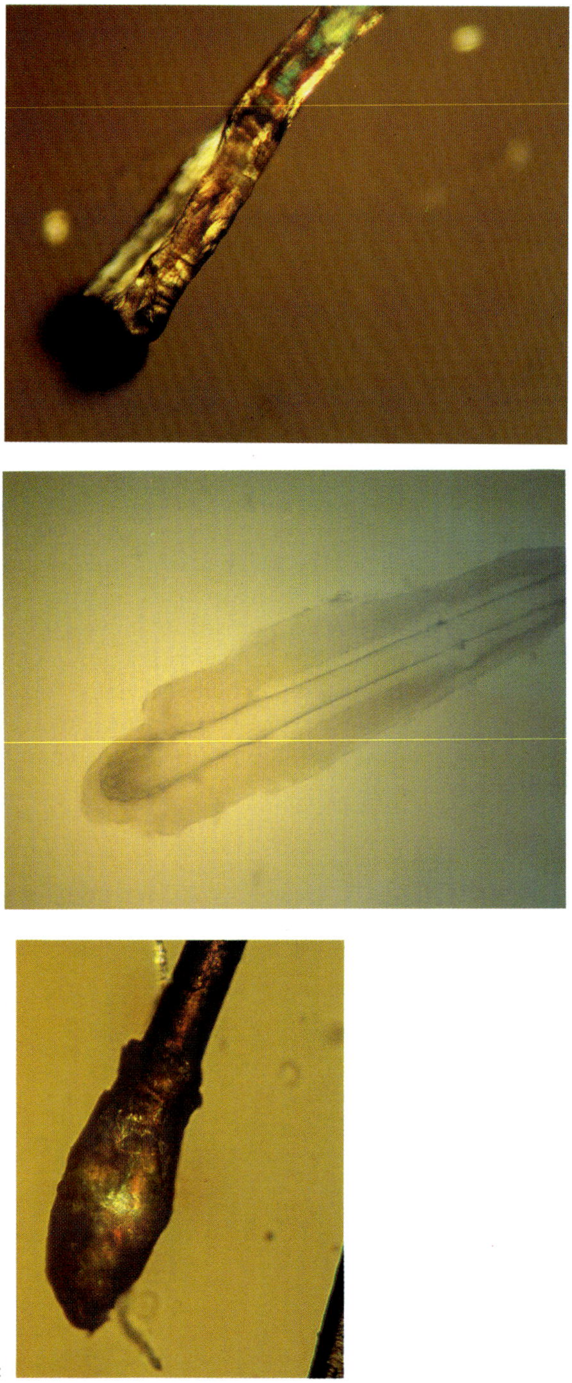

a b c

Photo 1a–c. Microscopic aspect of stages of bulb. **a** Aspect of anagenic hair. **b** Aspect of catagenic hair. **c** Aspect of telogenic hair

Cell differentiation then takes place at the upper part of this new bulb, which leads to the formation of new hair (melanogenesis, keratogenesis); this is the late anagenic phase. At the same time, the old hair is definitively shed, after which mitotic activity suddenly ceases. This is the catagenic phase.

Catagenic Phase

Also called the phase of regression, the catagenic phase lasts 2–4 weeks (mean, 3 weeks), during which involution of the lower two thirds of the follicle and of the bulb and papilla takes place.

Telogenic Phase

Also called the resting phase, the telogenic phase lasts 3–4 months. The follicle is now short, and its base (which terminates near the opening of the sebaceous gland) contains a rounded bulb at its lower end ("club hair") and is completely keratinised. Beneath this, a thin band of undifferentiated epithelial cells connecting the clubbed bulb to the atrophic papilla extends in depth to give rise to the new hair to follow in the anagenic phase, while the old hair in telogenic phase is ready to be shed.

In total, for a head of 100000–150000 hairs (over an average cycle of 3 years), 50–100 hairs are normally shed each day. Hair growth does not occur in a uniform manner, and the percentage of follicles in the different phases can be assessed by means of the trichogram.

Trichogram (Photo 2)

A trichogram consists in the microscopic examination, in a subject whose hair has not been washed for 3 days, of some 50 hairs taken from three scalp regions (vertex, temporal and occipital regions). This establishes the percentage of follicles in the different phases and the ratio of the number of anagenic hairs to that of telogenic hairs, i.e. the coeffi-

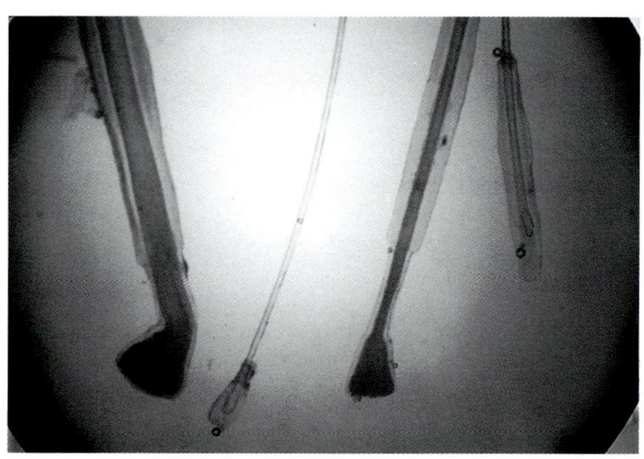

Photo 2. Hair bulbs in anagenic, catagenic and telogenic phases

cient of growth of the hair (normal values above or equal to 4). The usual findings in the young healthy adult [5] are:

- Anagenic phase: 80%–85%
- Telogenic phase: 10%–15%
- Catagenic phase: 1%–2%
- Dystrophic hair: < 15%–20%

Macrophotographic Examination

Phototrichogram. Based on the studies by Saitoh [32] in 1982, Bouhanna suggested the use of the term phototrichogram (PTG; Photo 3) [6] for a standardised method of macrophotographic study. The location of the area of the scalp to be analysed was determined by the intersection of two plastic strips directed toward the vertex from four fixed points of the face and micro-tattooed in indian ink [7]. The demarcation of an area of 0.5 cm^2 was made after application of a fenestrated strip marked in millimetres. Since 1986 Bouhanna has preferred the use of a circular aluminium frame with intersecting nylon threads which demarcate an area of 0.25 cm^2 [9]. Two photographs are taken at an interval of 3 days, at first on an unwashed and unbrushed scalp whose hairs have been cut at their emergence and then on a washed and brushed scalp.

Analysis and counting of the hairs on the successive macrophotographs of these areas [8] allows evaluation of:

- Density of the hair
- Number of hairs in the anagenic stage which have continued to grow
- Number of telogenic hairs which have stopped growing or which have fallen out during previous shampooing or brushing.

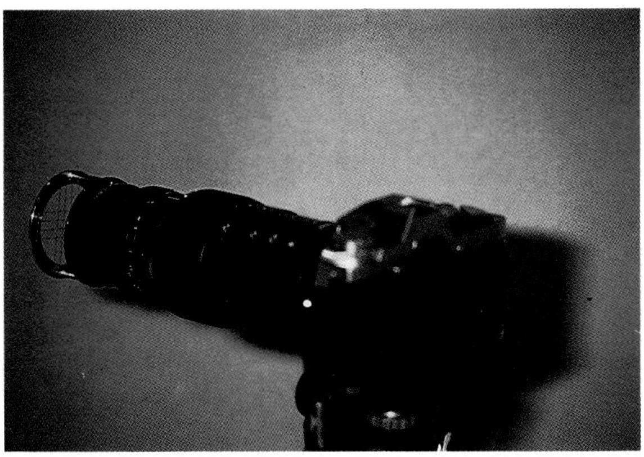
a

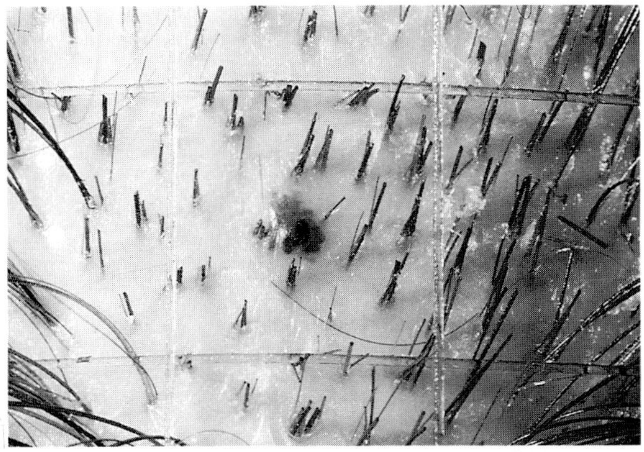
b

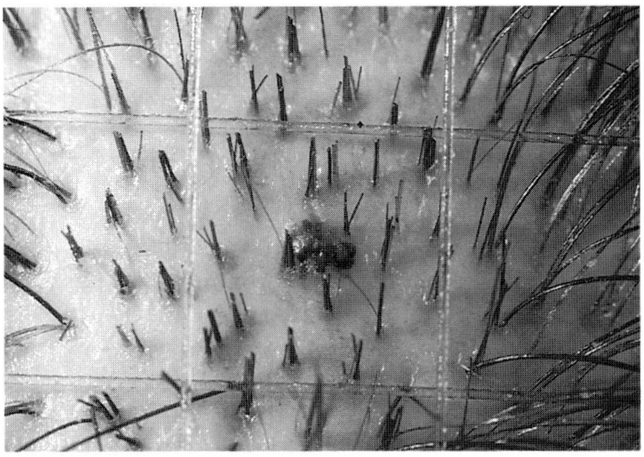
c

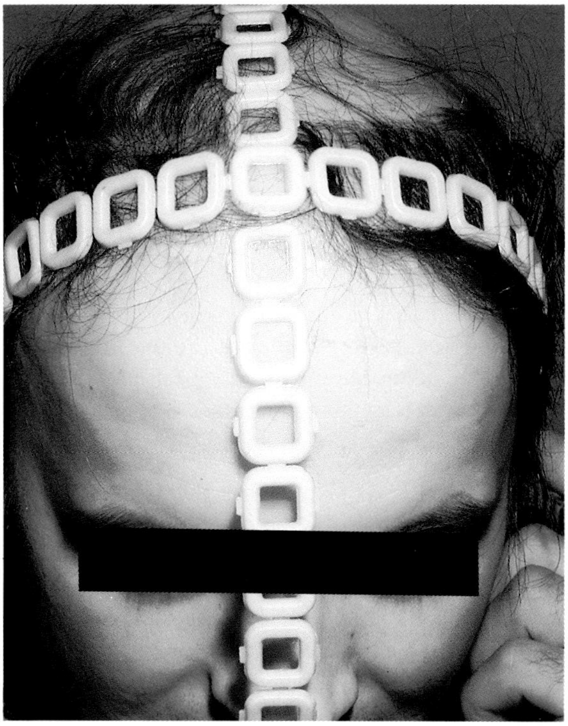
d

Photo 3a–d. Phototrichogram (Bouhanna). **a** Equipment for macrophotography. **b,c** Macrophotographs at 3 days' interval. **d** Location by strips

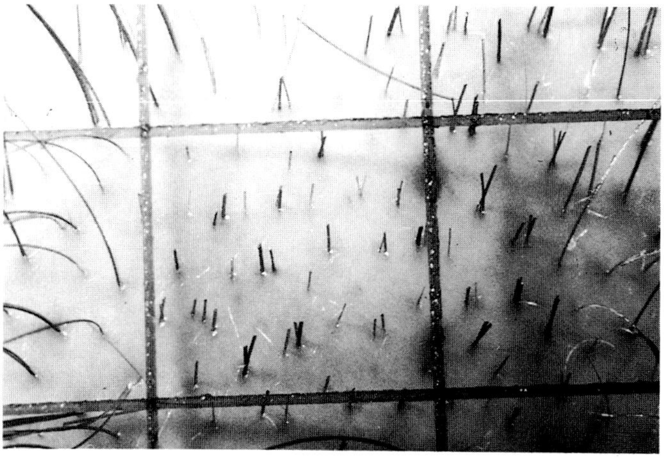

Photo 4. Tractiophototrichogram. Macrophotograph of area located by two tattooings. Remaining hairs counted after elimination of hairs susceptible to manual traction

This examination also allows assessment of the rate of growth and of increase in the diameter of the hair shafts [37, 39].

Tractiophototrichogram. In 1988 Bouhanna suggested a simplified phototrichographic method, the tractiophototrichogram (Photo 4) [10], which consists in eliminating the telogenic hairs by previous manual traction over a defined area of 0.25 cm^2. Macrophotography then allows the anagenic hairs remaining at this site to be counted. The ratio of anagenic to telogenic hairs thus obtained is considered pathological if it is less than 15. These simple and reliable macrophotographic studies allow verification of the presence and degree of hair loss. They can be repeated to assess the spontaneous course of the alopecic process or its response to treatment.

Factors Influencing Hair Formation

Age. In children, the amount of hair in the anagenic phase often exceeds 90%; after the age of 30, the percentage in anagenesis begins to fall [20] and the proportion in telogenesis increases [11].

Sex. In women, the percentage in anagenesis exceeds that in men [18].

Regions. In the adult, even if unaffected by baldness, the proportion of hair in telogenesis is higher in the anterior frontal region [35]. In addition to variations caused by age, sex and region (as monitored in the trichogram), many factors appear to be involved in hair growth, but their respective precise roles remain debatable.

Vascularisation. The role of vascularisation in the physiological state has never been objectively established [25]. However, certain observations concerning the increase in hair growth after the use of vasodilator agents (minoxidil) and the reduction of growth after circulatory decrease or interruption (grafts, flaps) seem to confirm its role [15]. At the follicle, acute major ischaemia impedes the adequate vascular supply of metabolites and thus endangers hair growth [36]. This explains the temporary loss of hair from grafts, but also at the margins of wounds closed under excessive tension or in certain flaps where vascularisation is limited (anagenic defluvium).

If the ischaemia is too severe and prolonged, there is necrosis of the bulb and therefore definitive alopecia.

Apart from this extreme case it should be noted that:

- Ligature of the arteries of the scalp (superficial temporal branches, occipital, posterior auricular) produces a change in vascular dynamics with a reduced supply of oxygen, which results in reduced activity of 5-alpha-reductase, thus explaining the frequent normalisation of seborrhoea in the areas concerned (and even a temporary slowing in hair loss).
- On the other hand, in the determination of baldness, it now seems established that the reduction in blood supply is a consequence and not a cause of baldness, the decrease in follicular activity adapting itself to the reduced metabolic needs.

Innervation. Certain clinical facts suggest that innervation influences hair formation, including increased hair in the area of a sympathectomy and alopecia from disruption of the capillary and hair cycle [26, 27] after a psychological shock. However, the present tendency is to regard hair growth not to be under direct control of the nervous system.

Hormones. Endocrine influences are much more definite, but not always identical, on the scalp hair and on other hairs [28]. Thus:

- The thyroid hormones contribute to the maintenance of biochemical activity in the anagenic phase and hypothyroidism leads to diffuse loss of scalp and body hair, which is lacklustre and fragile, though some hyperthyroid states also produce alopecia.
- There is hirsutism in Cushing's syndrome, but the adrenocortical hormones have no direct influence on hair growth.
- The sex hormones, on the other hand, play an important role [4]. Oestrogens retard growth rate during the anagenic phase, but prolong the duration of this phase; they also have an anti-androgenic action at the pilo-follicular receptors. Androgens, especially at puberty, induce the transformation from intermediate to terminal hair (see "The Modifications of Puberty" below); moreover, and quite paradoxically, development of the body hair and beard is stimulated, whereas in the regions genetically predisposed to androgenic alopecia (vertex, fronto-temporal recession) [1], androgens reduce the diameter of the hair shaft, the growth rate and the duration of the anagenic phase and may even lead to transformation into down (see "Role of Androgens in Male Baldness" below).

Metabolic Factors. As evidenced by certain alimentary imbalances and deficiencies, many factors are essential for keratogenesis and hair growth, particularly:

- Saccharides (energy source)
- Vitamin A, pantothenic acid and the B group of vitamins (riboflavine, pyridoxine), which are essential to oxidative processes
- Lipids and particularly essential amino acids, especially cystine and methionine
- Zinc, iron, copper, sulphur and phosphorus

Physical and mechanical factors essential for keratogenesis and hair growth include the following [40]:

- Depilation is involved only if performed on a hair in telogenic phase, which accelerates growth by reducing the duration of this phase.
- Certain traumas (such as surgery) have a stimulating effect on local mitotic activity, mediated by the prostaglandins freed by the damaged cells.
- The effects of massage are reported differently by different authors, but most regard it as growth stimulating.
- Sunlight and temperature have a stimulating action on hair growth only in a few individuals.
- Finally, cutting has no effect on hair growth.

Psychological Factors. Their role is not negligible; emotional shock and various neurotic disorders may provoke loss of hair.

Androgenic Alopecia

Baldness begins mainly in the androgen-sensitive follicles of the forehead and summit of the cranium [31]. The process is slow, and the anagenic phase becomes shorter and shorter at each cycle; consequently, the proportion of hairs in the telogenic phase increases, as can be objectivised by the trichogram in the frontal region (even before the appearance of obvious baldness).

The affected follicle becomes progressively smaller after a succession of cycles, thus leading to a reduction in diameter of the hair produced and ending by progressive involution with a fine down. At the follicle, all the other structures are also reduced in proportion to this "follicular miniaturisation" in a manner adapted to the reduced requirements [23] (reduced nerve plexuses and blood supply, persistent but quantitatively reduced enzymatic activity and keratogenesis). It should also be noted that these small follicles differ from those of the primary down of the newborn by the presence of the arrector muscle of the hair.

At a still more advanced stage, and in the bald areas, there remain only follicles of down which are non-pigmented and mostly in telogenic phase. Finally, alopecia develops only in hair follicles which have the genetic potential [34] to be inhibited by androgens during a certain androchronogenic period [29]. The converse process exists, i.e. the transformation of down into beard and hirsutism.

In women, alopecia tends to be less severe [16], more delayed, slower and more diffuse, probably because women have less circulating androgens.

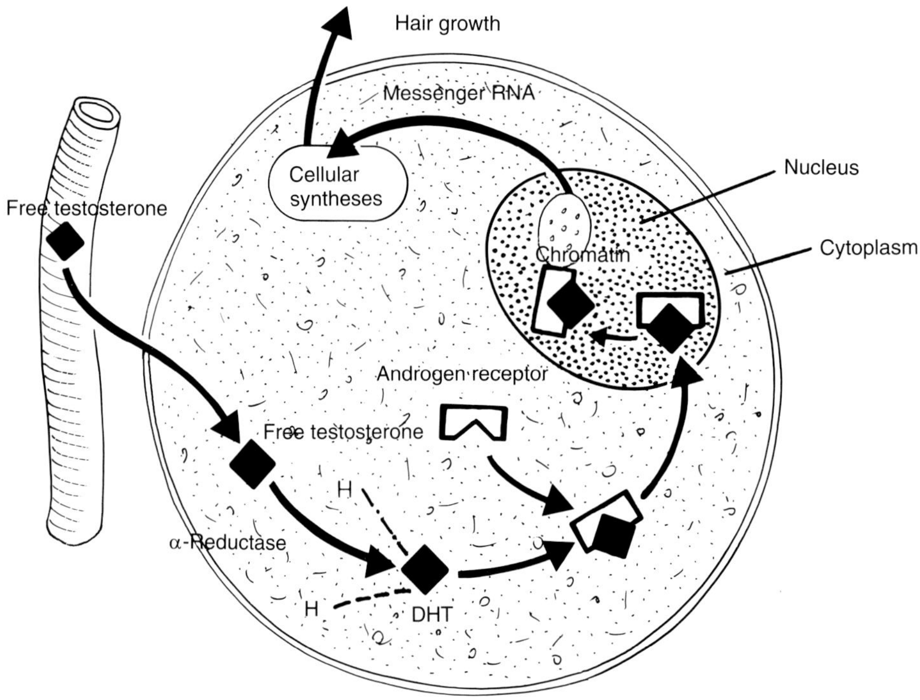

Fig. 2. Mechanisms of action of androgens on hair bulbs. DHT, dihydrotestosterone

Mode of Action of Androgens on Target Cells (Fig. 2)

Hormonal action is effected at the level of the follicle and mainly concerns the bulbar region, which is a site of active metabolic conversion [33]. Free testosterone penetrates the cell and is reduced to dihydrotestosterone (DHT) by the 5-alpha-reductase present in the sensory cells of the follicles. It is actually this DHT which is the hormone acting on the target cell in the papilla or matrix. The initial stage of baldness consists of its accumulation in the follicle.

In type 2 pseudo-hermaphroditism, characterised by a deficiency of 5-alpha-reductase, testosterone accumulates, there is a marked decrease of DHT and baldness does not develop. The DHT is subsequently bound to a cytoplasmic protein, which permits its transport to the nucleus, where it may then act. Finally, whereas DHT has a stimulating effect on sebaceous secretion, it has an inhibitory action on the follicular metabolism of the hair.

The prevention and early medical treatment of androgenic alopecia is based on the control of androgenic activity, since no genetic or chronological management exists. In women, the excess production of androgen decreases the fraction bound to proteins and increases the turnover.

Plasma Androgens

Increased production of plasma androgens may be reduced by corticoids and oestrogens; the latter stimulate the production of proteins fixed by the liver.

Local Treatment

Although many inhibitors of 5-alpha-reductase and of the binding of DHT to the target cells are known, there is as yet no clinically useful agent. Progesterone has only a partial and temporary action. In man, castration arrests, but does not reverse the process. Any reduction in circulating androgens necessary to lessen fall-out of hair gives rise to side-effects [14].

Reversibility of the process is possible, but at a price acceptable only by transsexuals: complete clinical castration, suppression of adrenal androgens, reduction of free androgens by increasing the globulins bound to the sex hormones, increase of thyroid hormones and oestrogens and local treatment to reduce 5-alpha-reductase and DHT.

Grafts on the Receptor Site and Hair Behaviour

In the majority of cases, baldness behaves in terms of dominance of the donor site; after the transplantation of grafts to a receptor site, the grafts continue their development independently as if they had never left their place of origin. This suggests that the mechanism of hair growth (as well as its programming in alopecia) exists essentially within the follicle itself, without direct dependence on local vascular and nervous factors.

Foetuses and Infants

During intrauterine life and in the very small child, several successive modifications occur in the hair cycles and the characteristics of the hair [30].

Hair Cycles

At the end of the fifth month of intrauterine life, the fine lanugo (the definitive stock of the first generation of hair) is completely formed and covers the entire skin surface area, including the head. At this stage, all the follicles of the scalp are in anagenic phase. Then, up to the seventh month of intrauterine life, the hair of the frontal and parietal regions rapidly enters into catagenic and then telogenic phase (ready to fall), while the lanugo of the occipital region still remains in anagenic phase. Five to six weeks before birth, the frontal and parietal regions begin to be covered with a second generation of hair, the down. Then, at the end of the first month of life, the hair in all regions enters into telogenic phase.

In the second month of the first year, and beginning with the third generation of hairs, each follicle has its own growth rhythm, leading to a desynchronisation of the hair cycles (mosaicism), as well as a prolongation of the phases of the cycle (with the usual timing already noted).

Hair Characteristics

The characteristics of the hair change as follows:

- First the silky lanugo, lacking pigment and medulla.
- Then the equally fine, soft down, often already a little more pigmented, but short (less than 1–2 cm).
- This is replaced quite rapidly by a more pigmented and thicker intermediate hair, with rapid growth in diameter occurring towards the third year.

Adolescents

During the years preceding puberty, the hair cycle and mosaic follicular activity are well-established, with 94% of the follicles in anagenic phase. At puberty, and in response to the androgens, a striking change takes place in terms of the characteristics of the hair, i.e. replacement of the intermediate by the terminal hair. This is very pigmented, thick, relatively long and contains a medulla [40]. This change may develop in a barely perceptible fashion or more suddenly when it is accompanied by a change in colour and/or form (waviness etc.). At this period, and to a greater or lesser degree according to the individual's genetic predisposition, there is also recession of the frontal hairline, especially at the fronto-temporal recession, and the androgens may produce the reducing effects already mentioned in the programmed regions (decrease of diameter and growth rate, even conversion into down etc.).

Old Age

In the elderly subject, it is the colour of the hair (whitening) which is the most noticeable feature. Apart from the phenomena of whitening, studies of elderly subjects have shown only minor variations in other parameters:

- The density of the follicles decreases only very slightly after the age of 50 years.
- The hair seems finer in the elderly.
- The growth rate decreases slightly and the anagenic to telogenic ratio decreases significantly with age, especially after 60 years.

Whitening appears physiologically with ageing, at a time probably genetically determined. In the Caucasian subject it usually appears around 35 years, and at the age of 50 half the population has greying of 50% of the hair. The phenomenon usually starts at the temples and then extends to the vertex and crown. This defect of pigmentation, with marked decrease in granular content due to reduction of melanocyte activity, is not entirely understood:

- Melanogenesis is probably arrested.
- Inhibition of tyrosinase activity in the bulb may be involved.

- Neural, vascular, hormonal and even auto-immune factors have also been suggested.

This phenomenon is generally progressive and irreversible, but observations of sudden whitening of the hair after emotional shock, for example, seem debatable and may rather be due to the loss of pigmented hairs which have been masking the white hairs.

References

1. Adachi K, Kano M (1972) The role of receptor proteins in controlling the action on the sebaceous glands of hamster. Steroids 19: 567–574
2. Allegra F (1968) Histology and histochemical aspects of the hair follicles in pattern alopecia. In: Biopathology of pattern alopecia. Karger, Basel, pp 107–128
3. Barman JM, Astore I, Pecoraro V (1964) Method, technic and computation in the study of the trophic state of the human scalp hair. J Invest Dermatol 42: 421–425
4. Bingman KD, Shaw DA (1973) Male pattern baldness and the metabolism of androgens by human scalp skin. J Soc Cosmet Chem 24: 523–536
5. Bouhanna P (1980) Anatomie et physiologie du cuir chevelu. Bull soc Med Paris 8(5): 132–135
6. Bouhanna P (1982) The advantage of phototrichogram in hair surgery. Communication at the International Advanced Hair Replacement Symposium, Birmingham, Alabama
7. Bouhanna P (1983) Phototrichogram: a technic for the objective evaluation of the diagnosis and course of diffuse alopecia. I: Montagna W et al. (eds) Hair and aesthetic medicine. Salus, Rome, pp 277–280
8. Bouhanna P (1985) The phototrichogram, a macrophotographic study of the scalp. Bioengineer Skin 3: 265
9. Bouhanna P (1987) The phototrichogram: an objective technique used in hair replacement surgery evaluation. In: Unger WP, Nordstrom RD (eds) Hair transplantation. Dekker, New York, pp. 837–883
10. Bouhanna P (1988) Le tractiophototrichogramme, méthode d'apprécation objective d'une chute de cheveux. Ann Dermatol Venereol 115: 759–764
11. Burch PRJ, Murray JJ, Jackson D (1971) The age-prevalence of acrus senilis, greying of hair, and baldness, etiological consideration. J Gerontol 26: 364–372
12. Cabane J (1980) Étude des variations de la formule pilaire à partir d'une nouvelle technique photographique du trichogramme. Bull Soc med Paris 8: 150–152
13. Caperan D (1973) La formule pilaire: son intérêt en pathologie générale et cutanée. Thesis, Besançon
14. Chadwick J, Mann WN (1950) The medical works of hippocrates. Blackwell, London/Thomas, Springfield, p 171
15. Chase HB et al. (1969) Hair growth cycles in subcutaneous implants. Anat Rec 164(3): 333–337
16. Degos R, Civatte J (1961) Physiologie et physiopathologie du cuir chevelu, classification des alopecis. Rev Praticien 11(19): 1919–1926
17. Fiquet C, Courtois M (1979) Une technique originale d'appréciation de la croissance et de la chute des cheveux. Cutis, Paris, pp 975–983
18. Ebling FJ (1987) The biology of hair. Dermatol Clin 5(3): 467–481
19. Guarera M, Ciullia MPA (1986) Quantitative evaluation of hair loss. The phototrichogram. J Appl Cosmetol 4: 61–66
20. Hamilton JB (1961) Male hormone stimulation is prerequisite and an incitant in common baldness. Rev Pract 11(19): 1919–1926
21. Hamilton JB (1951) Patterned loss of hair in man: types and incidence. Ann NY Acad Sci 53: 708–728
22. Hamilton JB (1958) Age, sex and genetic factors in the regulation of hair growth in man: a comparison of Caucasian and Japanese populations. In: Montagna W, Ellis RA (eds) The biology of hair growth. Academic, Orlando, pp 399–433
23. Hincky M (1981) Les alopécies. E.M.C. Dermatologie 12855/A10: 2
24. Kligman AM (1959) The human hair cycles. J Invest Dermatol 33: 307–316
25. Montagna W, Ellis RA (1958) The vascularity and innervation of human hair follicles. In: Montagna W, Ellis RA (eds) Biology of hair growth 10: 219–226
26. Munro DD, Darley CR (1979) Disorders of epidermal appendages. In: Fiztpatrick TB (ed) Dermatology in general medicine: textbook and atlas. 2nd edn, Mc Graw-Hill, New York, pp 395–418
27. Orfanos CE, Montana W, Stuttgern G (1981) Hair research status and future aspects. Springer, Heidelberg New York Berlin
28. Rook A (1965) Endocrine influences on hair growth. Br Med J 1: 609–614
29. Rook A (1970) Hair. Introduction to the biology of the skin. Blackwell, London, pp 164–174
30. Rothman S (1958) Introduction. In: Montagna E, Ellis RA (eds) The biology of hair growth. Academic, New York
31. Sabouraud R (1936) De la séborrhée – des états pré- et post-séborrhiques. Nouv Pract Dermatol VII: 44–52, 79–82
32. Saitoh M, Uzuka M, Sakamoto M (1970) Human hair cycle. J Invest Dermatol 54: 65–81
33. Schweikert HU, Wilson JD (1981) Androgen metabolism in isolated human hair roots. In: Orfanos CE, Montagna W, Stuttgen G (eds) Hair research. Springer, Berlin Heidelberg New York, pp 210–214
34. Snyder L, Yingling H (1935) Studies in human inheritance XII. The application of the gene-frequency method of analysis of sex-influenced factors, with specific reference to baldness. Hum Biol 1: 608–615
35. Szabo G (1958) The regional frequency and distribution of hair follicles in human skin. In: Montagna W, Ellis RA (eds) The biology of hair growth. Academic, New York, pp 33–38
36. Szasz TS, Robertson AM (1950) The theory of the pathogenesis of ordinary human baldness. AMA Arch Dermatol Syphilol 61: 34–48
37. Van Neste D, Lachapelle JM, Antonie JR (1989) Trends in human hair growth and alopecia research. Kluwer, Dordrecht
38. Van Sctott EJ, Reinertson RP, Steinmuller R (1957) The growing hair roots of the human scalp and morphologic changes following amethopterin therapy. J Invest Dermatol 29: 197–204
39. Will F (1986) Mise au point et applications d'une méthode d'étude du cheveu. Le phototrichogramme. Thesis, no. 253. Strasbourg, p 96
40. Zviak C (1986) The science of hair care. Dekker, New York

Male Baldness

It is impossible to write a book about male baldness without providing at least one definition. This seemed obvious at the start. However, experience and attention to the demands of patients obliged us to ask at just what point one may properly speak of baldness. Can normality of the hair be defined? And in relation to whom? Many patients come to consult us even when it is impossible to classify them as bald. These patients seek advice simply because the hair is a little sparse. This is manifested sometimes by simple fronto-temporal recession; in others the anterior frontal line is unchanged but the hair is sparse behind, a simple decrease in density compared with the crown. If such aspects cannot be considered as baldness, they have in common the fact that their owners will become bald in the years to come and that they already have the mental attitude of the bald; it is exactly as if the complex due to the malformation occurs before the malformation itself.

General Features

To understand the different aspects of baldness, several parameters must always be borne in mind. The ratio between the bald and hairy areas is certainly essential, and must be evaluated in as precise a manner as possible. This absence of mathematical rigour is the chief criticism to be made of the different classifications of baldness. The elasticity of the scalp varies and may considerably modify the therapeutic possibilities for an equivalent hairless area. The covering power of the existing hair itself depends on numerous factors:

- The density of the hair, which depends on the number of hairs per cm^2 and their thickness
- Hair type (stiff, curly, frizzy or crinkly)
- Colour (light hair adjusts better to a lack of uniformity)
- Length of the hair
- Cleanliness (dry, clean hair is much more bouffant than greasy or moist hair)

Any classification with therapeutic aims must take account of most of these parameters.

Ratio of Bald to Hairy Areas

The basic principle of the surgery of baldness consists in distributing the paucity of material as uniformly as possible, while sometimes favouring certain regions. This is possible only because of the elasticity of the skin, which allows expansion of the hairy area.

The ratio between the bald and hairy areas is therefore of vital importance. In our experience, when this ratio exceeds 1:2 baldness is no longer amenable to surgery.

It was seen, in the chapter on "Anatomy" (p. 14) that the total surface area of the scalp is 600–700 cm^2. In our opinion, 200 cm^2 is the maximum bald area that can be covered with any degree of cosmetic satisfaction. The use of skin expansion may permit this limit to be exceeded, which is certainly variable in terms of many factors, particularly the elasticity of the scalp. This area corresponds to an exposed cranium over an area some 10 cm wide and 20 cm long. As what we have called the bi-auricular distance (see "Anatomy") is fixed at 31–32 cm, a length of 10 cm for the hippocratic crown (HC) corresponds to such an extent of baldness (Fig. 1)[1]. In practice, therefore, this measurement by itself defines the degree of baldness. In such a case, the height of the crown measured in the nuchal region is on average 13–14 cm. One centimetre more or less in the height of this crown represents a very important difference, since it corresponds to an additional surface area of 40 cm^2 to be covered and at the same time to a decrease in the covering zone by the same amount. To take an example: if HC=10 cm, the bald area is

[1] Throughout this book the "crown", unless otherwise stated, refers to the "hippocratic crown", as shown in Fig. 1.

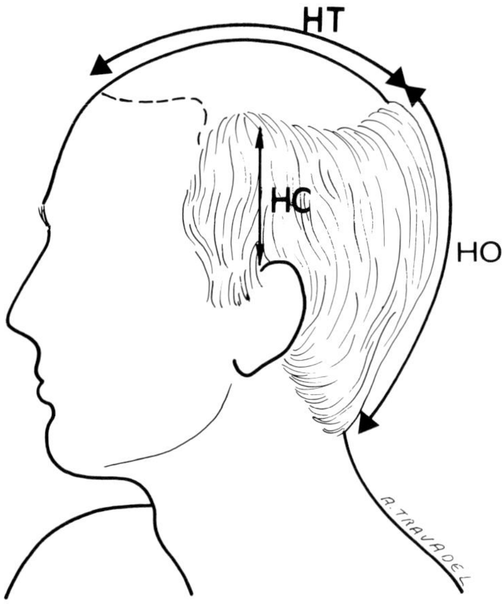

Fig. 1. Measurements. *HC*, height of crown; *HO*, occipital height; *HT*, length of vertex

Table 1. Changes in scalp elasticity with age

		Elasticity (%)		
		< 25 years	25–45 years	> 45 years
Elasticity	I	10	22	30
	II	75	62	59
	III	15	16	11

200 cm^2 and the covering zone 400 cm^2. If HC=9 cm, the bald area becomes 240 cm^2 and the covering zone 360 cm^2; the ratio of the bald area to the hairy area has changed from 0.5 to 0.66 (i.e. from 1:2 to 2:3), which is considerable.

Laxity of the Scalp

Laxity of the scalp is the second essential prognostic factor. Unfortunately, there is no scientific method of quantifying it. We have seen that elasticity increases statistically with age, which in our view represents an excess of skin rather than a true increase in elasticity of the scalp itself, but which is without any practical value (Table 1). We also know that elasticity is more important for vertical than horizontal mobilisation of the scalp and that it is less marked in the occipital than in the temporal region.

In practical terms, it is possible to assess the laxity of the scalp by palming it with both hands and mobilising it on the cranium. In the temporal region this mobilisation can be done between the thumbs. When mobility is nil, or virtually nil, only very narrow flaps less than 3 cm wide are possible, and reductions will not be attractive. In contrast, very great elasticity allows the fashioning of flaps up to 4 cm in breadth in the vertical direction and even 5 cm in the horizontal direction. In these same patients, reductions allow the excision of quite large bald areas; moreover, the elasticity of the scalp returns more quickly, allowing early reintervention.

Covering Power of the Hair

The covering power of the hair is the third important prognostic factor and depends on numerous parameters.

Hair Density

Clinically, hair density is a function of two variable and independent parameters:

Hair Thickness. This is more important in Blacks and Asiatics than in Whites. The diameter varies from 0.5 to 0.9 mm or even more. It will be seen that hair thickness becomes especially important when density is low.

Number of Hairs. The number of hairs per cm^2 defines actual density. It is normally 200–400 per cm^2 (see Photo 1a in "Anatomy"). In bald subjects this density is markedly diminished, especially in the transition zones. It may fall to 150 or even 80 in the hairy zone. It also diminishes regularly with age, particularly after 60 years.

If, by means of an expansion prosthesis, the hair-bearing area is doubled, the density will fall to 100–200, depending on the patient, which still gives a very good visual impression. A graft 4 mm in diameter carrying an average of 12 hairs (see Photo 1b in "Anatomy") will provide a maximum density of 100 hairs/cm^2 after a minimum of three or four implantation sessions.

Variable Factors

These fundamental factors are immutable, but in a given patient certain variable factors may be added and these are sometimes modifiable. The hair has a greater covering power when it is frizzier and is maximal in Blacks with crinkly hair. Here, a few grafts suffice to give the illusion of a covered cranium; naturally, this illusion will be more convincing when the hairs are longer. But, from an aesthetical point of view, stiff hair can be grown much longer than frizzy hair, which very quickly becomes unmanageable. Therefore patients should often be advised to let their hair grow somewhat and sometimes to have a permanent wave. Dry and clean hair is more bouffant than greasy, dirty hair. Therefore frequent shampooing as required is advised, especially as the frequency of shampooing has no influence on seborrhoea or the speed of relubrication of the hair.

We also feel that hair colour has little influence on its covering power. However, black or dark-brown hair is less tolerant of a non-uniform aspect than light or greying hair, which may be of some importance in the choice of surgical treatment.

Classifications

All the detailed and simplified classifications proposed hitherto are aimed at arranging each aspect of the clinical course according to the morphology of the hair loss. They take into account only the bald and hairy areas, which, as has been seen, does not suffice when planning treatment. However, they will be reviewed here for historical reasons. We shall then propose a personal classification, simpler to remember and employ, which is more applicable in planning treatment as it allows for the chief parameters previously mentioned and gives a better picture of baldness.

Morphological Classifications

Numerous classifications have been suggested since Beck's study in 1950 [3], carried out on 1000 male Caucasians, who were divided into two evolutional types (frontal and fronto-vertical baldness).

In 1951, Hamilton [15] brought out a classification based on the description of eight evolutional aspects and three subdivisions; he compared the incidence of baldness between Caucasians and Chinese. In 1972, Setty [21] simplified the classification into three aspects: totopilosis (equivalent to Hamilton's type I), indentatopilosis (types II–IV) and indentato-circulo-pilosis (types VI and VII), this last stage being subdivided into confluent and non-confluent.

Feit [14], Rook [18] and Norwood [17] suggested variants of Hamilton's classification. Blanchard [4] proposed a more precise classification with six evolutional stages determined by six measurements (Fig. 2a): the glabello-frontal, superciliary frontal, interparietal, fronto-vertical, helico-vertical and nucho-vertical distances.

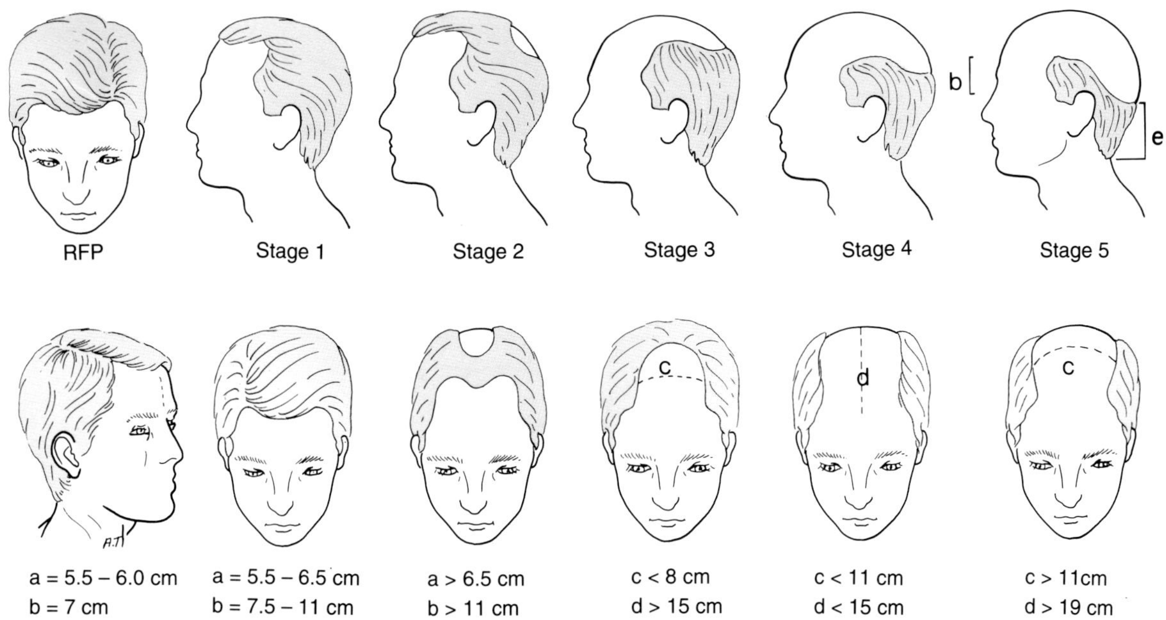

Fig. 2. a Blanchard's classification. *RFP*, frontal regression in puberty

Hamilton's Classification

Hamilton's classification (1951) [15] (Fig. 2b) serves as a standard for every classification proposed subsequently. It seems to us difficult to apply because it includes so many figural representations that it must be kept constantly at hand.

- Type I: no or little recession of the anterior frontal line (AFL).
- Type II: symmetric recession of the anterior frontal line resulting in two fronto-temporal areas of recession whose deepest point is 2 cm in front of a vertical line drawn from the external auditory meatus.
- Type III: the fronto-temporal areas of recession are deeper; hair loss at the vertex is associated with recession of the AFL.
- Type IV: the two anterior and posterior areas of hair loss are separated by a densely haired band.

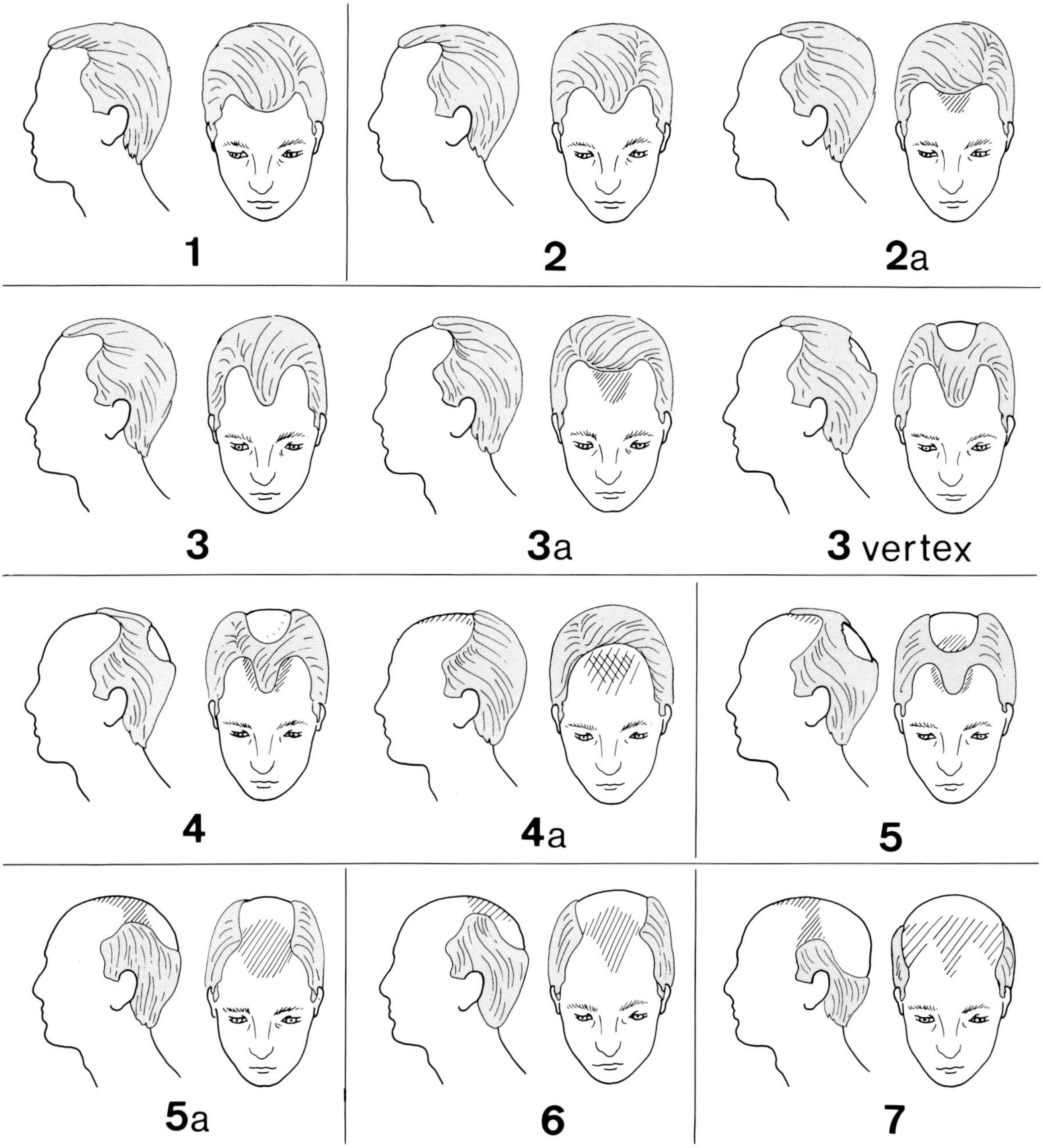

Fig. 2. b Hamilton's classification

- Type V: the hair-bearing band separating the two zones of hair loss is narrower and thinner.
- Type VI: the sparsely haired zones are completely confluent and extend towards the posterior and lateral regions.
- Type VII: extension of the hair loss is maximal. A hair-bearing crown persists and covers the lower temporo-occipital regions.

Bouhanna's Classification

Bouhanna's classification [6] (Fig. 3) distinguishes three schematic stages:

- Stage 1
  - Type a: symmetric recession of the frontal margin forming two temporal areas of recession of varying depth
  - Type b: sparseness at the cranial summit or vertex
- Stage 2
  - Type a: uniform recession of the frontal margin as far as the cranial summit
  - Type b: with associated vertex
- Stage 3: hippocratic baldness, the ultimate stage of alopecia, where only the temporo-occipital crown remains

Dynamic Classification of Dardour and Bouhanna

The diversity of surgical techniques and the difficulty in arriving at operative indications led us to try to include all the parameters, both morphological and dynamic, that affect the scalp and the hair itself. This classification includes for each heading a symbol followed by a number which indicates its situation. We decided arbitrarily to classify a case as "1" when the conditions are optimal, followed by "2", "3" and "4" as they deteriorate.

Stage

Stage grossly defines the severity of baldness [6]:

- Stage 0, normal hair
- Stage 1, simple fronto-temporal recession
- Stage 2, intermediate between stages 1 and 3
- Stage 3, cranial summit entirely hairless

Density

This classification allows a more precise approach, to be defined clinically for each region. We have seen that clinical density depends not only on the number of hairs per cm^2, but also on their thickness. We prefer to use this purely subjective assessment since counting the hairs and measuring their thickness is difficult in the consulting room. Moreover, the clinical aspect is ultimately more important in assessment. We therefore proceed from the best to worst case: "1" is normal density (200–400 hairs per cm^2), "2" signifies sparse hair (100–200 hairs per cm^2), "3" is very sparse hair (50–100 hairs per cm^2) and "4" signifies a smooth zone (less than 50 hairs per cm^2).

A density listed as 3 contraindicates the transplantation of cylindrical grafts but not of micrografts. An expander may stretch the scalp in such a way as to divide the density at the central zone of distension by 5–10. The degree of density should be noted in three regions (Fig. 4): frontal region (F), vertical region (T) and the hippocratic crown (C).

As an example, a subject listed as C1, F2, T4 will have a crown of normal density, a sparse but not bald frontal region and a completely smooth vertex. The density can be complemented by various measurements (Fig. 4):

- HC is the height of the crown above the ear, which, as we have seen, determines by itself the ratio between bald and hairy areas; as the interauricular distance is 30–32 cm, if HC=10 cm the breadth of the bald zone is 10–12 cm.
- HO is the height of the crown in the posterior occipital region.
- HT is the length of the vertex in its anteroposterior diameter.

This last measurement is only important when the patient has an isolated vertex while the frontal density is normal (F1). When the frontal region is also hairless, the measurement HT represents the distance between the summit of the crown behind and the theoretic limit of the mid-frontal line in front. The sum HO + HT is then around 33 or 34 cm. Conventionally, all these measurements apply only to adequately hairy areas and ignore any area covered with down.

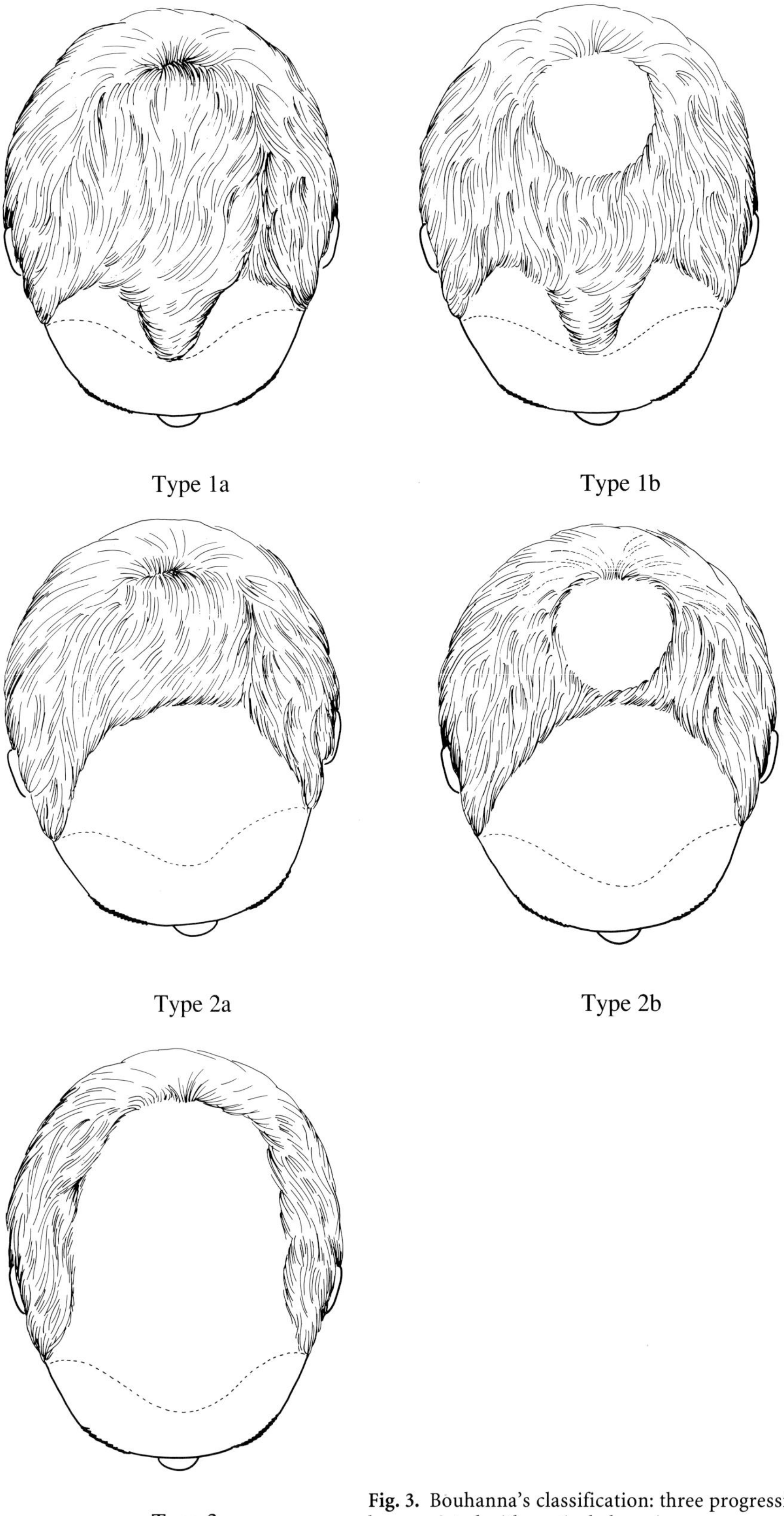

Fig. 3. Bouhanna's classification: three progressive stages, which may or may not be associated with vertical alopecia

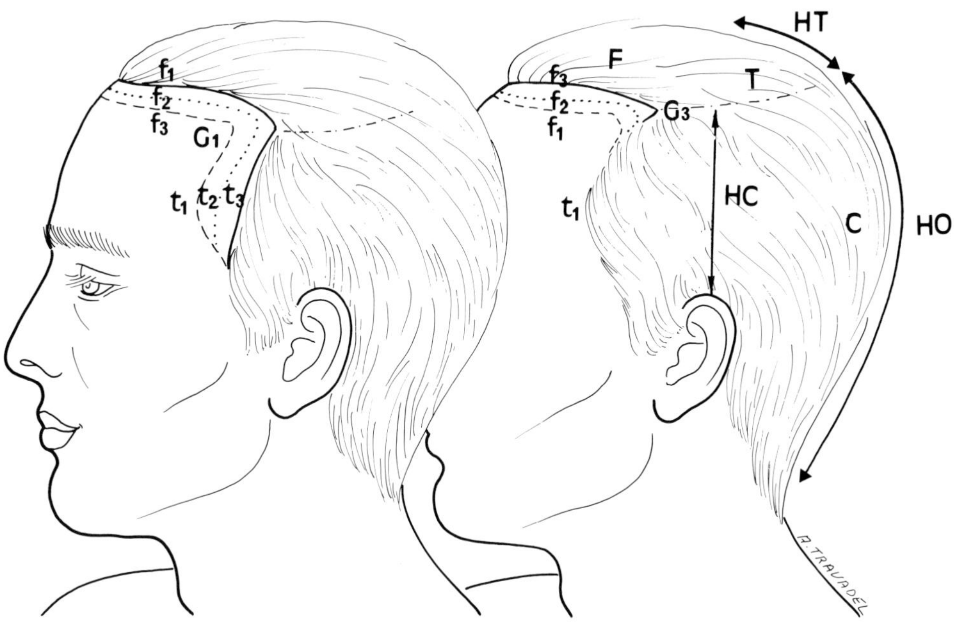

Fig. 4. Dardour-Bouhanna classification: regions and measurements

Laxity of the Scalp

Laxity of the scalp is the final important factor in the classification: "1" signifies very great laxity, "2" considerable laxity, "3" minor laxity and "4" poor or no laxity.

Other Factors

Other factors are less important and serve only to refine the therapeutic indications.

Base of the Fronto-temporal Recession (G)

Essentially, the base of the fronto-temporal recession recedes more as baldness advances; however, there are some rare individual variations:

- G=1: a vertical dropped from point G passes in front of the sideburn.
- G=2: it passes through the sideburn.
- G=3: it passes behind the sideburn.

Frontal Line

The position of the frontal line is denoted *f* (Fig. 4):

- *f*1=frontal line in normal position (10.5% of our patients)
- *f*2=recession of point G with frontal line receded between 1 and 2 cm (36.8% of our patients)
- *f*3=point G very receded or absent in cases F3 and F4 and frontal line receded by 2 cm or more (52.6% of cases)

Anterior Temporal Line

The position and recession of the anterior temporal line (*t*) is also an important factor and may modify certain operative indications (Fig. 4, Photo 1):

- *t*1=temporal line in anterior position (40.4% of patients)
- *t*2=temporal line in mid-position (50.4%)
- *t*3=temporal line in posterior position (9.2%)

For a more precise determination of *t*, it is preferable to choose a point on this line situated 10 cm above the ear. This point actually corresponds to point G, i.e. the base of the fronto-temporal recession. A vertical line dropped from this point passes:

- In front of the sideburn if *t*=1
- Through the sideburn if *t*=2
- Behind the sideburn if *t*=3

Sometimes *f* and *t* recede symmetrically, but this is not inevitable and our precise review shows that:

- If *f* is in place (*f*=1), the temporal line is in anterior or mid-position (*t*1 = *t*2 = 50%) at equality, but never posterior (*t*3 = 0).

a b c d

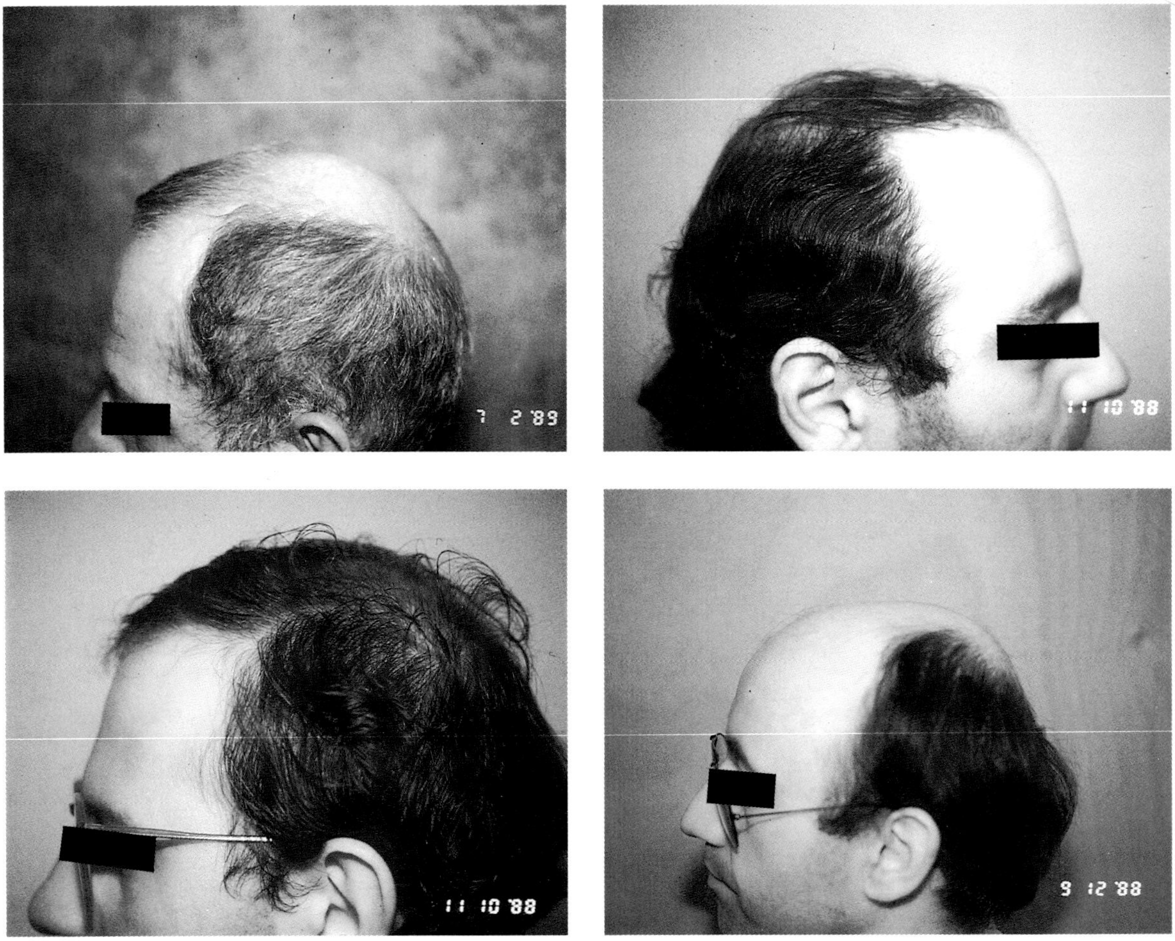

Photo 1a–d. Positions of anterior temporal line. **a,b** *t*1. **c** *t*2. **d** *t*3

- If f is slightly receded (f=2), t is in position 1 or 2 at equality, never in position 3.
- If f=3, t=1 in 20% of cases, t=2 in 70% and t=3 in 10%. These statistics simply indicate that the frontal line recedes before the temporal line and not simultaneously. Even in very hairless patients, the temporal line is rarely very posterior.

Aspect of Hair

Whether stiff, curly, frizzy or crinkly, the aspect of the hair is due to the configuration of the keratin chains. Long hair, waved or frizzy, has the maximum covering effect both in situ and at a distance. Crinkly hair has a covering effect only in situ, which gives preference to grafts rather than flaps.

Colour

Very dark hair may have an artificial and unpleasing appearance at the frontal line after transplantation of cylindrical grafts, especially if the light skin of the subject accentuates the contrast. Very fair or greying hair, on the other hand, is more tolerant.

Thickness

Thickness is assessed clinically. Although already mentioned in the assessment of clinical density, this measurement should be taken into account. The diameter of the hair shaft varies to give three stages:

- E1=very thick hair (diameter in excess of 80 μ)
- E2=medium hair (diameter between 60 and 80 μ)
- E3=fine hair (diameter between 40 and 60 μ)

Thick hair, especially when dark, is unsatisfactory for the performance of cylindrical grafts; micrograft transplantation is indicated.

Rate of Growth in Each Region Considered

The rate of hair growth varies markedly between different people. This factor is vital when considering the indications for operation. Thus, the covering effect and the possibility of masking are directly linked to the possibility of growth of the transplanted or transposed hair. This growth is on average 1 cm a month. The subject's history allows a rough assessment in terms of the periods between visits to the barber (once a month on average). A ranking can be made either roughly, in terms of the frequency of hair-cutting ("1", once a month; "2", once every 2 months; "3", once every 3 months) or in a more precise fashion by the measurement of hair growth in successive macrophotographs taken at intervals of 3 days. This classification thus gives a simple and very faithful picture of the baldness under study.

Examples

Stage 2 Baldness. This subject has type C1 F3 T3 baldness (Photo 2). As far as the primary factors are concerned, HC=11 cm, HO=16 cm, S=2. As for the secondary factors, E=2, *f*=3, *t*=1, G=2; the hair is black and stiff. This patient has a moderately severe degree of baldness. The crown is normal. Hair on the forehead and vertex is very sparse. The height of the posterior hair-bearing zone is 16 cm. The height of the crown above the ear is 11 cm, signifying that the vertex is some 9 cm in breadth and that the ratio of bald to hairy areas is acceptable, given that elasticity at S2 is very correct. The fronto-temporal areas are well receded, the temporal line is in the anterior position and the frontal line is very receded indeed (over 2 cm). The hair thickness is medium. Being black and stiff, the hairs have good covering power provided they are left rather long.

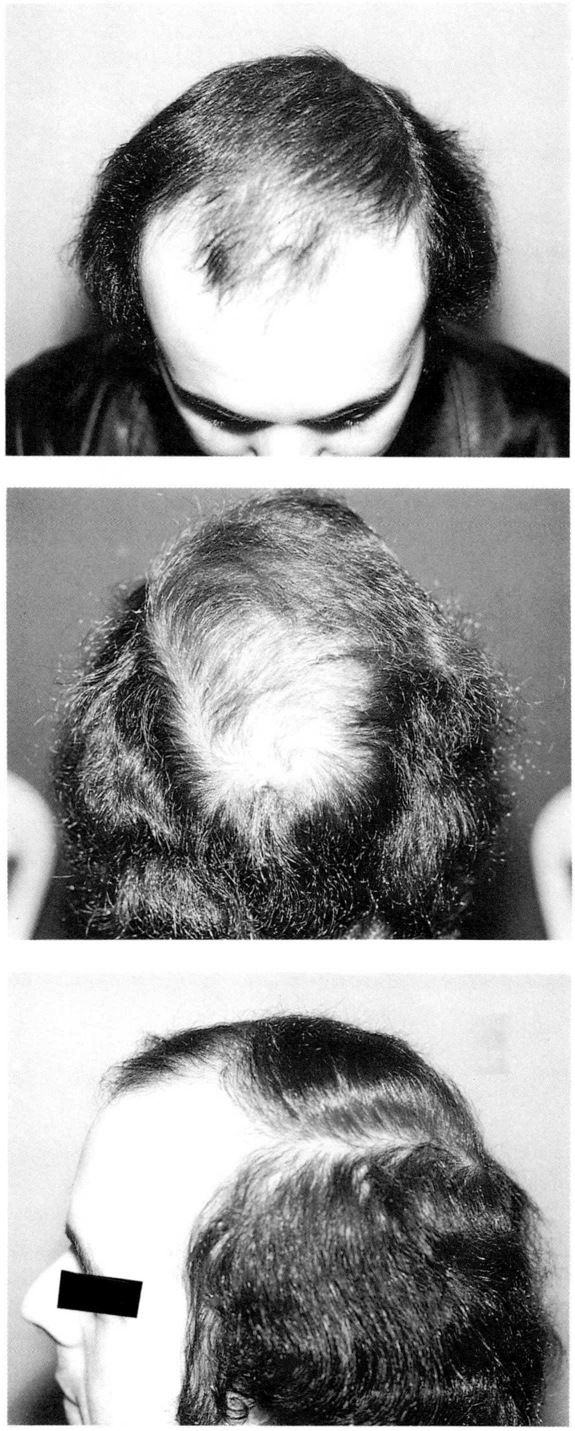

a

b

c

Photo 2a–c. Stage 2 baldness: C1 T3 F3 G2 *f*3 *t*1, HC=11 cm, S=2

Stage 3 Baldness. This subject has type C1 F4 T4 baldness (Photo 3). The variables are as follows: HC=10 cm, S=2, G=3, *f*=3, *t*=–1. This patient has severe baldness. The crown is of normal density, the forehead and vertex are completely smooth, which implies the absence of fronto-temporal recession (G3) and a frontal line (*f*3), but the temporal line is in the anterior position (*t*1). The height of the crown (HC) is 10 cm, which permits the hope of suitable coverage, especially as the laxity of the scalp is satisfactory (S=2).

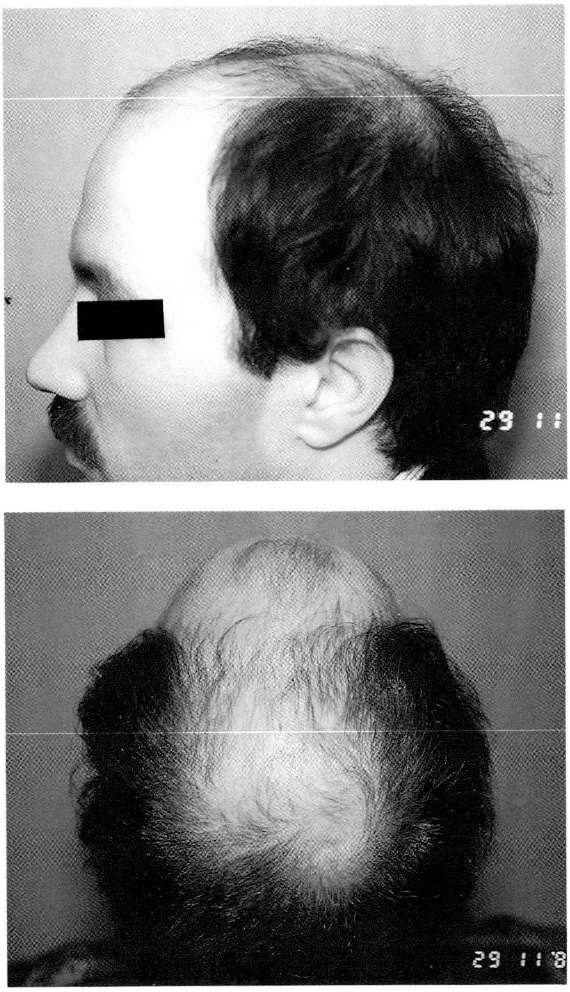

a

b

Photo 3a,b. Stage 3 baldness: C1 T4 F4 G3 *f*3 *t*1, HC=10 cm, S=2

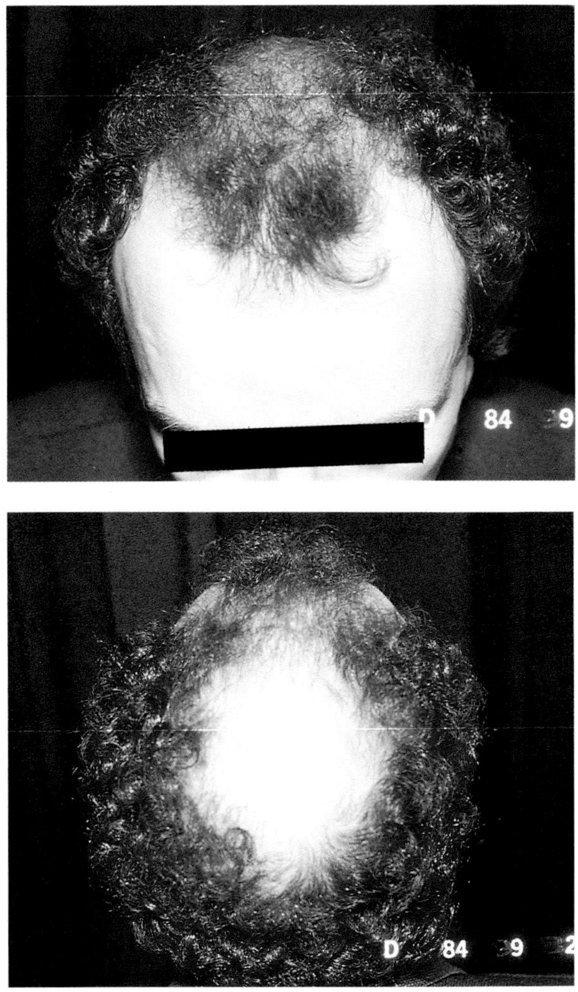

a

b

Photo 4a,b. Stage 2 baldness: C1 F2 T4 G2 *f*2, HC=12 cm, HO=16 cm, HT=8 cm

Stage 2 Baldness. This subject has type C1 F2 T4 baldness (Photo 4). The variables are as follows: HC=12 cm, HO=16 cm, HT=8 cm, G=2, *f*=2. This patient has moderate baldness. The frontal region is slightly affected, whereas the vertex is completely smooth. The height of the crown (12 cm) indicates a good ratio of bald to hairy areas. The height of the crown behind is 16 cm, which is correct, but the distance HT is 8 cm, indicating a vertex too large to be covered by a classical transverse reduction. G=2 and *f*=2 indicate minor fronto-temporal recession and frontal line (less than 2 cm).

Stage 2 Baldness. This subject has type C1 F2 T3 baldness (Photo 5). There is minor baldness with slight frontal thinning and marked thinning of the vertex, which is, however, not completely smooth.

Stage 1 Baldness. This subject has type C1 F2 T1 (Photo 6); *f*=2 and *t*=2. There is commencing baldness with a moderate decrease in hair density and only minor recession of the frontal and temporal lines.

Comparison of the Classifications of Bouhanna, Hamilton and Dardour

Table 2 summarises the relationships between the classifications. It shows that all the cases described by Hamilton can be found in our own classification, but that the converse is not true. It also confirms that some important factors are not represented in Hamilton's classification, especially:

- The hair density in each region
- The position of the temporal line *t*

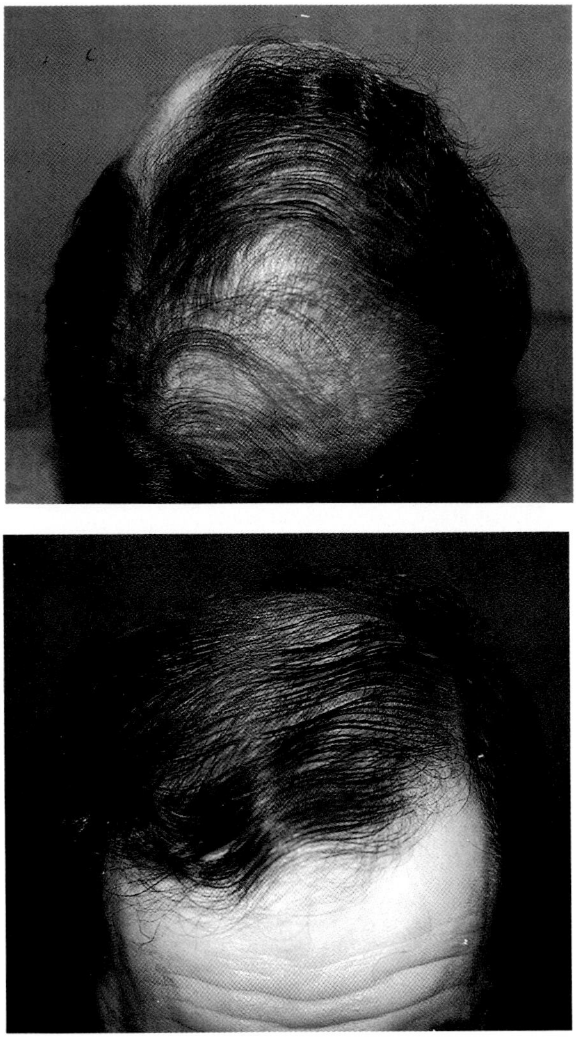

Photo 5a,b. Example of baldness C1 F2 T3

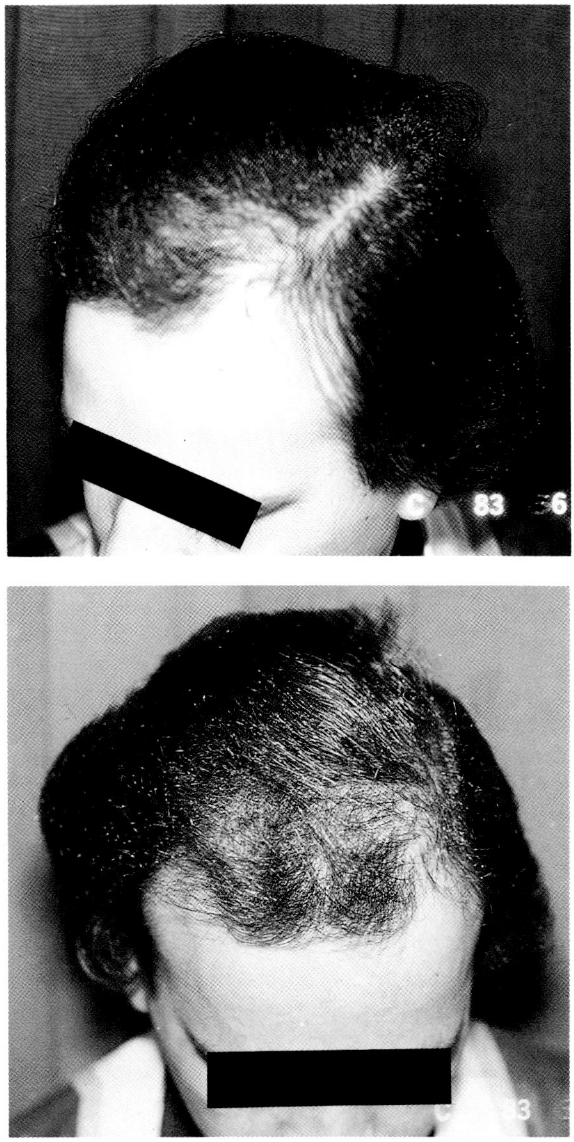

Photo 6a,b. Example of stage 1 baldness: C1 F2 T1 *f2 t2*

Table 2. Comparison of classifications

Bouhanna (Fig. 3)	Hamilton (Fig. 2)	Dardour (Fig. 4)			
Stage Ia, Ib	Stage I	C1 T1	F1	G1 f2	
	Stage II	C1 T1	F1	G2 f3	
	Stage IIa	C1 T1	F3	G3 f3	
	Stage III	C1 T1	F1 (F2)	G3 f3	
	Stage IIIa	C1 T1	F4	G3	
	Stage III vertex	C1 T2 (T3)	F2 (F1)	G3	
	Stage IV	C1 T2 (T3–T4)	F2 (F3)	G3	
Stage IIa, IIb	Stage IVa	C1 T1	F4	G3	
	Stage V	C1 T3 (T4)	F4 (F3)	G3	
	Stage Va	C1 T3 (T4)	F4	G3	HC>12 cm
Stage III	Stage VI	C1 T4 (T3)	F4 (F3)		HC=10 cm
	Stage VI	C1 T4	F4		HC<9 cm

- The laxity of the scalp S
- The exact height of the crown (HC), though we know that this by itself determines the ratio of bald and hairy areas
- The covering power of the hair
- The rate of growth of the hair

Temporal Course

Apart from the "fixed" aspect of the baldness discussed in the previous chapter, there is a dynamic aspect which is important to grasp as it is one of the prognostic factors. The trichogram, as well the other supplementary studies, are certainly factors in assessing age changes, but they cannot predict the fate of the region studied in the long term, i.e. after 10 years. Population studies show that there are peaks in the evolution of baldness which allow us to distinguish two types: juvenile and late-onset baldness.

Juvenile Baldness

Fortunately more rare, this carries a worse prognosis. These are the cases which lead to "inoperable baldness", i.e. those where the height of the residual crown does not exceed 6–8 cm and where the frontal and vertical regions are completely smooth. This type of baldness begins very early, sometimes at around 16 or 17 years and is established between 20 and 25 years. An hereditary factor is evident in virtually all these cases [19]. Apart from these extreme cases, juvenile baldness usually starts at 20–22 years and its acute phase is over by the age of 25–30 years, the age at which it stabilises [13]. Thus there seems to be a relationship between early age of onset and severity.

Late-Onset Baldness

Late-onset baldness begins between 35 and 40 years, and it too is established in a few years. The prognosis is usually better. The height of the hippocratic crown is greater, between 10 and 12 cm, and even if there is a decrease in clinical hair density (stage 2 or 3) in the frontal and vertical regions, these are rarely completely smooth (stage 4). As will be shown, in these cases the transposition of a well-placed flap often suffices to produce a very satisfactory result. The prognosis of late-onset baldness is therefore better than that of juvenile baldness.

Age-Related Changes

Apart from these two evolutional peaks in baldness, there is always in almost the entire population a progressive thinning of the hair with age, with decreased density and thickness. This of course leads to an increased incidence of baldness in the population, estimated at 80% after the age of 70 or 80 years. Unlike juvenile baldness, where the crown always has a normal density, here there is often a marked thinning of the hair in this region, which, apart from age-related vascular problems, makes the outcome of operation more uncertain. In our series of operated patients we have found this progress of baldness with age (Table 3):

Table 3. Incidence (%)of baldness by age

		<25 years	25–45 years	>45 years
Baldness	I	40	15	11
	II	50	39	30
	III	10	46	59

- Before the age of 25 years, 40% of patients have stage 1 baldness, 50% stage 2 and 10% stage 3.
- Between 25 and 45 years, only 15% are at stage 1, 30% at stage 2 and 46% at stage 3.
- After 45 years, 11% are stage 1, 30% stage 2 and 59% stage 3.

From this it emerges that a major development takes place between the second and third decades.

Factors Determining the Course of Baldness

There does not seem to be any factor either promoting or restraining the natural progress of male baldness. However, certain factors may influence the rate of growth and the fall of hair. We have noted the effect of these factors on pilogenesis in the previous chapter, but they exert their effect diffusely and are not localised to the cranial summit; they cannot reproduce the aspect of androgeno-genetic baldness.

Genetic Factors

Family studies have long demonstrated the determining role of heredity, though the exact mode of transmission is not yet entirely elucidated. An autosomal dominant mode with variable and incomplete penetrance [19] seems likely, transmission being effected by both men and women (though often not expressed because of hormonal influences). The current trend is to consider baldness as the outcome of the interaction of several genes, i.e. of multi-factorial heredity. However, Orentreich states that baldness is controlled by a single dominant autosomal sex-linked gene and influenced by numerous factors limiting the expression of the trait. However this may be, genetic determinism cannot act in the absence of androgens and only after a certain age.

Age

The age of onset of baldness (always after puberty) is genetically determined. The follicle is progammed to become receptive to the influence of certain hormonal fractions at certain ages, earlier or later. The rate of progress of alopecia varies with time.

Androgens

The determinant action of androgens has often been noted. Hippocrates had already remarked on the absence of baldness in eunuchs, women and children. The injection of male hormones in castrated or eunuchoid subjects provokes baldness, but only in genetically predisposed subjects, and the progress of the baldness ceases when treatment stops. Castration of the normal man interrupts the development of baldness, but does not lead to regrowth of hair. However, the presence of androgens is necessary, though insufficient:

- In the feminising testicle (male genotype and female phenotype) there is a normal or even elevated level of androgens, but the receptor tissues are insensitive to testosterone or to 5-alpha-dihydrotestosterone; thus there is no alopecia, nor any development of secondary sexual characteristics.
- In male baldness, the serum testosterone level is normal, but there is a particular receptivity of the follicles in certain scalp regions in genetically predisposed individuals.

The stereotyped topography of baldness at the forehead and vertex has never been properly explained. As we have seen, it seems that the mechanism is to be found within the follicle itself in genetically determined regions, but the exact regulation of this special receptivity (whose stigmata are an increased activity of 5-alpha-reductase and an accumulation of dihydrotestosterone in the sensory follicles) is still unknown, and some aspects of androgen metabolism in these follicles have yet to be disovered [3].

It has been seen that the role of the androgens predominates and that other hormones have no influence [18]. The corticoid and thyroid hormones can affect the hair if excessive or insufficient, but this involves body hair rather than the scalp and always diffusely.

The conjunction of these different factors has been shown by a study of identical twins reported by Hamilton. One of them had been castrated before puberty and retained abundant hair at the age of 40; his uncastrated brother became progressively bald over a period of 20 years. At the age of 40 the castrated twin received injections of testosterone and became as bald as his brother in less than 6 months. Thus, the expression of the gene was operative over time, though not expressed in the absence of the essential hormonal influence.

Other Causes of Alopecia

Primary Alopecia in Women

In women the process of baldness is similar to that in men. Progressive thinning of the vertex is suggestive, despite the persistence of a frontal margin [16] (Photo 7). Onset is usually later [10], with increased hair loss between 25 and 40 years. Progress is less rapid and is indicated more by a diffuse thinning of varying severity (Ludwig's classification) (Fig. 5) which is often more marked at the summit. Hormonal disorders should sometimes be sought by endocrine assessment. In the premenopausal woman, it is always important to consider possible hormone substitution treatment [9].

Acute Diffuse Alopecia [8]

Acute diffuse alopecia occurs after certain physical insults (rapid weight loss, feverish illnesses, surgical

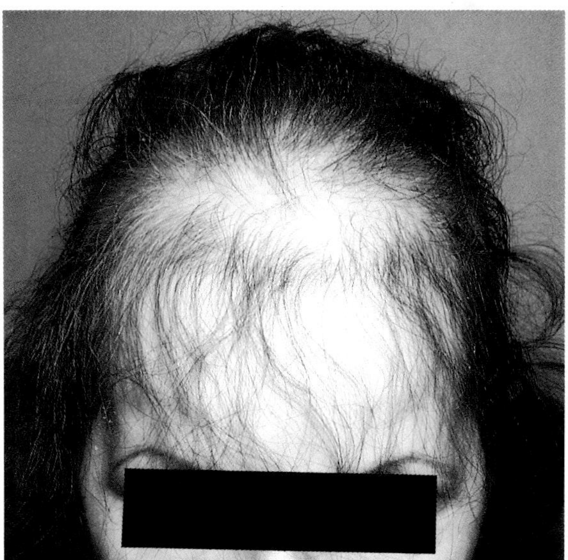

Photo 7. "Feminine" type of alopecia in menopausal woman

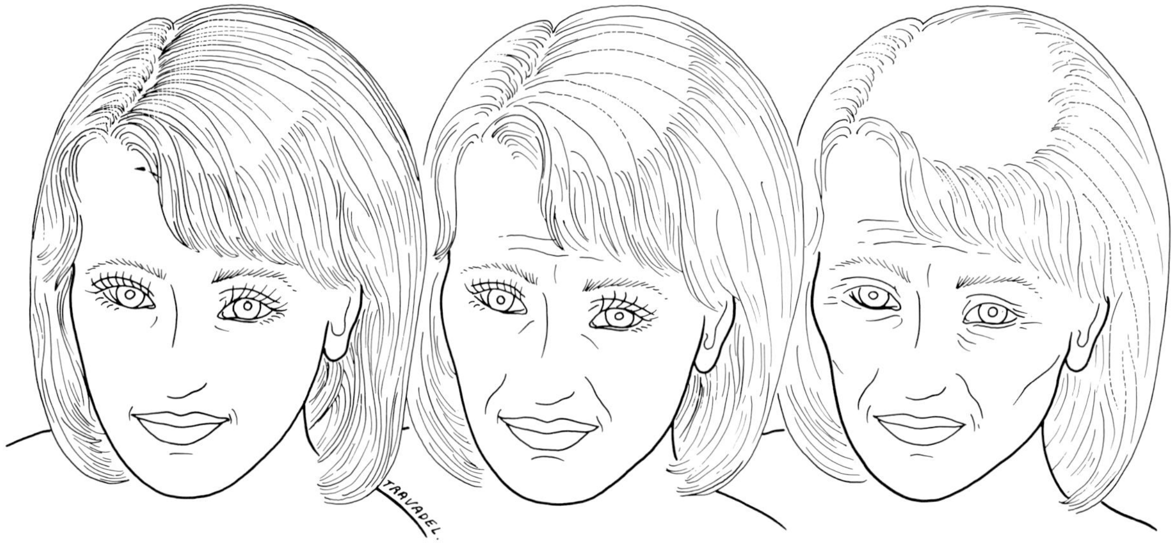

Fig. 5a–c. Ludwig's classification. **a** Stage 1: oval moderate alopecia of vertex with long axis anteroposterior, situated 2–3 cm behind frontal zone of implantation, which is unaffected. **b** Stage 2: clear alopecia with short grey or white hair, situated 1 cm from frontal zone of implantation. **c** Stage 3: near-total alopecia of vertex, but with preservation of thin frontal band of hair

procedures, post-partum), psychological influences (stress, emotional shock) or chemical factors (sometimes after stopping oestrogenic contraception) and especially during anti-mitotic treatment (cyclophosphamide, methotrexate). It is often reversible.

Among the various forms of acute temporary hair loss [12], it is important to note the anagenic defluvium, which is a loss of hair in the anagenic stage found during alopecia areata and especially as a sequel to surgical procedures. This loss occurs during the 2–3 weeks following the operation and spontaneously regresses in 2–3 months, whereas telogenic effluvium is an acceleration of the cycle towards the telogenic phase, ending in massive hair loss. It may be manifested following illness or pregnancy and usually occurs during the 3 months following the event.

Diffuse Chronic Alopecia

The causes of diffuse chronic alopecia may be hormonal in origin (various thyroid, adrenal, pituitary or genital syndromes) or even metabolic [1] (unstabilised diabetes) or nutritional [11] (dietary deficiency, malabsorption).

Alopecia areata

Alopecia areata is quite a common disorder [1], most often affecting subjects between 20 and 40 years of age. It is evidenced by the often abrupt development of a very regular, round or oval plaque of alopecia. Its course is unpredictable and, after a phase of extension and then of stability, regrowth may occur after several months, sometimes with depigmented hair; in other cases, other areas may appear on the scalp, or even at the beard, eyebrows and eyelashes. More rarely, and maximally, there may be an alopecia leading to total baldness, where the potential for more or less total regrowth is unpredictable.

In the phase of extension at the periphery of the alopecic plaque, typical hairs of the "exclamation mark" type may be observed. The exact cause is not clearly known: there may be familial factors or sometimes a precipitating stress, while more recently the presence of peribulbar lymphocytic infiltration has suggested the possibility of an auto-immune mechanism.

Traumatic Alopecia Without Skin Damage

Traumatic alopecia not associated with wounds is actually secondary to prolonged ischaemia of the hair bulbs:

- Occipital alopecia in the infant
- After a haematoma of the scalp
- After prolonged compression, as during general anaesthesia of long duration

Repetitive mechanical traction (trichotillomania), often in children, sometimes in women, often produces alopecic plaques in the temporal or retorauricular regions [20].

Congenital Alopecia

Congenital alopecia is more rare, more or less incomplete and sometimes associated with other (particularly cutaneous) dystrophies. Quite different is the alopecia caused by a nevus, particularly the sebaceous nevus of Jadahsson, or by a subcutaneous angioma.

Alopecia with Skin Damage

Post-traumatic Alopecia

Post-traumatic alopecia may be accidental (injury or avulsion of the scalp) or may occur after tumoral excision (epithelioma etc.) or due to cosmetic injury: excessive traction by combs or hot irons, hair-clips, chignons, or over-tight plaiting [7]. It may also occur after lifting procedures. In this case it may appear:

- In the early sequelae (temporal alopecia, which is however usually limited and transient). The responsible mechanism may be vascular (excessive tension, smoking) or traumatism of the hair bulbs by too superficial a dissection. For this reason, we advise that the dissection should always be performed under the fascio-epicranial plane at this level.
- Secondarily, in the form of a dehiscent smooth and broadened scar within the hair cover, particularly visible in subjects whose temporal hair is already sparse.

After Burns or Irradiation (Radiodermatitis)

Alopecia after burns or irradiation is of infective origin (favus, impetigo, folliculitis etc.) or may even be due to dermatological conditions (scleroderma, chronic lupus erythematosus, lichen planus, the pseudo-alopecia of Brocq).

References

1. Bartosova L, Jorda V, Stava Z (1984) Diseases of the hair and scalp. Karger, Basel
2. Bergfeld WF, Redmond GP (1987) Androgenetic alopecia. Dermatol Clin 5(3): 491–500
3. Beck CH (1950) A study on extension and distribution of the human body hair. Dermatologica 101: 317–331
4. Blanchard D, Blanchard G (1984) Proposition d'une approche topograhique de la transplantation capillaire et de la reduction tonsurale. ann Chir Plast Esth 29(2): 152–161
5. Bouhanna P (1976) Le cuir Chevelu: les alopécies définitives et leurs traitements. Thesis, Paris
6. Bouhanna P (1977) Conduite à tenir devant une alopécie séborrhéique masculine. Med Act 4(5): 131–133
7. Bouhanna P (1985) Alpécie androgénétique dite séborrhéique. Bull Esth Dermatol Cosmet 5: 19–25
8. Bouhanna P (1986) Guide diagnostique des alopécies. Bull Esthet Dermatol Cosmet 14: 19–24
9. Bouhanna P (1988) les alopécies de la femne ménopausée. Reproduction humaine et hormones 1(1): 33–41
10. Bouhanna P (1989) les alopécies de la femme jeune. Gynecol Obstet 218: 18–20
11. Burke KE (1989) Hair loss. Post Grad Med 85(6): 52–77
12. Caserio RJ, Hordinsky MK (1988) Disorders of hair. J Am Acad Dermatol 19(5): 895–903
13. Degos R, Civatte J (1961)Physiologie et physiopathologie du cuir chevelu, classification des alopécies. Rev Pracitien 11(19): 1919–1926
14. Feit LJ (1969) Pathogenic classification of male pattern baldness. New innovation in surgical techniques. Int Surg 51(1): 58–67
15. Hamilton JB (1951) Patterned loss of hair in man: types and incidence. Ann NY Acad Sci 53: 708–728
16. Ludwig E (1977) Classifications of the types of androgenetic alopecia (common baldness) occurring in the female sex. Br J Dermatol 97: 249–257
17. Norwood OT, Shiell RC (1984) Hair transplant surgery, 2nd edn. Thomas, Springfield
18. Rook A, Dawber R (1986) Diseases of the hair and scalp. Blackwell, Oxford
19. Salamon T (1968) Genetic factors in male pattern alopecia. In: Baccareda et al. (eds) Biopathology of pattern alopecia. Karger, Basel, pp. 39–49
20. Steck WD (1979) The clinical evaluation of pathologic hair loss with a diagnostic sign in trichotillomania. Cutis 24(3): 293–5, 298–301
21. Setty LR (1970) Hair pattern of the scalp of white and negro male. Am J Phys Anthropol 33: 49–56
22. Unger WP (1978) Hair transplantation. Dekker, New York

Psychological Aspects

Hair as symbol and hair as adornment are the two poles whose evolution through the ages explains the psychological factors in male baldness.

Role of the Fur in Animals

In animals the primary function of the fur is as a covering to protect against cold, even though it may also appear as a remarkable adornment. But there is nothing here that usefully compares with man. Further, it is convenient to distinguish between head and body hair, different in their appearance, density and distribution. The hair of the head exists only on the scalp and nowhere else. While the beard approaches it in its density, it differs in being much frizzier and less amenable to styling.

History and Symbolism of Hair in Different Ages and Countries

We do not know whether baldness existed among prehistoric men, nor how they managed. It is certain that the first symbolic evocations of the hair are found in the Bible. In "Leviticus" 19: 27 it is said: "Ye shall not round the corners of your heads, neither shalt thou mar the corners of thy beard." This last rule explains why Hassidic Jews let their hair and very long sideburns grow. They make them into plaits and curls, which combine both aspects, hair as symbol and as adornment.

The story of Samson (in "Judges") certainly makes a greater impression on the imagination. The Bible says that an angel sent by God had announced the forthcoming birth of Samson to his mother and counselled her "never to take a razor to his head", as he was to be a Nazarite, consecrated to God from his mother's breast and to life. In "Numbers" 6:2 we are told that the Nazarite was to vow himself to the Lord and in 2:5 that as a sign of his allegiance to God he must not cut his hair: "There shall no razor come upon his head" and later: "For the halo of the Lord is upon his head". Therefore Samson lost his strength with his hair, for "God had withdrawn Himself from him" and he did not regain his strength until after his hair had regrown. Popular imagery, in particular, preserved this myth of the hair as symbol of strength and virility, not to mention the symbolism attached to the mane of the lion, the king of beasts and the most powerful.

In the same way, throughout the ages, shaving has been a sign of servitude, humiliation and degradation, which deprived those subjected to it of their status as a man or woman. From antiquity slaves were shaven, and Julius Caesar had the conquered Gauls shaved before sending them to Rome as slaves. In the Merovingian period, to cut the hair of a king was to remove his virility and his right to reign (the Salic Law).

These symbolic practices recur in more recent epochs. For the North American Indians, to scalp a dead enemy was to inflict the supreme degradation, to deprive him of his human status, to deny him access to the "eternal prairies". Similarly, after the Second World War, the women who had had relationships with the Germans were shaved before being exposed to public scorn. Humiliation and submission are similar concepts, and it is probably as a sign of submission to God that the monks of the Middle Ages shaved their vertex, to be compared with the shaving of Hassidic women and the concealment of the hair of nuns under their veils.

Beside this symbolic aspect of the hair, the significance of which has remained the same throughout ages and countries, there is the concept of hair as ornament which, in contrast, has varied in different periods and parts of the world. Hair as adornment has also existed since antiquity, and we need no further confirmation than the decorative and very voluminous hair styles of the Egyptians of the new Empire. The history of hair as an ornament in man revolves around four parameters: long hair, short hair, styled hair and dishevelled (or often pseudo-dishevelled) hair. It is difficult to define what it is, at each epoch, that determines the length or sophistication of coiffures. Taken at random, we have the Romantics with long disordered hair, the short-haired Romans, and the same under the Empire and in the decade of 1950–1960, which doubtless corresponds to periods of prosperity. The sophisticated periwigs of the courts of Louis XIV and Louis XV evoke the Sun King and his splendour.

It seems that the more civilised a nation is, the more attention it devotes to its hair, and that savage peoples are more dishevelled. It is interesting to note in recent years fashions have changed so rapidly that they have finished by overlapping, the next appearing before the last has had time to die, this overlap being accentuated by the rapidity of travel, the mingling of men and civilisations and the fact that progress is not simultaneous in different countries.

Finally, the hair being one of the factors in ornament on a par with clothing, it has served to demarcate certain social groups. Thus the eccentrics have used coiffure to stand out from the rest, to shun the norm. The long hair of the hippies, the bizarre modes of shaving the hair in punks, as well as dyeing it in bright and gaudy colors, are a method of letting others know at first glance that one is different, rather than a form of exhibitionism. And yet, while there can be no doubt that the coiffure evolves with the caprice of fashion, it is more difficult to determine the driving forces which evolve in cycles in relation to numerous factors: the degree of civilisation, periods of prosperity or recession, political ideas etc.

Finally, we cannot conclude this short chapter without mentioning the coiffure as a secondary sexual characteristic, treated differently at different epochs and in different civilisations. Long hair worn freely down the back was worn by young girls until the Middle Ages; today it rather suggests the uncouth symbol of a certain sexual liberation. Although, as has been seen, men have worn long hair at different periods, the two sexes have always been distinguished by different hair styles, except in the very recent epoch when unisex was the fashion in both clothes and hair-style. But let us note that baldness has never been the fashion.

Present-Day Psychology of Baldness

The preceding reflections may help us to some extent in understanding why the bald are so obsessed about their condition. This must have been the case even in antiquity, since the Egyptians in 1500 BC proposed very sophisticated preparations intended to cause hair regrowth; in the light of their ingredients it must certainly have taken real motivation to use them.

Quite often, in aesthetic matters, the complex due to a malformation may be explained by the fact that the patient deviates from the norm represented by the majority. But the bald are so numerous that it is difficult to apply this rule to them. We tend rather to think that the bald man feels different from the male archetype as we know it, which explains the apparent paradox that only men can be bald. Contact and discussion with our patients have led us to compare male baldness with the absence of breasts in women; their attitude, their motivation, their postoperative reactions are similar. The woman without breasts feels herself not to be a real woman, and her motivation is such that she is not very demanding as to the results of a corrective operation; even when the implanted prostheses are too firm, she prefers to keep them rather than ask for their removal. The bald man feels himself diminished, he is ill at ease. Questioning bald patients reveals a loss of self-confidence, a feeling of exclusion from social life, which is a source of timidity, a feeling of inferiority. There is also an obsessive fear of the gaze of others and even of one's own gaze (many bald men avoid mirrors). Baldness is then experienced as a shameful disease, a handicap to be concealed. The study of symbolism shows us that baldness is to be interpreted in terms of a narcissistic wound, like a form of mutilation, and even of a sexual mutilation. Thus one can better understand the feeling of shame already mentioned, and this explains the diminution of the personality and its consequences: fear of the looks of others and then of mirrors. The motivation is such that the bald man accepts procedures that are sometimes painful, or unpleasant and repeated, and that he is not himself very demanding about the quality of the end-result, less so than his friends and even than the surgeon himself. For us this is an undeniable test of the importance of the psychological effects of a malformation. Such a motivation cannot be entirely explained by the effect produced on the opposite sex; women are not averse to bald men or at least pretend not to be.

The symbolism of hair and hairdressing through the ages certainly helps to understand how the bald man, through his archetypes, resents his baldness. But two supplementary factors provide a better understanding of this reaction: the attitude of society and the cosmetic factor.

Social Attitudes

Social attitudes tend rather to consider the bald man as suffering from an infirmity making him, like the hunchback, a figure of fun. He is in fact the target of easy mockery and often of derogatory puns. There is an easy tendency to caress a bald head as if it were a billiard ball; this is often associated with a certain degree of disdain, as when a man one wishes to put down is called "small and bald", as if these two qualifications denied him the status of a proper man. The role of the juvenile lead has never been played on the screen by a bald man (Yul Brynner was not bald but had his head shaved deliberately). The only young bald actors are those with roles as comics or cuckolds. It is impossible to imagine James Bond bald. This social attitude buries the bald man in a certain isolation, in a solitude which prevents him from discussing his problem. He is misunderstood, and even if the doctor listens to him he cannot shoulder the anguish of his patient.

Cosmetic Effects

The cosmetic effect of baldness is far from negligible. One needs to have a very handsome face and a perfectly round head to compensate for the burden of baldness. It is a matter of common observation that a man is always handsomer and always seem younger with his hair than without. Not only does baldness make men ugly, but it also ages them, which is unacceptable in our epoch. We do not claim that all bald men are ugly, but that a man of whatever nature always appears handsomer and younger with his hair; so it is understandable why he seeks to keep it by any means, even if some women pretend, for personal reasons, to like bald men. But they are very rare.

Even in ageing, the hair retains its importance. Greying hair has its charm; it shows experience. When it is abundant and thick as well, it is readily compared to the mane of an old lion; it symbolises the combination of strength and experience, i.e. wisdom. When handsomeness is added, it is perfection for the discriminating. How do bald men react in terms of these factors?

We believe that no man is indifferent to his baldness, but that reactions vary with the individual:

1. Some make up for this, or compensate, usually in their work, where they find the potency lost by their lack of hair. Others compensate by sublimation in art, which in a way is also a source of power. Others compensate by their attitude or their mode of dress: by wearing their remaining hair very long, by being bearded, by eccentric clothing or by completely shaving their heads, which is much more rare.
2. However, the majority of bald men do not compensate. They can do nothing and remain harassed by all the consequences and effects this may provoke in everyday life. Some try to correct their baldness, but it is a long road to travel, whether they wear a hair-piece or resort to surgery. Sometimes, at the outset, there is an attempt to rationalise this complex; the bald man seeks a remedy because he wishes to be smart or sometimes, so he says, for the sake of his wife and children.

   In the next stage, baldness is experienced as an illness; the patient speaks of diseased hair, of tendencies to exacerbations, and this disease leads to a search for treatment, initially using special shampoo and then medicated lotions. After this comes the visit to the doctor and then the dermatologist.

   Faced with their impotence or the inefficacy of treatment, he then resorts to hair institutes. Thus each stage leads to its quota of the resigned who give up or the rebellious who persevere, and the further one goes the more subjects there are who experience their baldness as a kind of infirmity, like the loss of a part of the self, an amputation. It is only then that some take the final step: a hair-piece or surgery. Each solution has its advantages and disadvantages, and the final choice is the outcome of several factors: degree of baldness, financial means, profession, fear of operation, appearance desired and constraints accepted. But even then, the choice of hair-piece is never entirely satisfactory, for it is often felt to be a kind of cheating with its corollary, the fear of being unmasked.
3. Finally, a very small proportion of the bald never think about their baldness and live normally, without complexes, without sublimation or compensation and without constraints. It is important not to alert them to these potential problems.

Medical and Cosmetic Treatment

From Antiquity to the Present Day (From Empiricism to Inefficacy)

The first publication concerning the treatment of baldness is an Egyptian manuscript from the eighteenth dynasty (1580 BC). The author recommends a mixture composed of equal parts of the fat of the lion, hippopotamus, crocodile, snake and ibex. He also recommends the guts of fishes, the genital organs of the bitch and a mouse cooked in grease until it is rotten. These magic formulae may remind us of the placental extracts and fresh cells of today. But the fact is that, while the bald have failed to accept their fate ever since antiquity and have been easy prey for charlatans, and while certain current treaments do for a time normalise hair loss, the only visible and durable results are those obtained by surgery.

Modern Treatments

Seborrhoea and Dandruff

Currently, proper hygiene of the scalp should provide clean hair without dandruff or seborrhoea if the treatment is suitable and repeated often enough. Sebaceous secretion develops at puberty in varying degrees depending on genetic predisposition and on the increase in androgen secretion, first by the adrenals and then by the gonads. The concept of hyperseborrhoea, which is strictly relative and individual, seems to be aggravated by stress, environmental pollution and the abuse of detergent shampoos. Hyperseborrhoea makes the hair heavy, greasy and sometimes itchy.

The pullulation of micro-organisms may induce the development of a squamous erythema called seborrhoeic dermatitis at the scalp margins and behind the ears. This dermatitis may also affect the external auditory meatus, the middle facial and the middle thoracic regions. It is important to stress the absence of any relationship between the degree of baldness and the severity of seborrhoea and dandruff. Treatment essentially relies on lotions, shampoos and conditioners; there is a current trend to avoid excessively detergent shampoos. They are used gently at the rate required according to the degree of soiling and the speed of relubrication of the hair (best to wash beforehand and several times a week if need be). As for dandruff, treatment also relies on repeated application of appropriate lotions and shampooing, the agents most used being germicides and keratolytics. In all cases, a shampoo without aggressive cleansing agents is advised. The simultaneous use of two shampoos whose tensioactive agents may be incompatible should be avoided. The frequency of shampooing has no effect on sebum production; washing or the tensio-active agents of a shampoo make it possible to "wet" the dirt encrusted in the sebum surrounding the hair and thus to eliminate it in the rinse. These tensioactive agents are of ambivalent structure (partly lipophilic, partly hydrophilic) and so may be divided into four groups: anionic, cationic, amphoteric and nonionic, the latter having no electrical charge and considered as the gentlest of the detergents.

Apart from the classical washing shampoos or cosmetics (for dry, greasy, fine or brittle hair), there are shampoos for specific treatment:

- Anti-dandruff: based on cade or coal-tar or undecylinic acid, pyridine-thione, octopyrox or econazole.
- Anti-seborrhoeics: based on Panama wood, sulphur derivatives or mild washing agents.
- Dry shampoos: powders of starch rice, maize, silica or lycopodium. They absorb the sebum and are got rid of by vigorous brushing. Lotions and creams containing the active agents listed above may also be used.

Hair Loss

Vitamin Therapy and Other General Treatments

Vitamins [7] are often prescribed and have the advantage of being perfectly well tolerated; they are advised for moderate hair loss, especially biotin and pantothenic acid (preferably by intramuscular injection). This may be combined with the administration of sulphurated amino acids (cystine) in courses of 2 months repeated over time. The local use of other chemical or physical agents (ultraviolet rays, ozone etc.) has given no objective results.

Lotions

Lotions applied locally once or more a week are very well tolerated and much used by the public. They lead to normalisation of hair loss in 55%–70% of cases, usually in 8–12 weeks. They are composed of vitamins B5-B6-H, sulphurated amino acids, tissue extracts, sulphated polysaccharides (trichosaccharides, trichopeptides), rubefacients (nicotinic acid) or various plant extracts. They are recommended for moderate hair loss. Local intradermal multi-injections of vitamins B5 and H and of placental extracts are sometimes prescribed weekly for 6 weeks. The American Food and Drug Administration (FDA), in a report from 1981, decided that a product supposed to encourage hair growth or arrest its loss should be proved to be not only harmless but also effective. In this context, after analysing reports dealing with the products most often used – amino acids, ascorbic acid, benzoic acid, biotin (vitamin H), oil of jojoba, lanoline – the FDA proposes simply to ban all these products and not to approve any of them because of the lack of proof of their efficacy. At present it seems that only minoxidil satisfies any of these criteria. It may reasonably be said that certain treatments may be considered acceptable, having a delaying action on the natural course and by normalising major hair loss occurring periodically during an individual's life-time.

Minoxidil

Minoxidil (2,4 diamino-6-piperidino-pyrimidine-3-oxide) in the form of a lotion for local application seems to be the first molecule with proven activity on male baldness by stimulating hair growth. However, the enthusiasm aroused by this recent finding must be tempered by objective analysis of the results, selection of subjects and conditions of use. This agent, a powerful peripheral vasodilator, has been in use for over 10 years orally for the treatment of arterial hypertension, during which application of a solution of minoxidil was found to have a stimulating effect on hair growth in androgenic alopecia with a recognisable time pattern: possible exacerbation of the process of hair loss for the first 4 weeks, then normalisation of loss between the fifth and eighth weeks, reported by most authors, and increase in diameter of the intermediate hair (atrophic but not yet downy hair more than 1 cm long and 40 μm in diameter) in 8–16 weeks [14, 19–21] (Photos 1, 2). These favourable effects of minoxidil on hair loss and on the covering effect by increasing the hair shaft diameter have been monitored by various supplementary studies: histological examination [8], macrophotography and phototrichography [3, 4]. The histological studies have verified hypertrophy of the follicles with increased diameter of the hair

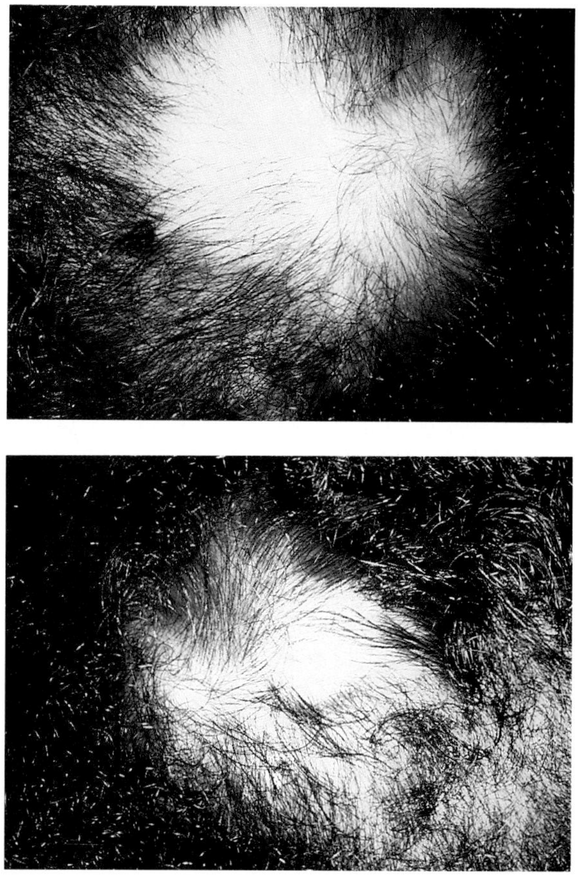

a

b

Photo 1a,b. Vertical alopecia **a** before and **b** after treatment with 2% minoxidil

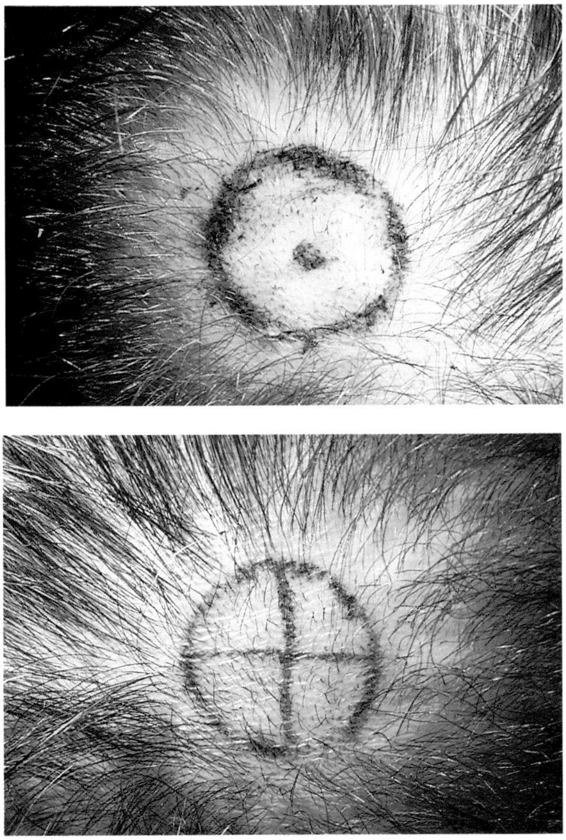

Photo 2a,b. Macrophotographic aspects a before and b 9 months after minoxidil treatment

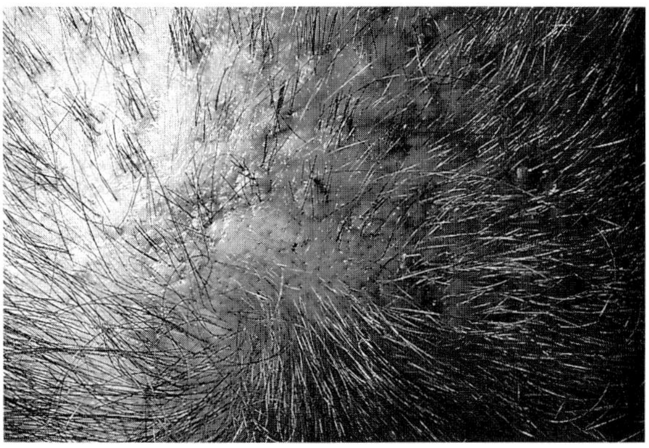

Photo 3. Identification by central tattooing for macrophotographic monitoring of grafts

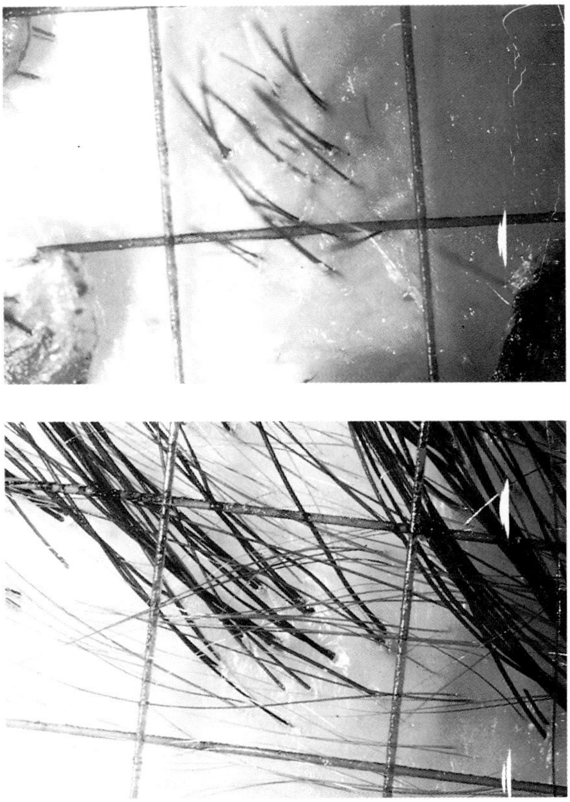

Photo 4. a Persistence of hair growth on graft at third week. b Persistence of hair growth on graft at third month

shafts [18]. This phemonenon appears from the eighth week of application and there is a correlation with the serum levels of minoxidil [15].

A twofold hypothesis has been proposed: stimulation of passage of the hair from the telogenic to the anagenic phase and prolongation of growth in the anagenic phase. Studies counting target zones of the scalp 2.5 cm in diameter have reported a cosmetically valid "regrowth"; but this may actually be a covering effect due to increase in shaft calibre, giving the hair a bulkier aspect. Thus there is hypertrophy of the follicles and hair shafts without multiplication of their number. The favourable results given by various writers are from 4% to 30% [6, 9, 10, 17]. The average effective concentration of minoxidil is 2% [11]. The minimum effective concentration is 1% and efficacy is not much improved by a 3% lotion. Efficacy appears to reach a plateau after 1 year [12]; 2–4 months after cessation of treatment the process of abnormal hair loss reappears and the hair shaft diameter decreases.

Mode of Action of Minoxidil

The action of minoxidil is based essentially on increase in blood-flow and cell mitosis [16–22]; there is no influence on testosterone metabolism. Other hypotheses include:

- Inhibition of prostaglandin formation in cultures of human keratinocytes

- Inhibition of synthesis of lysyl-hydroxylase in cultures of human fibroblasts
- Promotion of potassium flow into the smooth muscle fibres of the vessel walls

Effects of Minoxidil Lotion on Hair Grafts [6]

Bouhanna carried out a study on 16 volunteer patients aged from 25 to 52 years with androgenic alopecia of types III–VI (in Hamilton's classification) which monitored the effects on the grafts of a 2% minoxidil-based lotion. Local twice-daily treatment of the receptor area was begun 1 month before the operation and resumed for the following 3 months, with a 3-week break. Sixty-four 4-mm grafts removed with a motorised punch were inserted in orifices of 3.5 mm in diameter. In each of the 16 patients; four grafts identified by tattooing were monitored using a macrophotography system on days 0, 30 and 90. Classically, 2–4 weeks after transplantation, all the hairs fall out and regrow after 3–5 months. Contrary to the opinion of some authors, this loss of the graft hairs is an anagenic and not a telogenic defluvium. We have not found any report of the continuance of hair growth on the grafts without preliminary hair loss. The use of minoxidil before and after transplantation using the programme given above allowed us to note the continuance of hair growth in 71% of the grafts 30 days after transplantation and hair loss of less than 50% in 84% of the grafts 90 days after the operation.

In conclusion, local application of minoxidil seems to allow continuance of growth of hair grafted at the anagenic stage. Therefore, its use seems essential during transplantations to permit better progress of the grafts.

Side-Effects

Local and general tolerance of the 2% lotion studied in over 2000 subjects has proved satisfactory [13]. Pruritus and local transient erythemato-squamous irritation in 2%–3% of cases, allergic eczema (0.8%), hypertrichosis of the face and neck (1%) and, more generally, flushing (2%) and headache (1%) have been noted, with variations in arterial pressure and pulse (0.1%), but without any electrocardiographic changes.

Hormonal Treatment in Women

Hormonal assessment is essential if clinical hyperandrogenism is suspected, to guide possible appropriate hormonal treatment. Actually, serum hormone levels are usually normal. Local and general treatments are based on the same principle as those advised in men [2]. Any androgen administration should be forbidden (anabolic hormones, pills containing derivatives of 19-nortestosterone). Cyproterone acetate (androcur) combined with oestrogens (estraderm-estrogel) is prescribed after consultation with the gynaecologist. The anti-androgenic effect of this treatment will normalise hair loss in a few months and reduce the seborrhoea often associated with it.

References

1. Baden HP, Kubilus J (1983) Effect of Minoxidil on cultured keratinocytes. J Invest Dermatol 81(6): 558–560
2. Bonerandi JJ, Bouhanna P (1987) Les alopécies androgénétiques et leurs traitements: place du Minoxidil. Impact no. spécial, juin, « Les alopécies », pp 19–25
3. Bouhanna JF (1987) Étude objective de l'action du Minoxidil topique sur le processus de chute des cheveux, dans l'alopécie androgénétique. Thesis, Nice
4. Bouhanna P (1988) Le tractiophototrichogramme: méthode d'appréciation objective d'une chute de cheveux. Ann Dermatol Venereol 115: 759–764
5. Bouhanna P (1989) Topical Minoxidil used before and after hair transplantation. J Dermatol Surg Oncol 16(1): 50–53
6. Devillez R (1985) Topical Minoxidil therapy in hereditary androgenic alopecia. Arch Dermatol 121: 197–202
7. Goldsmith LA (1980) Vitamins and alopecia. Arch Dermatol 116: 1135–1136
8. Headington J, Novak E (1982) Histological findings in androgenic alopecia treated with topical Minoxidil. Br J Dermatol 107 [Suppl 22]: 20–21
9. Kopersky JA, Orenberg EK, Wilkinson DI (1987) Topical Minoxidil therapy for androgenetic alopecia: a 30-month study. Arch Dermatol 123(11): 1483–7
10. Mortimer CH, Rushton H, James KC (1984) Effective medical treatment for common baldness in women. Clin Exp Dermatol 9: 342–350
11. Olsen E, Weiner M, Delong E et al. (1985) Topical Minoxidil in early male pattern baldness. J Am Acad Dermatol 13: 185–912
12. Olsen E, Delong E, Weiner M (1986) Long term follow-up of men with male pattern baldness treated with topical Minoxidil. J Am Acad Dermatol 15(1): 30–37
13. Rietschel R1, Duncan SH (1987) Safety and efficacy of topical Minoxidil in the management of androgenetic alopecia. J Am Acad Dermatol 16: 677–685
14. Roberts J (1987) Androgenic alopecia: treatment results with topical Minoxidil. J Am Acad Dermatol 16(3): 705

15. Schupack JL, Kassimir JJ, Thirumoothy T et al. (1987) Dose-response study of topical Minoxidil in male pattern alopecia. J Am Acad Dermatol 16: 673–676
16. Storer J, Brzuskiewicz J, Floyd H, Rice J (1986) Topical Minoxidil for male pattern baldness. Am J Med Sci. 291(5): 328–333
17. Tosti A, Querzoca M, Caponeri GM, Minghetti G, De Padova MP, Veronesi S (1985) Minoxidil for local application in the treatment of alopecia. J Ital Dermatol Venereol 120(3): 223–225
18. Uno H, Cappas A, Schlagel C (1985) Cyclic dynamics of hair follicles and the effect of Minoxidil on the bald scalps of stumptailed macaques. Am J Dermatopathol 7: 283–297
19. Vanderveen E, Ellis C, Kang S, Case P (1984) Topical Minoxidil for hair regrowth. J Am Acad Dermatol 11: 416–421
20. Vanderveen EE, Ellis N, Kang MPH et al. (1984) Topical Minoxidil for hair regrowth. J Am Acad Dermatol 11: 416–421
21. Vermorken AJM (1983) Reversal of androgenic alopecia by Minoxidil lack of effect of simultaneous administered intermediate doses of cyproterone acetate. Acta Derm Venerol 63: 268–269
22. Weiss V, West D (1985) Topical Minoxidil therapy and hair regrowth. Arch Dermatol 121: 191–192
23. Zappacosta AR (1980) Reversal of baldness in patients receiving Minoxidil for hypertension. N Engl J Med 303: 1480–1481

Hair-Pieces

The use of hair-pieces is a non-surgical procedure which supplies the patient with additional hair. To this extent, a hair-piece often constitutes an alternative to the various surgical solutions. In fact, we believe that it should be used more often as a method to complement the surgical repertoire, a mixed programme combining a hair-piece with surgery, giving excellent results in the treatment of major baldness. Enormous progress has been made in recent years in the field of hair-pieces as regards both their composition and their conception. Very many hair-pieces are currently commercially available. Their main differences relate to:

- Type of hair used
- Base on which the hair is implanted
- Mode of fixation of the hair-piece

Types of Hair Used

Natural Hair

The main advantage of using natural hair is the natural appearance and the fact that waving is as easy as with normal hair. This allows the use of shampoos and a hair-dryer. However, there is one great disadvantage, which is rapid deterioration with time. The hair becomes discoloured in sunlight and requires dyeing after 6–12 months. The hairs split at their ends and lose their natural laxity. To obtain the desired colour, it is usually necessary to dye it, which makes it even more brittle.

Artificial Hair

Many kinds of fibres are used in artificial hair. They often permit a natural appearance after waving and conditioning, but in practice frequent conditioning is necessary and should be done by a professional. Waving remains stable for about a month, even after shampooing. The fibres always retain their original colour. They deteriorate with time but less rapidly than natural hair. The chief flaw is the fact that few fibres give the textural feel of natural hair.

Bases for Implantation

Wide-Meshed Net

The hair is sewn on a wide-meshed net after having previously been fixed on a thread. The advantage is that the prosthesis is very aerated and the scalp can easily be washed without removing the hair-piece. The disadvantage is that when the hair is somewhat dirty and greasy, it becomes raised in ridges by the effect of the wind and acquires an unnatural appearance.

Close-Meshed Net

Close-meshed nets often have the aspect of a tulle on which the hairs are attached one by one. They can be fastened, stuck on, or fastened and stuck. The tulle usually has a nylon base. Aeration of the scalp is relative and its washing may require complete or partial removal of the hair-piece, but distribution of the hair is more uniform.

"Microskin"

"Microskin" is a very thin transparent sheet of nylon on which the hairs are fixed, usually by gluing. The distribution of the hairs is very uniform. When they are raised, the aspect of the base is very similar to that of the normal scalp, which is seen by transparency. However, aeration of the scalp is very poor and even promotes a certain maceration. Washing must therefore be very frequent and the hair-piece has to be completely removed each time.

Mode of Fixation of the Hair-Piece

Adhesives

The oldest method of fixing hair-pieces is by gluing, the hair-piece having several adhesive patches on its inner aspect. The procedure is easy but allergies are common. The glues or gums can be replaced by a double-sided adhesive, with the same risks of allergy. These two types of fixation have the disadvantage of being relatively precarious and do not allow the wearer to practice sport or sea or pool bathing.

Weaving

The prosthesis may be sewn on a thread, which is itself fixed to the patient's hairs by means of a braid. This braid is made of three linen threads which are braided, taking a lock of hair as the fourth thread. A lock of hair is thus caught every centimetre and ensconced in the weave. Fixation of the hair-piece is very firm, but it is necessary to perform a tightening-up about every month, since the hair grows and the hair-piece then becomes loose. This procedure has the disadvantage of provoking in the long term a progressive peripheral traction alopecia, and this alopecia, which is transient to begin with, may become permanent with time.

Microspots

The hair-piece may be fixed by microspots; several locks of hair are knotted to the hair-piece and fixed in place by a spot of glue. The glue may provoke allergies and the retightening necessary every month requires cutting the hair to which the glue has been applied, since there is no solvent capable of dissolving it. Again, this procedure presents the same risks of traction alopecia as the previous method.

Grips

Fixation by hair grips has the disadvantage of being too precarious. The small grips are flat and 1 cm long, and six or seven are needed to keep a hair-piece in place.

Surgical Fixation

Surgical fixation has now been virtually abandoned by most surgeons because of the excessive number of infections it causes. The surgeon fixes a thread on the scalp, a thread of nylon, steel or gold wire, and the hair-piece is then sewn on this thread. This procedure is very attractive, but the fixation thread always ends up by becoming infected or by cutting the hair because of the permanent traction it exerts.This procedure is therefore contraindicated. Another procedure has been described, which consists of making tunnels 2 or 3 cm long under the scalp and lining their inner aspect with a split skin graft. The results in practice are disappointing.

Advantages of Hair-Pieces

Hair-pieces have, of course, the value of not requiring surgical intervention. Apart from artificial implants, to which we shall return, it is also the only procedure which allows augmentation of the number of hairs. To this extent, it is the sole treatment possible for major baldness where the crown height is less than 8 cm.

Disadvantages of the Procedure

The chief of this procedure is the careful and permanent maintenance of the hair-piece, which moreover has to be changed quite often. In particular, there is the worry of having properly styled hair so as to ensure that the hair-piece is not conspicuous. Specifically, the meshes must always mask the anterior frontal line as it is impossible to simulate this line correctly with any kind of hair-piece. This is the main reason why the combination of surgery and hair-piece may be an excellent solution in some cases.

Surgical Techniques: History, Anaesthesia and General Principles

History

The history of the surgery of baldness is marked, in the first half of the twentieth century, by certain tentative autoplasties, which are often overlooked [29, 31, 49, 65]. Then, after Orentreich's report in 1959 [47], at which time the work of Okuda [46] (published in 1939) was still unrecognised, the technique of scalp grafts developed. As for the so-called pathogenic surgical treatments, these have never been more than palliative and ineffective procedures.

The considerable progress in reparative surgery and a better anatomic and physiological understanding of the scalp led to a renewal of flap surgery for baldness [22, 23], but it was mainly the reports and articles by Juri [27] which served as the point of departure for the development of scalp flaps. However, certain imperfections of this procedure stimulated research into flaps in which the hair direction was better adapted to the fronto-temporal line [11, 17, 40]. At the same time, the principle of repeated excisions described by Morestin in 1911 [37] seems to have been rediscovered for the surgery of vertical reduction [9, 66, 67].

Recent years have seen enormous progress in reparative surgery of the scalp as a result of the use of expanders, though their future in the cosmetic surgery of baldness seems limited to very restricted cases. Today it is possible to refine and specify the indications for the different techniques that can be successfully performed.

Pathogenic Interventions

Pathogenic interventions were intended to act on the tension of the scalp and on its vascularisation (and therefore on the supply of androgens). In fact, they have never been of proven efficacy in the treatment of male baldness. Pathogenic interventions include the following:

- *Galeotomy.* This was initially proposed by Pincus in 1875 [52] and then taken up by several workers, including Schein [61], Young [69], and Szasz and Robertson [64].
- *Galeoplasty.* This was described by Feit in 1969 [22] and combines three incisions of the galea with stripping of this layer and vascular ligations.
- *Ligature of the superficial temporal vessels.* This procedure aims at reducing seborrhoea and was performed by Maréchal in 1975 [35].

Vertical Reduction

The technique of vertical reduction was derived from the general principles of repeated excisions initially described by Morestin in 1911 [37] and taken up later by Davis in 1919 and Sistrunk in 1927. But it was probably Correa-Iturraspe and Arufe [16] who first applied this principle to reconstructive surgery of the scalp. It was not until 1977 that Blanchard and Blanchard [9] reported a series of 100 patients in whom they had performed repeated fusiform excisions, essentially longitudinal and paramedian, at intervals of 4–6 weeks. The technique really took off at the International Symposium on Hair Transplantion at Lucerne in 1978, where the Blanchards described their technique, Stough and Webster presented a fusiform reduction technique sometimes combined with an "M" design at the occiput, and Sparkuhl reported his work and introduced the term "scalp reduction".

In April 1978, Unger and Unger [67] reported a series of 60 patients who had undergone fusiform scalp excisions (2–4 cm × 15–20 cm) and described other reduction designs: shaped like a "C", "U" and "J" (not very effective) and like a "Y" and "T" (risk of apical necrosis). They specified the indications and detailed the technique in their book. Then, in 1980, Bosley reported one of the largest series, with 749 cases [10]. In 1980, Alt presented his technique and gave a historical review [2]. In 1984, Nordstrom [42] assessed the kinetics and the "stretch-back" of the scalp after vertical reduction. In 1984, Marzola [36] proposed a "comma-shaped" excision and the advance of a sliding parietal flap combined with very major occipital stripping.

In 1986, Brandy [13] published a report on the biparietal-occipital (BPO) flap, which used complete stripping of the entire scalp. Manders et al. [34] used the principle of simple reduction combined with bilateral expansion. In 1989, Dardour [19] reported lifting of the scalp, which is a wide reduction of the Brandy type combined with two vertical flaps at the same operative stage and which allows simultaneous coverage of the fronto-temporal recession and the vertex.

Grafts

At the beginning of the nineteenth century, animal studies demonstrated the possibility of performing autografts of hair-bearing areas, and Dom Unger suggested the use of this type of treatment to correct baldness. At the end of the century, the uncertain results of transplantation of autografts of the scalp in post-traumatic alopecia led to preference being given to the transposition of flaps. In 1930, Saragona proposed a method for insertion of hair-roots which was repeated in 1943 by Tamura for grafting on the female pubic area. In 1939, the Japanese dermatologist Okuda [46] described the transposition of scalp autografts of 2–4 mm in diameter, removed by punch and inserted at smooth regions of the eyelids, scalp and moustache after preliminary forage with the same instrument. His treatment seems to have been used mainly for the correction of wound alopecia.

In 1953, Fujita grafted the eyelid regions of lepers with scalp fragments carrying two to ten hairs, inserting the grafts after perforation of the receptor zone with a large needle or scalpel tip. He used this technique to correct various wound alopecias. In 1959, Orentreich [47] referred to the possibility of cosmetic surgical correction of androgenic alopecia by transplantation of autografts removed with a cylindrical instrument of 4 mm in diameter. He reported his technique and contributed very largely to popularising this method, which was then modified by many authors. Ayres [4] advised punches of different sizes. Seltzer [62] used an electric motor. Arouette suggested an occipital and frontal haemostat. Vallis [68] used long strips (5–9 mm) to reconstruct a new anterior frontal line. In 1976, Nataf et al. [40] recommended the removal of fusiform grafts (15–30 × 5 mm) embedded in anterior incisions.

Norwood and Shiell [44] gave a detailed account of the technique of cylindrical grafts in their book Hair Transplant Surgery in 1984. They greatly developed and refined the graft technique, in particular the method of calculating the follicles on each graft, the technique of grafting scar tissues and the technique of micrografts. Bouhanna [12] recommended mini- and micrografts with long hairs by cutting up removed strips.

Scalp Flaps

In 1908, Tillman [65] suggested the use of transposition flaps fashioned at the edges of the vertex and applied to it like the spokes of a wheel. In 1919, Passot [49] was the first to recommend transposition of flaps to cover a bald area, either with a flap raised in the temporo-occipital zone and rotated 90° forward on a temporal pedicle or with two temporo-occipital flaps on an occipital pedicle transposed into a sagittal paramedian position at the apex of the bald area. Lamont [29] treated baldness of the vertex by the transposition of temporo-occipital flaps in two stages:

- In the first stage he prepared two transverse temporo-occipital flaps with an anterior pedicle aligned on the superficial temporal artery.
- In the second stage, a week later, the two flaps were transposed into the smooth frontal region.

Some months later the hair of these flaps concealed the persistent smooth area and the grafted donor areas.

Limburger [31] used similar flaps, but with a posterior pedicle, whose direction after transposition was no longer transverse but sagittal. For Z-plasties he decreased the vertical diameter in some patients. Feit [22] described a bi-lobed flap, already used by Esser and by Zimany for the repair of losses of skin substance of the face. This temporal flap allows partial coverage of the anterior fronto-temporal line.

In 1972, Juri reported his prepared parieto-occipital flap for reconstruction of the anterior frontal line. Then, in 1975 [27], he elaborated on his technique, mentioning that his research had been stimulated by the work of Correa-Iturraspe and Arufe. He described the principle of his temporo-parieto-occipital flap intended for frontal baldness, prepared in two separate stages at an interval of 1 week. The author even recommended, for more severe baldness, the use of a second, contralateral, flap and even of a third flap. He reported 400 cases with an analysis of the results. In 1978, J. Juri, C. Juri and Arufe [28] described a transposition flap for occipital baldness.

Following J. Juri's first report, several authors published their results and their attempts to modify or simplify the Juri flap:

- Elliot [21] used shorter temporal flaps than those of Juri, not requiring previous preparation, but needing to be bilateral to cover all of the frontal line.
- Heiburger suggested rotation of a Juri flap in a single stage after Doppler localisation.
- Kabaker proposed some refinements of the technique and a somewhat different design from that of Juri.
- Stough and Cates compared and combined with flaps other techniques adapted to baldness (grafts, reductions); they proposed a temporo-parietal flap not much different from that of Juri with a single preparation 10 days earlier.

At the same time, French workers proposed a transposition flap on a superior pedicle intended to give a more natural appearance to hair growth at the anterior frontal line:

- In 1976, Nataf and Bouhanna [11, 40] proposed a long vertical temporal flap on a superior parietal pedicle, with counterflow in the superficial temporal vessels and with subdermal embedding of the anterior border, transposed for frontal alopecia. The technique was progressively refined [39]; its course is preferentially retroauricular in its long variant and requires two preparatory stages (1 month later and then 3 months later).
- Further, Nataf [38] also proposed a forward transposed flap for the vertex.
- Dardour [17] also suggested a counterflow flap raised in the temporal region, but not so long and curved forward above the ear, in a single-stage procedure.

In 1981, to correct the direction of hair growth (towards the back), J. and C. Juri described two new flaps:

- A temporo-parieto-occipital flap folded in its distal portion at the frontal region
- A free temporo-parieto-occipital flap anastomosed with the other side

Ohmori [45] also used free scalp flaps for male baldness (temporo-occipital or occipito-temporal flaps).

Expansion

In 1957, Neumann [41] published the first case of skin expansion, using an inflatable latex balloon with an external valve for reconstruction of an ear, but his report was largely ignored and the procedure failed to become popular. It was essentially due to Radovan [54] that the technique really developed in 1976. Other authors developed it further, e.g. Austad [7], Argenta [6], Manders [33], Sasaky [59]. The properties of expanded skin have been examined in numerous experimental studies:

- In 1982, the Ann Arbor team of Pasyk and Austad looked into the anatomopathological aspects.
- In 1984, Sasaki and then Pasyk-Cherry and Austad specified the vascular qualities of expanded flaps.
- In 1986, Austad et al. [7] showed that there was a genuine gain during the expansion and that it derived not only from the traction but also from cell multiplication.

Recent studies [55] allowed assessment of the area increment. Currently, several teams are researching procedures permitting rapid expansion, automatic expansion etc., but the technique of filling still remains much as in the original procedure. Expansion in reconstructive scalp surgery has rapidly become a method of choice and really made its name in the 1980s, under the guidance of Manders [33]. Other authors have aided promotion of this method:

- Argenta [4, 5] used it to repair a major congenital aplasia in 1984 and then for a wound alopecia in 1985.
- Shively [63] used this method in the separation of two Siamese twins joined at the cranium.
- In 1986, several workers also used the method [30].

Currently, the indications are widely extended to wound alopecias and for certain giant nevi.

As far as male baldness is concerned:

- Manders [32] codified his method in 1985, using techniques of differential expansion so as to obtain bilateral ascent and advancement of the hair-bearing zones.
- In France, Ozun [48] has been using an expander since 1986 before the transposition of a superior pedicled parieto-temporal flap; he then combines another expansion for a contralateral flap or an advancement of vertical reduction type.
- In 1987, different authors also used the expander before flap transposition, varyingly combined with the vertical type of reduction advancements:

Adson et al. [1] used an expander plus a Juri flap and a temporal flap; Anderson et al. [3] used an expander plus a Juri flap and/or a vertical reduction).

- In 1988, Norstrom [43] reported the use of a crescent-shaped expander, allowing transposition of a Juri-type flap, and then inserted a second, banana-shaped expander for vertical reduction.
- In 1988, Dardour [18] published a report on the use of two expanders allowing the use of a vertical preauricular flap and a contralateral reduction.

Other reports will follow, and it is to be hoped that they will add further to the growth of interest in these techniques.

Anaesthesia

Anaesthesia is an important part of the procedure and should be designed to give maximum support to both patient and surgeon. Each patient will have to undergo several operative stages, and pain is certainly one factor which may lead to cessation of treatment by a fearful patient. The type of anaesthesia chosen for the surgery of baldness depends not only on the routines of anaesthetist and surgeon and on the operation itself (nature, duration and patient position), but also on the subjects's general health (including previous history, medication, handicaps etc.) and his psychological state. The well-informed patient will have preferences based on the advantages and disadvantages of the different methods. Some will dread general anaesthesia, while others ask for it so as to see, hear and feel nothing during the procedure. Local anaesthesia must always be conducted with every necessary precaution, as it carries no less risk than general anaesthesia with intubation.

All these factors are assessed at the routine pre-anaesthetic examination. The history and paraclinical investigations relate especially to the detection of allergic or neurological factors (especially convulsions) which might complicate local anaesthesia. It is also important to check for disorders of cardiac rhythm and the electrocardiogram (ECG) because of the risk of exacerbation by local anaesthetic agents and adrenaline. Arterial hypertension should also be looked for. The patient must avoid the use of aspirin in the days leading up to the operation and during the following week. If he or she is on anti-coagulants, careful testing is indicated. In general, when cessation of such treatment is impossible, we regard flaps and reductions as contraindicated. The risk of haematomas with grafting seems less serious.

Glaucoma should be routinely sought and contraindicates the use of atropine in premedication. Certain other drugs will suggest caution and may have to be discontinued well in advance, e.g. the monoamine oxidase inhibitors. Laboratory studies are naturally routine: complete blood count, blood group, blood urea and blood sugar and the ionogram with emphasis on the search for disorders of coagulation (bleeding time, coagulation time, prothrombin level, kaolin-cephalin time). If necessary in doubtful cases, more thorough investigations for subclinical haemophilia should be carried out; failure to recognise it may have dramatic results after constructing a flap. When this assessment is entirely normal we do not usually prescribe preoperative medication with anti-vitamins K or antibiotics, nor do we, as some do (W. Unger), impose a special diet. Some of our colleagues reserve human immunodeficiency virus (HIV) testing for high-risk subjects such as drug addicts, homosexuals and those with infected partners or those transfused before August 1985 or transfused in high-risk countries (Africa, Haiti, the Antilles). However, we tend to perform it routinely.

Local Anaesthesia

Local anaesthesia is the type of anaesthesia most often chosen by the patient. In nervous patients a light sedative may be given on the eve of operation. Premedication is very important in our opinion. Apart from the advantage of calming the patient's anxiety before the operation, it helps to avoid very common perioperative incidents such as vagal malaise and convulsions. When the patient has to be hospitalised for a flap or a major reduction, we use "heavy" premedication, which has the advantage of completely "disconnecting" the patient and sometimes even of producing complete amnesia for the procedure itself. An hour and a half before the operation, the patient is given a suppository of secobarbital (Nembutal; 120 mg) or of Dolosal. It may be replaced by a tablet of diazepam (Valium; 10 mg). Forty-five minutes beforehand, the premedication is supplemented by an intramuscular injection of atropine (0.5 mg) and alimemazine (1 mg). The patient rests in a quiet place and is verbally reassured before and during the procedure. An intravenous line is established.

The different local anaesthetics are chosen in terms of their advantages and disadvantages, as determined by the surgeon's routine, the nature of the patient and of the procedure, as well as the desired effect.

Esteriform Agents

Procaine (Novocaine) acts quite rapidly (10–20 min), but its duration is limited to between 45 and 90 min, as it is rapidly metabolised. It is ideal for surface infiltration. Solutions at 0.5%, 1% and 2% are used, with or without a vascoconstrictor; the maximum dose is 50 mg (60 mg with adrenaline).

Tetracaine (Pontocaine, Amethocaine) acts slowly (20–30 min), but lasts longer (3–6 h), as it is slowly metabolised; 0.5%–2% solutions are used and the maximum dose is 100 mg.

Amide Derivatives

Lidocaine (Xylocaine-Lignocaine) acts rapidly (2–5 min), but its duration is limited to 1–2 h. There are 0.5%, 1%, 2%, 4% and 5% solutions, with or without adrenaline (1/100000, 1/200000). In practice, Xylocaine 1% with adrenaline is the agent most commonly used, in a dilution of 1:2 or 1:3 depending on the patient. This dilution is adequate to obtain the desired anaesthetic and vasoconstrictor effect. The maximum dose is 200 mg without a vasoconstrictor (i.e. 60 ml of 1% Xylocaine).

Mepicavaine (Scandicaine) acts rapidly (5–10 min) and is long-acting (1½–3 h). Solutions of 1%, 1.5% and 2% are used. The maximum dose is 300 mg without and 600 mg with a vasoconstrictor.

Buvicaine (Marcaine) acts very slowly (20–30 min) but over a very long period (3–6 h); the solutions used are 0.25%, 0.50% and 0.75% and the maximum dose is 175 mg.

Remarks

Very often, the great advantages of 1% Xylocaine are made use of, but during a long procedure it may be combined with an agent such as Marcaine, which also ensures good postoperative analgesia. However, one must beware of the cumulative toxic dose in terms of the proportion of the two agents. Finally, it is useful, whenever possible, to add a vascoconstrictor such as adrenaline, which has the advantage of reducing bleeding and prolonging the local action of the anaesthetic; it is contraindicated by arterial hypertension, cardiopathy and coronary insufficiency. Especially in the scalp, the amounts needed for infiltration are often very large and sometimes near the maximum dosage, and it is important to use a dilution of a half or a third with normal saline.

Prevention of Complications and Accidents with Local Anaesthetics

The pre-anaesthetic consultation should be careful, in the knowledge that the main contraindications are known allergies to local anaesthetics, especially disorders of cardiac conduction, whereas neurological and psychological antecedents remain relative contraindications. Equipment for monitoring and resuscitation must always be available (see below). Finally, and especially, the norms for premedication, infiltration technique and maximum dosages must be strictly adhered to.

Possible Complications

Complications are usually a minor vagal type of malaise: lipothymic tendency, pallor, anxiety, nausea, perhaps headache. If severe, these may amount to actual vagal shock, with bradycardia and hypotension. They are usually attributable to the emotionality and anxiety of the patient and are usually prevented by proper premedication. Treatment includes stopping the infiltration, elevating the lower limbs with the head down, oxygen by mask and intravenous injection of 1 mg atropine. With these measures there is usually a rapid return to normal.

Allergic Incidents

Allergic incidents are rare and apply to the esters (procaine and its derivatives, or tetracaine). There may be a rash, Quincke's oedema, at worst anapylactic shock. Treatment includes stopping the infiltration, oxygen by mask, ensuring airway patency and intravenous injection of Soludecadron (4-mg ampoule, repeatable).

Toxic Accidents

Toxic accidents are linked to overdosage or over-rapid entry into the general circulation. The risk is lessened by dilution of the concentrations used.

Neurological Accidents

Neurological accidents are initially manifested by a phase of general malaise, with:

- Nausea, severe headache, visual and auditory hallucinations
- Confusion and difficulty in speaking
- Nystagmus
- Shivering, which may end in convulsions

A phase of depression may follow, with drowsiness or even coma, and at worst apnea and cardiovascular collapse. The treatment is Valium by intravenous injection and the usual measures for cardiorespiratory resuscitation.

Cardiovascular Accidents

Cardiovascular accidents include brady- or tachycardia, perhaps pallor, hypotension or even collapse with cardiac insufficency, the treatment of which consists of resuscitation measures with cardiac massage in the event of collapse. Most accidents with local anaesthetics can be avoided by:

- Rigorous pre-anaesthetic consultation aimed at detection of possible contraindications, such as known allergy to local anaesthetics, disorders of heart rhythm, neurological history
- Good selection and proper information of the patient
- Proper premedication
- A rigorous infiltration technique, always with an eye to the toxic dosage and the use of dilutions, if need be
- Finally, monitoring and the necessary technical precautions

Anaesthetic Equipment

Monitoring

Monitoring is the province of the anaesthetist (pulse, blood-pressure, ECG), and resuscitation depends on an installed venous line and drugs:

- Cardiovascular analeptics: neosinephrine (2-ml ampoule intramuscularly), adrenaline (1-mg ampoule)
- Anti-convulsants: diazepam (2-mg ampoule intramuscularly or intravenously), atropine (1 mg), Soludecadron (1 ml, 4 mg, intramuscularly or intravenously), Mayo cannulae, manual respirator, oxygen supply, tongue forceps, sucker, high molecular weight infusions and isotonic glucose saline

Infiltration Equipment

The infiltration equipment includes syringes and needles. Syringes should be of small bore (5 and 10 ml), since they are easier to handle if the pressure exerted by the operator is small, particularly in superficial infiltration; syringes of the Genia type are useful as they remain sealed and do not become disconnected, thus allowing high-pressure injection for superficial infiltration (see below). It is best to use very fine needles of the hypodermic type (0.5 mm) and diameter (30 gauge).

Infiltration Technique

The infiltration technique is very important. Apart from the anaesthesia it induces, it also has to prepare the planes of stripping and allow the surgeon to work in a virtually bloodless field.

Rules. It is classically necessary to aspirate before infiltration, a manoeuvre mainly practised near the great vessels (superficial temporal) and with nerve blocks. The essential principle is that of creeping infiltration, always progressing in the direction of stripping. To obtain the initial analgesia, the infiltration is gentle and gradual. It is preceded by antiseptic shampooing and preoperative marking with a felt pen or indelible ink.

The Different Stages. These are adapted to the particular case. Usually, it is useful to begin with a nerve-trunk block, which provides regional anaesthesia from the outset (Fig. 1):

- In front, for the forehead: the supra-orbital nerve at the junction of the inner and middle thirds of the superior orbital margin, about 3 cm from the midline, combined with anaesthesia of the medial frontal nerve, infiltrating towards the root of the

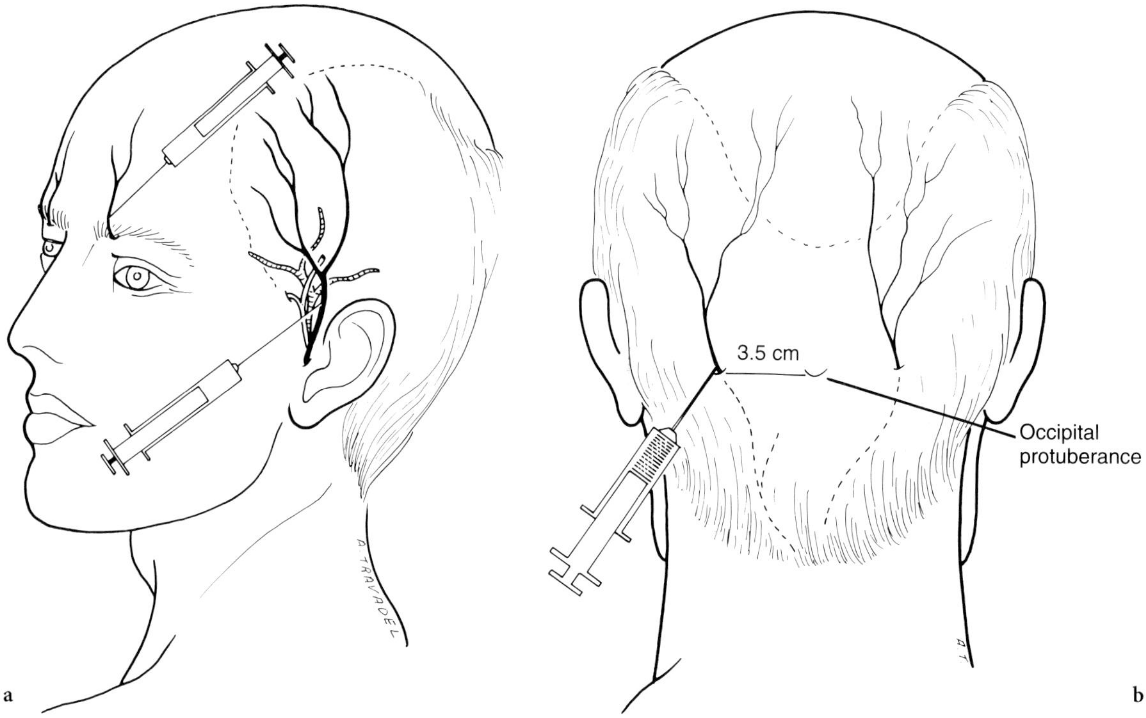

Fig. 1. **a** Anaesthesia of supra-orbital and auriculo-temporal nerve trunks. **b** Anaesthesia of trunk of occipital nerve (of Arnold)

nose on a vertical line passing slightly medial to the medial canthus. The anaesthesia obtained covers the entire anterior frontal region.

- Laterally: the auriculotemporal nerve, just under the skin between the external auditory meatus behind and the superficial temporal vessels in front. The anaesthesia obtained covers the lateral supra-auricular region.
- Laterally and posteriorly: the superficial mastoid and auricular branches of the superficial cervical plexus are injected along the posterior border of the sterno-cleido-mastoid muscle, 3–4 cm below the mastoid. The anaesthesia obtained covers the upper cervical region, below the external occipital protuberance.
- Behind, at the nuchal region and occiput: the greater occipital nerve (of Arnold; 2 cm below and lateral to the external occipital protuberance). The posterior branches of C3, a little below the protuberance, but more medial and nearer the mid-line. The anaesthesia obtained covers the entire occipital region and vertex.

This loco-regional infiltration may be supplemented by coronal infiltration at the periphery of the operative zone. Central infiltration allows subgaleal stripping (possible infiltration with normal saline, with or wihout adrenaline).

Finally, we always supplement the anaesthesia with superficial intradermal infiltration along the path of the incisions, which produces vasoconstriction of the subdermal plexus, thus diminishing bleeding from the margins of the incisions.

General Anaesthesia

General anaesthesia may be preferred by some fearful patients or merely for those who demand it or because the procedure requires it. The method is determined by the anaesthetist's preference and always includes premedication and intubation. It is combined with infiltration by the same method described for local anaesthesia, which has the advantage of reducing anaesthetic requirements, reducing bleeding and facilitating stripping.

General Principles of Scalp Surgery

Before embarking on surgery of the scalp it is essential to be acquainted with its rules and regulations. These derive primarily from the general rules of plastic surgery, particularly as regards flaps, grafts and the filling of losses of substance. They are also

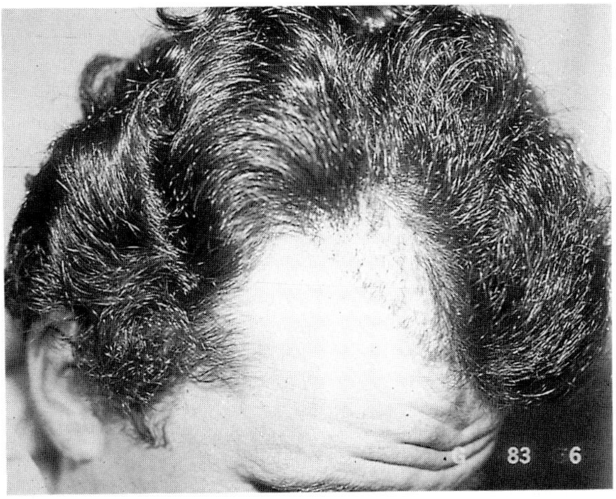

Photo 1. Total early alopecia on a flap (anagenic defluvium)

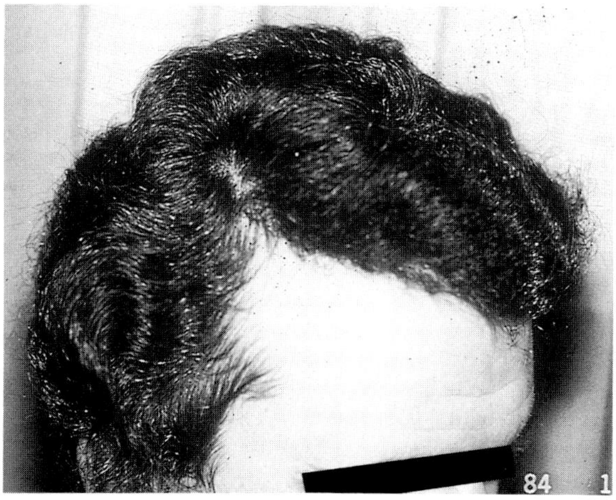

Photo 2. Complete regrowth of hair after several months

related to the specific properties of the scalp itself, the presence of appendages that must be preserved, i.e. the hair bulbs, the presence of a specific circulation and the galea.

Hair Bulbs

The hair bulbs are skin appendages which require a good blood supply for their survival. Even temporary ischaemia will lead to loss of the hair, which will not occur at once but during the 3 weeks following the ischaemia (anagenic defluvium) (Photo 1). When the circulation is rapidly restored, the bulb survives and a new hair replaces the fallen one. It begins to develop towards the sixth week, but several months are needed for it to reach a few centimetre (Photo 2). If the ischaemia is more severe, the bulb will die and the hair cannot regrow. This necrosis of the bulb occurs before skin necrosis, so that a definitive ischaemic alopecia is possible without skin necrosis.

In our first reported series of flaps, 15% of operated patients had presented with alopecia without necrosis at the first month. At the sixth month, 5% of the patients retained a definitive alopecia, i.e. regression had occurred in two thirds of the cases. The application of minoxidil before or after the operation may perhaps decrease the incidence of this anagenic defluvium or, if it occurs, promote regrowth of the hair. When the ischaemia is even more severe and prolonged, it leads to a skin necrosis which ends in loss of skin substance. In the scalp this skin necrosis forms a black, parchment-like plaque. Surgical ablation of this plaque leaves a raw area which one is often tempted to cover with a graft.

In general, we believe that it is preferable to leave in place this crust, which acts as a dressing, and to perform gradual marginal excision once or twice a week. Thus healing and epidermisation occur gradually, such that complete excision of the eschar coincides with the end of healing. The result is a plaque of cicatricial alopecia which, thanks to contraction of its margins, is reduced by 30%–50% in relation to the original necrosis. The advantages of this guided healing compared with a graft of split or full-thickness skin are many. It avoids surgical intervention (Photo 3). It avoids taking a graft and the inevitably unaesthetic sequel. It avoids the need for dressings, which are a great nuisance on the scalp, and leads to a smaller scar thanks to marginal contraction.

Tension of Closure

Tension of closure is a prime factor in the quality of a scalp scar, as emerges from the preceding analysis. In a study dealing with 156 flaps, we monitored the quality of the scar at the donor area in relation to the tension applied to close it. One month after the operation we observed a very extensive alopecia around the scar in 41% of patients where the donor site was under very great tension, whereas it was only 4% when closure tension had been minimal. The figures thus obtained may be considered as definitive at the sixth month. Thus, when closure tension was only minor, 96% of patients had a perfect scar, 4% had slight alopecia and none had marked alopecia. In contrast, when the closure tension was very considerable, 15% of patients had a very alopecic scar and 26% moderate alopecia, i.e. in all, 41% of

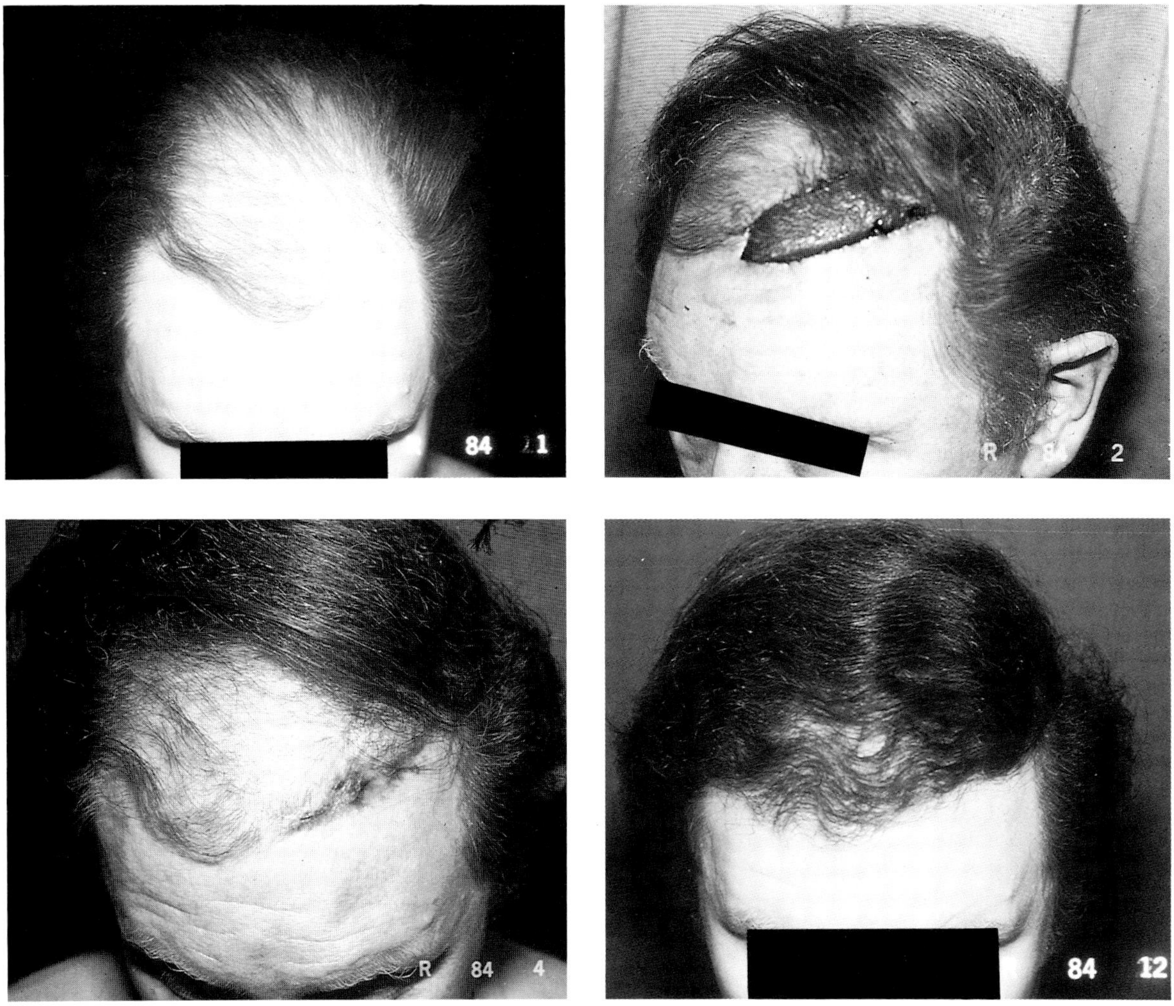

Photo 3. **a,b** Stage 3 baldness, necrosis of a flap over 5 cm. **c** Result after spontaneous healing. **d** End-result after correction by three fusiform grafts

scars were of poor or moderate quality (which corresponded to 41% of very poor quality scars after 1 month), whereas 59% of these patients still had a scar of excellent quality (see Table 9 in "Flaps", p. 140).

Closure in Two Layers

In our study, closure in two layers did not lead to any improvement in the quality of the scars compared with single-layer closure. Nor did skin closure by interrupted sutures, continuous sutures or intradermal sutures produce any significant cosmetic difference. On the other hand, the use of metal staples affords undeniable and fundamental progress in the quality of the scars. By their very nature (Photo 4) they eliminate the factor of supplementary ischae-

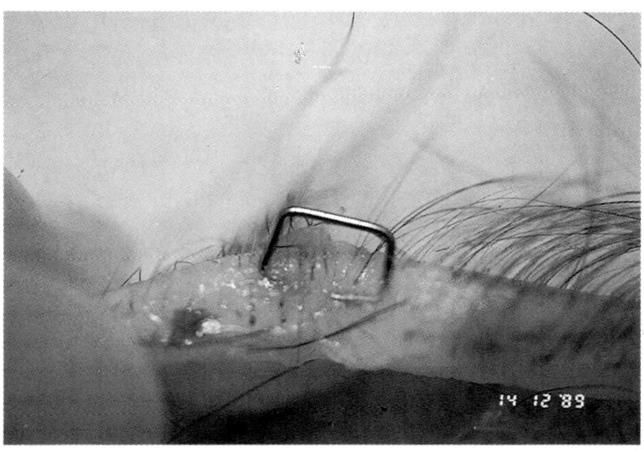

Photo 4. Staple closure in three layers. The staple bridges over the skin and prevents ischaemic necrosis of the margins. Note that the staple does not reach the galea

mia of the hair bulbs at the sutures. Furthermore, though the staples do not traverse the galea, we can report that reconstruction of the deep layer was still unnecessary. Removal of the staples is normally done between the eighth and tenth days. There is no point in leaving them longer except when there is excessive tension, and even then for no longer than 15 days.

Flaps and Grafts

A flap survives on its vascular pedicle. Depending on the type of vascularisation, there is a distinction between flaps centered on a vascular pedicle (artery and vein), i.e. axial flaps ("pattern flaps") and flaps surviving on the subdermal plexus ("random flaps"). An axial flap is always more reliable than a flap surviving on the subdermal plexus. In other words, it allows a much higher ratio between the length and breadth of the pedicle.

This ratio varies with the extent of the blood supply of the region considered. Classically, from 2 at the abdomen, it is on average 5 at the scalp, where a pedicle of 3 cm permits a flap of 15 cm. In practice, we have observed variations from 3 to 8 depending on the area. Thus, we have successfully constructed flaps 16 cm long and 2 cm wide in children. Conversely, in the adult smoker we have seen flaps 3.5 cm wide necrose after the 9 or 10 cm in length. Of course, all these figures are only of statistical value, and therefore they imply the need in everyday practice for using an adequate safety margin. It is possible to increase the flap ratio by autonomising it ("delayed flap"). Thus an axial flap of 4 cm may reach 28 cm or more on the scalp if autonomised.

The essential mechanism of autonomisation of flaps has not yet been clearly demonstrated, but its efficacy is beyond doubt. This can be done in one or two stages. It consists of partial section of the flap margins, with or without stripping of the distal extremity, and suture in situ without displacing the flap. This produces modifications of the blood-flow which are maximal and definitive around the fourth day. In theory, it is possible to autonomise a flap 4 days before its transfer. In practice, most authors wait for some 8 days, some a little longer. Thus a flap survives with a reduced blood-flow, which derives only from its pedicle for a certain period. It is therefore essential to protect the pedicle from any incautious trauma, both preoperative (section of the galea close to the pedicle, closure under tension) and postoperative (compressive dressings or haematoma underlying the flap).

Between the 15th and 21st days, the flap has been revascularised from the margins of the receptor area, and it is then possible to divide its pedicle without risk. Thus it is quite possible to perform tonsural reductions or grafts close to the pedicle of a flap, provided of course one has waited the necessary 3 weeks. Conversely, when there is a scar close to the pedicle of a projected flap, it is preferable not to construct it.

Naturally, every type of flap described in plastic surgery to fill in losses of substance can be used at the scalp. However, in practice, those most used are long transposition flaps with a narrow pedicle. When such a flap is insufficiently vascularised it is its extremity that will necrose, leading to definitive alopecia. But we have seen that there are cases where the ischaemia is limited, ending with a temporary alopecia of the flap. Hair loss is not then immediate, but occurs at around 3 weeks after the operation.

Every surgeon who constructs scalp flaps must be aware of this situation, so that he may reassure his patient (and himself) on the prognosis of certain secondary alopecias. The fine down which appears on the flap towards the sixth week is the first sign of complete regrowth.

Unlike flaps, grafts are completely detached from their donor site and survive by imbibition at the receptor site. There is therefore a sort of race between the time taken by revascularisation and the onset of necrosis. It is evident that a graft has more chance of taking if it is small.

We are not concerned here with thin split-skin grafts and full-thickness grafts; the grafts used in the surgery of baldness are composite grafts, i.e. they include the epidermis, the dermis and the hypodermis with its appendages. Thus it is less certain that they will take. This will be easier if the graft is small and the receptor site well vascularised. There is always a certain degree of temporary ischaemia of some days, which explains the constant hair loss on the grafts, whereas this is very rare in flaps. Again, if the graft has been revascularised soon enough, the bulbs will survive and the hair regrow; if not, the alopecia will persist. This explains why it is common to see grafts on which only some hairs have regrown, giving a very unpleasing appearance.

The farther a bulb is from the margins, the less chance it has of being revascularised; 2.5 mm seems to be the maximum tolerable distance. Thus, cylindrical grafts have a good take up to 5 mm in diameter, and the strips of Vallis can be very long but must not exceed 4 mm in breadth. The same applies to fusiform grafts, whose length may reach 2 cm but whose breadth must not exceed 4 mm.

Direction of Implantation of Grafted Hair

In our view the direction of implantation of grafted hair is of cardinal importance in terms of the final cosmetic result. We saw in the chapter on "Anatomy" (p. 4) that the hairs have a radiating implantation away from a central point at the vertex. It is essential to respect this implantation, particularly in the frontal region where the hair must grow forward except in certain cases (see "Indications"). Failure to respect this rule during placement of a flap leads to a frontal scar, which is always difficult to camouflage, and to a striking lack of naturalness (Photo 5). This also applies when placing grafts, which must have the direction of implantation of the receptor area.

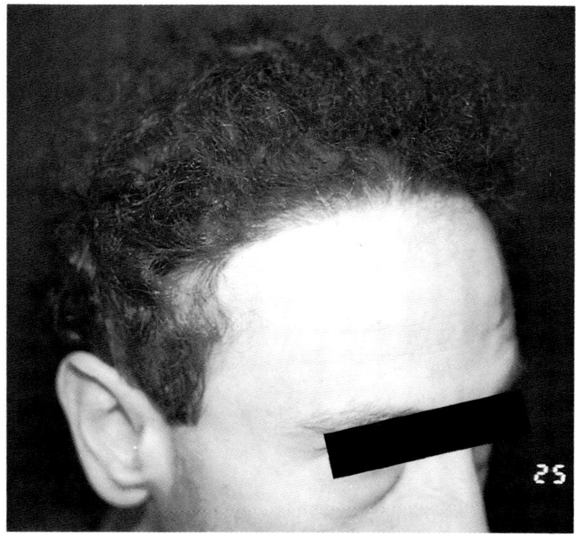

Photo 5. The anterior scar of a Juri flap attracts attention because the hairs grow backward

Scalp Incision

Incision of the scalp should always be made with a scalpel, parallel to the hair bulbs. This also applies to grafts, to the fashioning of flaps and of reductions. Failure to observe this rule leads to a loss of hair bulbs along the scars, often confused by some inexperienced surgeons with secondary broadening of the scars. This is a source of repeated and ineffective procedures.

Position of Scars

The position of scars (Fig. 2) in relation to the direction of implantation of the hair bulbs is very important. A scar parallel to the axis of the hairs is always more visible than one perpendicular to this same axis. Thus, at the crown, and in the parietal and occipital regions, horizontal scars are always less obvious than vertical ones. A horizontal scar is easily concealed by the overlying hair, which will spontaneously tend to arrange itself over it. In contrast, a vertical scar will only be covered by the hair if this is carefully styled, preferably in a direction different from the natural axis of the hairs (Photo 6).

In the extreme, a scar may become permanently obvious, even if it is very fine, when the hairs grow in a divergent manner on either side of its axis. This situation may occur:

- After excision of a scalp zone situated in an intermediate region surrounded by two zones where the hair grows in different directions: the posterior parietal region (Photo 7) and the vertex. This is

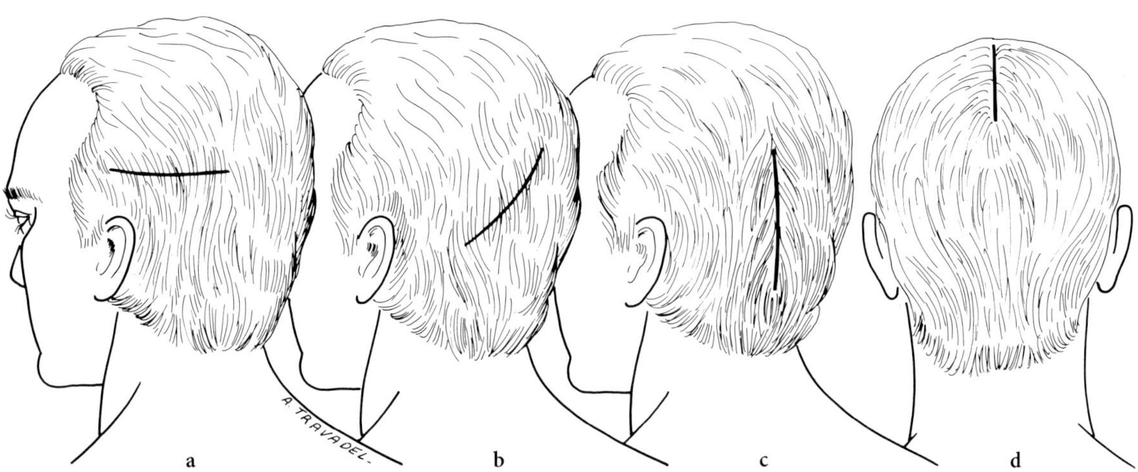

Fig. 2a–d. Situation of scars in relation to direction of implantation of hair-bulbs. **a** Excellent. **b** Correct. **c** Moderate. **d** Poor

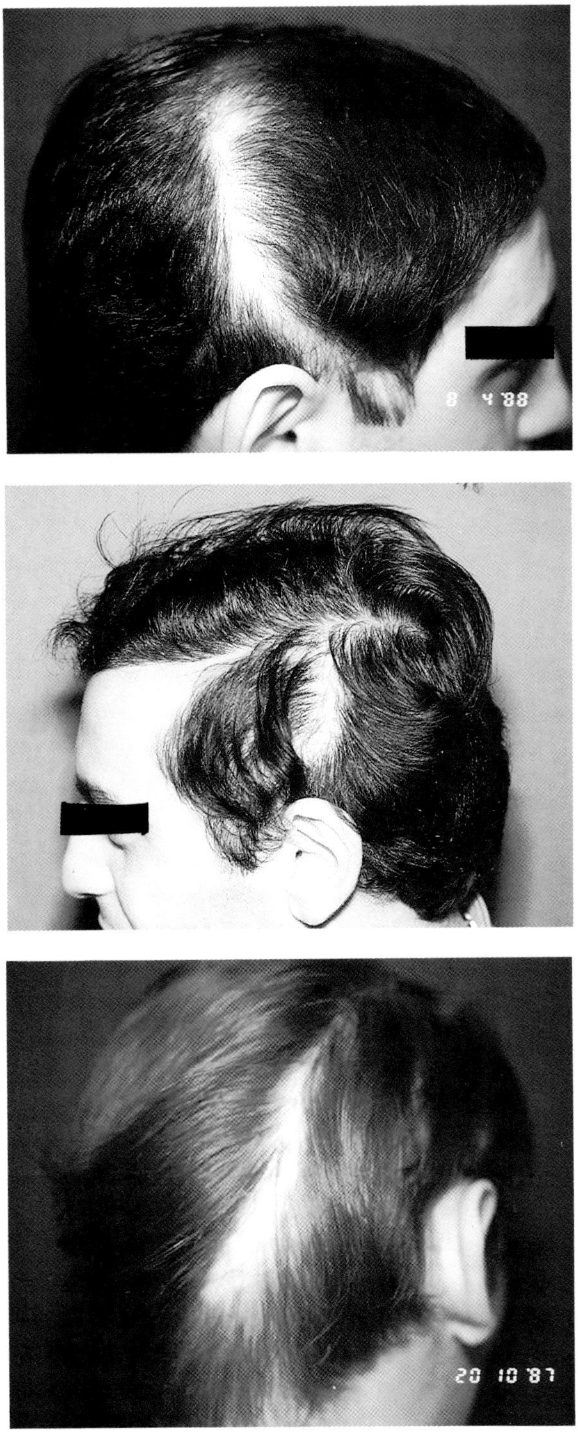

a

b

c

Photo 6a–c. Scar from raising of flap: the vertical portion is more evident than the horizontal portion, whereas the scar is of the same quality throughout its length. **c** Vertical scar in the occipital region which is more or less difficult to conceal

why we believe that it is always preferable to respect the region of the crown, when it is still present, particularly during a tonsural reduction.
- After the placement of a flap in which the axis of the hair is different from that of the hairs in the receptor site. This is one reason why we avoid using flaps to cover the vertex; the vertex is a zone of radiating implantation, and the hair growth on the flap cannot be satisfactory in relation to the receptor site.

However, correction of such a permanently visible scar is possible. It is not achieved by simple excision and suture, which would lead to the same outcome, but by a series of Z-plasties which transform the straight scar into a zigzag and which modifies the direction of hair implantation on either side of the scar (Photo 7). One or two sessions of micrografting, if correctly orientated, may give good results. The scar at the anterior margin of a flap can be improved by the technique of de-epithelialisation with embedding of the hairy margin under the smooth frontal skin (Fig. 3).

Infiltration of the Scalp

Infiltration of the scalp has three aims: local anaesthesia, lessening of bleeding and firming-up of the scalp. We refer the reader to the section on "Anaesthesia" (p. 59f.) for details of this infiltration. We simply recall here the fact that adrenalised 1% Xylocaine diluted to 1:3 suffices to produce the anaesthetic and haemostatic effect required. To facilitate stripping of the scalp, the infiltration must be made beneath the galea. However, most bleeding in the scalp is encountered in traversing the skin. To minimise this and provide easy haemostasis, it is therefore essential to perform superficial dermo-epidermal infiltration along the line of the incision. Blanching of the skin as the infiltration proceeds confirms its efficacy. Thus, during the incision, only the large vessels bleed and their haemostasis is easier. Lastly, infiltration produces induration of the site on removal of the grafts, allowing forage parallel to the axis of the hair bulbs.

Stripping the Scalp

The scalp must always be stripped under the plane of the galea in the space of Merkel. As this plane is virtually avascular, stripping is very easy and can be made with any instrument; our own preference is for large curved scissors. None of the strippers invented

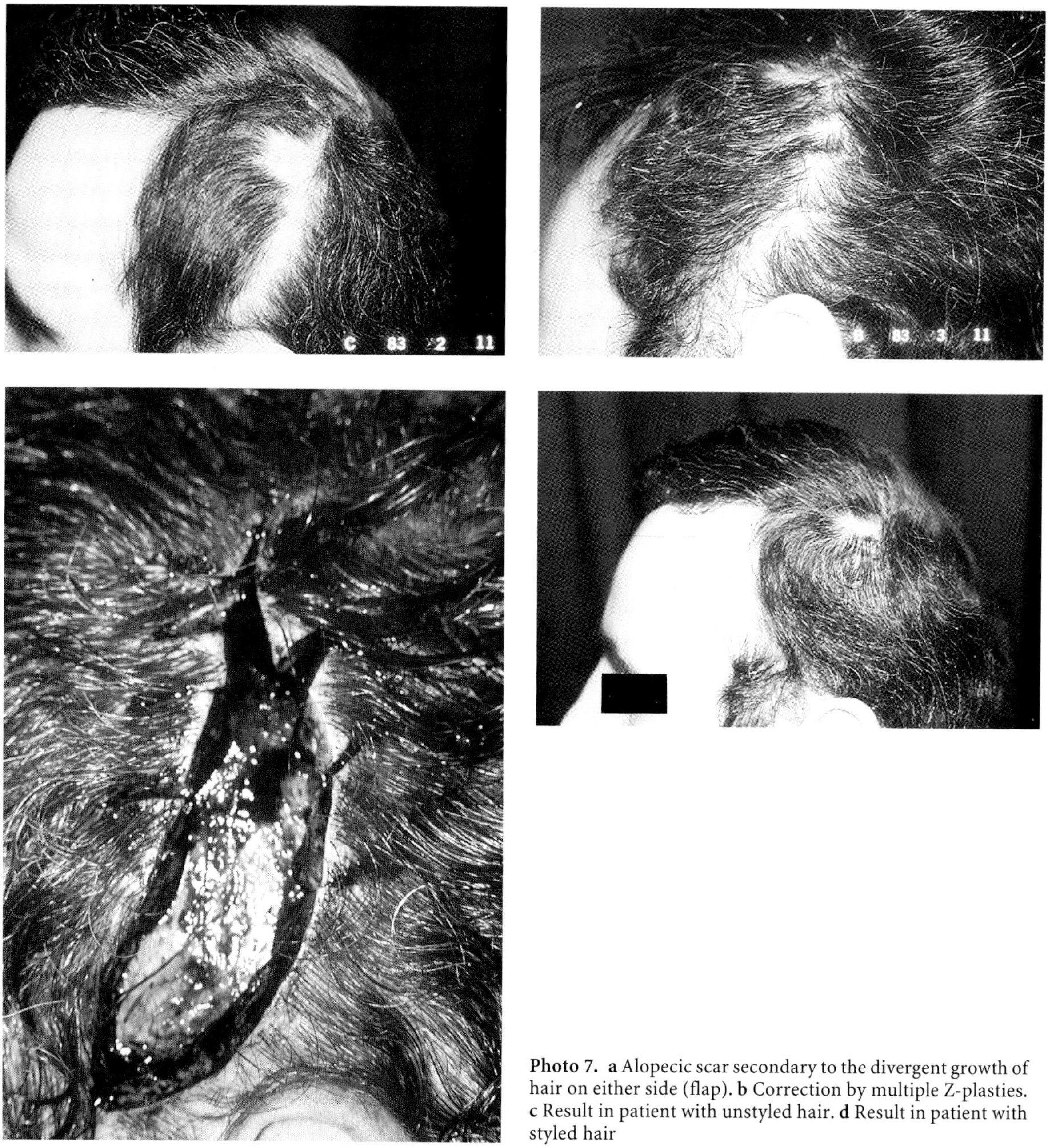

Photo 7. **a** Alopecic scar secondary to the divergent growth of hair on either side (flap). **b** Correction by multiple Z-plasties. **c** Result in patient with unstyled hair. **d** Result in patient with styled hair

seem of great use, as they have to be changed every time it is necessary to divide adhesions to continue the stripping. In peripheral zones the stripping must be carried on under the muscle plane at the periosteal level. This is the only way of avoiding the vessels that travel within the muscles. However, at the attachments of the occipital muscle at the superior curved occipital line, a change of plane is necessary for the simple reason that there is no longer any galea here. We discuss this further in the chapters on "Reduction Procedures" (p. 148ff.) and "Flaps" (p. 115ff.).

In addition, preservation of the galea acts as an excellent protection against excessive tension on the suture line. If it is excised or incised, as well as always sacrificing several vessels, it allows considerable stretching of the scalp. This leads to stretching of the underlying vessels and thus their partial or total obliteration, a source of secondary alopecia on the overlying flaps. We believe that incisions of the galea are permissible only for closure of the donor site of a flap in difficult cases.

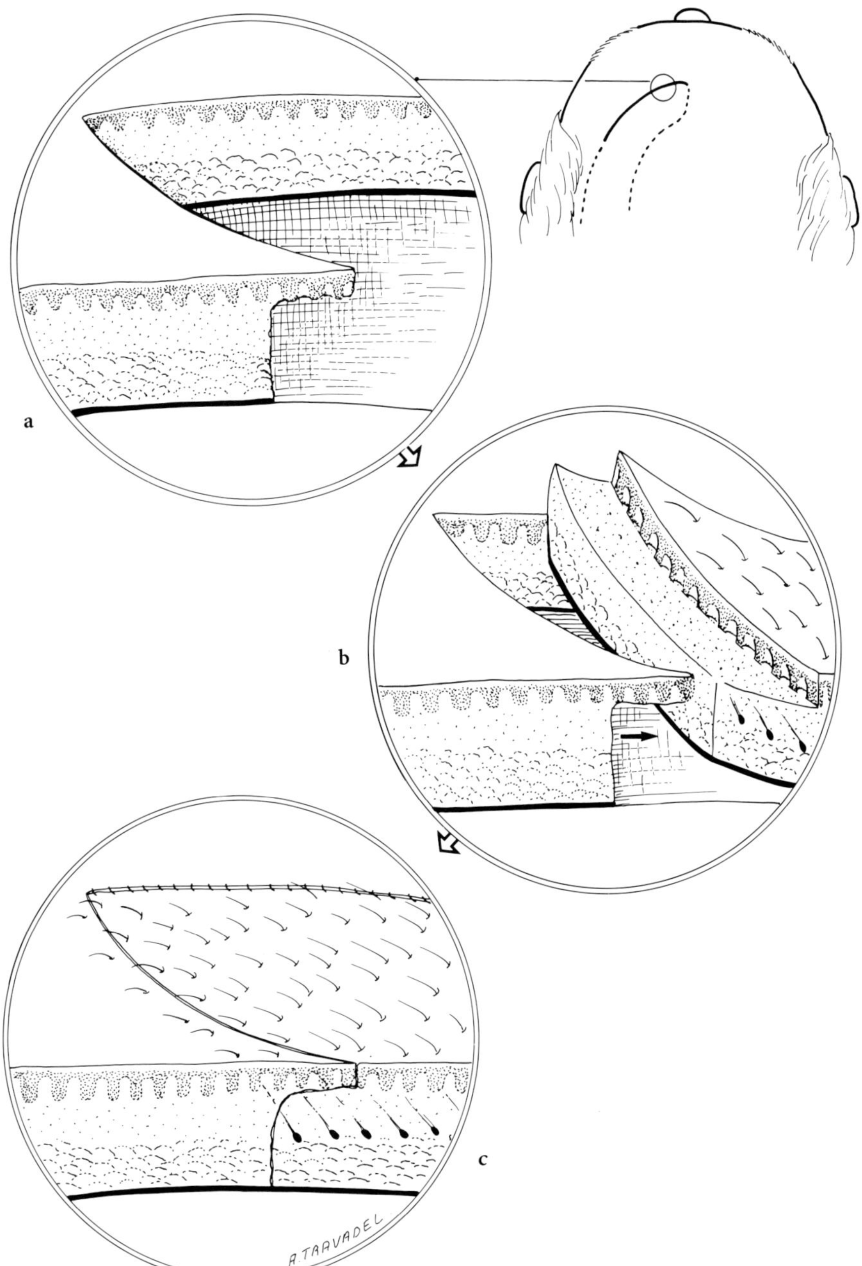

Fig. 3a–c. De-epithelialisation and embedding of anterior border of flap. **a** Frontal zone. **b,c** Epidermal denudation of flap (according to Nataf)

Marginal Haemostasis

After incision of the scalp, two types of vessels are damaged:

- The arteries and arterioles which travel in the supragaleal plane. These bleed in spurts and their lumen is obvious; they need to be dealt with.
- The capillaries and arterioles which travel in the hypodermis have a less obvious lumen. When the scalp has not been infiltrated they cause general oozing; on the other hand, when the line of incision has been properly infiltrated with a vasoconstrictor agent, only a few large vessels will bleed. These are visible enough to allow haemostasis, which we think advisable. Diathermy certainly sacrifices some of the hair bulbs, but this sacrifice is minimal and better than risking a haematoma, which is always more damaging to the peripheral bulbs

through the tension and ischaemia it produces, not to mention the increased risks of infection.

Galeotomy

Galeotomy may be necessary in some cases, particularly for closure of the donor site of a flap. To be effective it must be total, and the incision must split the entire thickness of the galea to reveal the underlying fat. In this case, the vessels travelling in contact with the galea are often divided, and careful haemostasis then becomes essential. Galeotomy, on average, allows a gain of between ½ and 1 cm during closure of a loss of substance. The risks entailed have been stated above. This is why we believe that it should be avoided in vertical reductions, where the excision must be made as required and closure must be without undue tension.

Anagenic Defluvium

Anagenic defluvium is the accelerated loss of hair secondary to practically all operations on the scalp. This hair loss is reported by the patients in the weeks following operation. It is clearly related to the trauma of the procedure, or more exactly to the temporary ischaemia it produces. This hair loss is always transient and regresses without complications. It is possible that it may be lessened if not suppressed by pre- and postoperative minoxidil.

Infection

Infection is rare (<5% in our series) in the scalp because of its excellent blood supply. This fact justifies not using postoperative antibiotics routinely. While true infection is rare, "mini-sepsis" at the sutural apertures is commoner. Such infection is not serious, but does destroy the peripheral hair bulbs and may therefore lead to alopecic scars. In the case of autografts, this mini-sepsis is very serious as it may lead to partial or total destruction of the bulbs. The most effective method of preventing this risk is certainly the use of staples, as well as postoperative hygienic measures.

Postoperative Management

Postoperative management is very simple but very important. As infection is rare, routine postoperative antibiotics are not justified in our view. However, to combat the mini-sepsis which destroys the hair bulbs locally and leads to alopecia round the scar, we request our patients to wash their hair with shampoo 48 h after operation and to perform frequent rinsing, every day if need be. Crusting is then uncommon.

In the case of a haematoma, evacuation of the clots is urgently indicated after the removal of one or two sutures. This will prevent compression and ischaemia of the overlying scalp. It also prevents secondary infection. If closure has been made with excessive tension, scabs will form under the scar, due to ischaemic necrosis of the margins. Only frequent washing will prevent infection beneath these scabs, which fall off spontaneously after 2–3 weeks, leaving an alopecic scar whose extant varies with the degree of ischaemia.

References

1. Adson MH, Anderson R, Argenta LC (1987) Scalp expansion in the treatment of male pattern baldness. Plast Reconstr Surg 79/6: 907–914
2. Alt TH (1980) Scalp reduction as an adjunct to hair transplantation. J Dermatol Surg Oncol 6: 1011–1018
3. Anderson RD (1987) Expansion-assisted treatment of male pattern baldness. Clin Plast Surg 14/3: 477–479
4. Argenta LC (1984) Controlled tissue expansion in reconstructive surgery. Br J Plast Surg 37: 502–529
5. Argenta LC (1985) Advances in tissue expansion. Clin Plast Surg 12/2: 159–171
6. Argenta LC, Marks MJ, Grabb WC (1983) The use of tissue expansion in head and neck reconstruction. Ann Plast Surg 11: 31
7. Austad EA, Thomas SB, Pasyk K (1986) Tissue expansion: dividend or loan. Plast Reconstr Surg 78/1: 63–67
8. Ayres S (1970) Hair transplantation. In: Epstein-Thomas E (ed) Skin surgery. Thomas, Springfield, pp 453–508
9. Blanchard G, Blanchard B (1976) La réduction tonsurale (détonsuration); concept nouveau dans le traitement chirurgical de la calvitie. Rev Chir Esth L Franc 4: 5–10
10. Bosley LL, Hope CR, Montroy RE (1979) Male pattern reduction (M.P.R.) for surgical reduction of male pattern baldness. Curr Ther Res 25: 281–287
11. Bouhanna P (1976) Le cuir chevelu: les alopécies définitives et leurs traitements. Thesis, Paris
12. Bouhanna P (1989) Greffes à cheveux longs immédiats. Nouv Dermatol 8/4: 418–420
13. Brandy D (1986) The Brandy bitemporal flap. Cosmet Surg
14. Cherry GW, Austad ED, Pasyk KA (1983) Increased survival and vascularity of random skin flaps elevated in controlled expanded skin. Plast Reconstr Surg 72: 680
15. Converse JM (1964) Reconstructive plastic surgery. Saunders, Philadelphia, pp 1087–1088
16. Correa-Iturraspe M, Arufe HN (1957) Plastic surgery in partial definitive alopecia of the scalp. Plast Reconstr Surg 20: 417

17. Dardour JC (1983) Treatment of male baldness with a one stage flap rotation. In: Transactions of the VII Congress of Plastic Surgery, Montreal, 26 June–1 July 1983, pp 680–681
18. Dardour JC (1988) Utilisation d'une prothèse d'expansion dans le traitment de la calvitie masculine. Ann Chir Plast Esth XXIII/4: 347–349
19. Dardour JC (1989) Les réductions de tonsure. Principes et innovation: le lifting du scalp. Ann Chir Plast Esth 34/3: 234–242
20. Dufourmentel C, Mouly R (1959) Chirurgie plastique. Flammarion, Paris
21. Elliot RA (1977) Lateral flaps for instant results in male pattern baldness. Plast Reconstr Surg 60/5: 699–703
22. Feit LJ (1969) Pathogenic classification of male pattern baldness. New innovations in surgical techniques. Int Surg 51: 58–67
23. Flemming RW, Mayer TG (1981) Short and long scalp flaps in the treatment of male pattern baldness. Arch Oto Laryngol 107/7: 403–408
24. Fleming J (1965) Surgery for baldness: a case report. Can J Surg 8: 400–403
25. Ginestet G, Frezières H, Dupuis A (1967) Chirurgie plastique et réconstructive de las face. Flammarion, Paris, pp 8–9
26. Harii K, Ohmori K, Ohmori S (1974) Successful clinical transfer of 10 free flaps by microvascular anastomoses. Plast Reconstr Surg 53/3: 259–270
27. Juri J (1975) Use of parieto-occipital flaps in the surgical treatment of baldness. Past Reconstr Surg 55/4: 456–460
28. Juri J, Juri C, Arufe HN (1978) Use of rotation scalp flaps for treatment of occipital baldness. Plast Reconstr Surg 61/1: 23–26
29. Lamont ES (1957) A plastic surgical transformation – report of a case. West J Surg 65: 164
30. Leonard AG, Small JO (1986) Tissue expansion in treatment of alopecia. Br Plast Surg 39: 42–56
31. Limburger S (1959) Die operative Behandlung des Haarverlustes. Medizinische 35: 1559
32. Manders EK, Friedman M (1985) The treatment of male pattern baldness utilizing a differential expander. Annual meeting of the ASAPS, Boston
33. Manders EK, Graham WP (1984) Alopecia reconstruction by scalp expansion. J Dermatol Surg Oncol 10: 967
34. Manders EK, Au VK, Wong RKM (1987) Sclap expansion for male pattern baldness. Clin Plast Surg 14/3: 469–175
35. Maréchal R (972) Alopécies séborrhéiques – traitement par ligature des artères. Presse Med 4: 257–259
36. Marzola M (1984) An alternative hair replacement method. In: Norwood OT (ed) Hair transplant surgery, 2nd edn. Thomas, Springfield, pp 315–324
37. Morestin (1911) La réduction graduelle des difformités tégumentaires. J Chir (Paris) 8: 509–511 (reprinted in Plast Reconstr Surg 42: 163)
38. Nataf J (1981) Particular techniques of hair transplantation. In: Orfanos CE, Montagna W, Stutten G (eds) Hair research status and future aspects. Springer, Berlin Heidelberg New York, pp 655–659
39. Nataf J (1984) Surgical treatment for frontal baldness: the long temporal vertical flap. Plast Reconstr Surg 74: 628
40. Nataf J, Elbaz JS, Pollet J (1976) Étude critique des transplantations du cuir chevelu et proposition dúne optique. Ann Chir Plast 21/3: 199–206
41. Neumann CG (1957) The expansion of an area of skin by progressive distension of a subcutaneous balloon. Plast Reconstr Surg 19: 124–128
42. Nordstrom R (1984) Stretch-back in scalp reductions for male pattern baldness. Past Reconstr Surg 71: 411–426
43. Nordstrom R (1988) Tissue expansion and flaps for surgical correction of male pattern baldness. Br J Plast Surg 41: 154–159
44. Norwood OT, Shiell RC (1984) Hair transplant surgery, 2nd edn. Thomas, Springfield
45. Ohmori K (1980) Free scalp flap. Plast Reconstr Surg 65/1: 42–49
46. Okuda S (1939) Clinical and experimental studies of transplantation of living hairs. Jpn J Dermatol Urol 46: 135–138
47. Orentreich N (1959) Autografts in alopecia and other selected dermatological conditions. Ann NY Acad Sci 83: 463–479
48. Ozun G (1986) Traitement de la calvitie par expansion cutanée. 31st National Congress of the SFCPRE
49. Passot R (1920) Les autoplasties esthétiques dans la calvities. Presse Med 23: 222–223
50. Passot R (2930) Un cas d'autoplastie esthétique du cuir chevelu pour calvities. Presse Med 48: 408
51. Pellegrini (1986) The history of hair in facial plastic surgery. Hair replacement. REA Norstrom Spring 2/3: 167–177
52. Pincus J (1950) Cited in Szasz and Robertson. Arch Dermatol 61: 34–48
53. Ponten B (1963) Tissue expansion in soft tissue reconstruction. Plast Reconstr Surg 74/3: 482–492
54. Radovan C (1984) Tissue expansion in soft tissue reconstruction. Plast Reconstr Surg 74/3: 482–489
55. Rappard JHA et al. (1988) Surface-area increase in tissue expansion. Plast Reconstr Surg 825: 833–839
56. Rees TD (1980) Aesthetic plastic surgery. Treatment of baldness. Saunders, Philadelphia, pp 865–899
57. Rook A, Wilkinson DS, Ebling FJG (1968) Textbook of dermatology, vol 2. Blackwell, Oxford, p 1383
58. Rook A, Dawber R (1986) Diseases of the hair and scalp. Blackwell, Oxford
59. Sasaki GH (1982) Vascular changes during tissue expansion. PSEF Symposium on Soft Tissue Expansion, Ann Arbor
60. Sasaki GH, Pang GY (1984) Pathophysiology of skin flaps raised on expanded pig skin. Plast Reconstr Surg 74: 59
61. Schein M (1903) Über die Entstehung der Glatze. Wien Klin Wochenschr 40: 1862–1864
62. Seltzer AP (1969) Reconstructive surgery of hair transplantation by improved motorized technique. Int Surg 51/4: 353–359
63. Shively RE, Bermant MA, Buchjolz RD (1985) Separation of cranio-pagus twins utilising tissue expanders (case report). Plast Reconstr Surg 76/5: 765–773
64. Szasz RS, Robertson WM (1950) A theory of the pathogenesis of ordinary human baldness. Arch Dermatol 61: 34–48
65. Tillman H (1908) Cited in: Bryant JD, Buck AH. American practice of surgery, vol 4. Wood, New York
66. Unger WP (1978) Hair transplantation. Dekker, New York
67. Unger MG, Unger WP (1978) Management of alopecia of the scalp by a combination of excision and transplantation. J Dermatol Surg Oncol 4: 670–672
68. Vallis CP (1967) Surgical treatment of the receding hairline. Plast Reconstr Surg 40/2: 138–146
69. Young MW (1948) Anatomical and pathological factors in senile alopecia. Ant Rec 100: 728

Autografts

General Principles

Definition

A graft is a tissue or collection of tissues completely detached from the organism and subsequently repositioned. Unlike a flap, a graft retains no vascular attachment but survives by imbibition. The vascularisation of the receptor site is therefore an essential factor determining the survival of a graft. The size of the graft is the second factor that influences the survival of a graft: the larger it is, the less the chances of its survival.

Classification

Depending on the thickness of the removed skin fragment, the following can be distinguished:

- Thin (split-skin) grafts, which include only the epidermis (a few microns) without transgressing on the basal layer. If the latter is damaged the risks of keloidal scarring are considerable. These grafts never comprise any skin appendages, whether hairs or glands. The chances of these grafts taking are certainly the best. The taking of thin grafts on the scalp has been particularly well described in the context of major burns with a restricted skin stock.
- Full-thickness grafts, which include the basal layer and hypodermis. Usually, full-thickness grafts are scrupulously defatted before being positioned. At the scalp, however, the fat is left in place as it is here that the hair follicles are situated.
- Composite grafts, which include several different tissues (skin, muscle etc.).

Depending on their size and shape, grafts can be classified as:

- Cylindrical, removed with a punch. Their maximum size is 5 mm, as we have already seen in the chapter on "Surgical Techniques" (p. 63) that, above this diameter, ischaemia of the follicles is too severe and that the hairs do not regrow (Photo 1).
- Spindle-shaped (fusiform) grafts, which may not exceed 4 mm in breadth for the same reasons; their average length is 2 cm.
- Strip grafts, which are 2–3 mm wide and may reach 5–10 cm in length.

According to the number of hairs contained in each graft, the following may be distinguished:

- Micrografts, which contain one or two hairs
- Minigrafts, which contain three to five hairs
- Conventional grafts, which include more than six hairs.

We may recall that a graft of 4 mm can carry on average eight to 25 hairs.

In practice, more importance is attached nowadays to the number of hairs per graft than to their diameter. Mini- and micrografts are increasingly being used, whereas punch grafts are finding fewer and fewer indications. Clearly, several grafting sessions (at least three or four) at the same receptor site are required to obtain a satisfactory density, which in

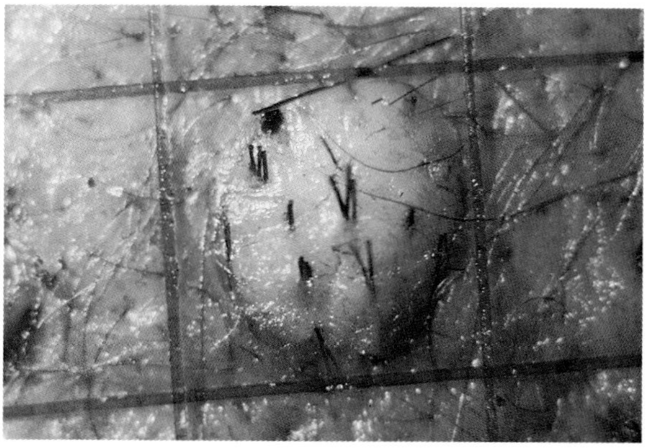

Photo 1. Grafts at recipient site immediately after transplantation, showing number of hairs implanted and their single or multiple emergence from the skin orifices

every case will be much less considerable than that obtained with a flap.

Harvesting Grafts

We have already seen in the preceding chapter how grafts take on the scalp. Initially, the hairs fall out with the scabs and regrow subsequently. The new hair begins to appear at the third month and continues to grow at the rate of 1 cm a month on average. Therefore, 3 months is the minimum interval required between two sessions.

Factors Influencing the Survival of a Graft

Some factors that influence how well a graft takes relate to the operator:

- The size of the grafts: the smaller the graft, the greater its chances of survival.
- Manipulation of the grafts: this must be as atraumatic as possible, taking special care not to crush the follicles with the dissecting forceps and not to let them dry out too long in the air.

Some factors depend on the patient:

- Vascularisation of the receptor site: tolerance is known to be very important here, since it may be possible to position micrografts on a burn scar.
- The postoperative management is very important; microsepsis, which destroys the follicles, must always be prevented. Rather than antibiotics, which we sometimes give, we insist that our patients undergo frequent and early shampooing (48 h).

Donor Area

Where the transplantation of hair grafts is concerned, one of the most important factors is assessment of the donor area. Apart from any cosmetic considerations, the patient's motivation and his state of health, three features must be carefully assessed by the surgeon [1]:

- The increase of hair loss and the possible extent of baldness
- The quality and density of the hair at the donor area
- Camouflage of the donor area

Measurements and Assessment

The potential donor area is obtained by multiplying the length of the area by its breadth. Since a graft of 4 mm in diameter has a surface area of 0.125 cm^2, it is easy to calculate the number of grafts available in the event of total removal.

If the distance between the two external auditory meatuses or the breadth of the donor area is on average 28 cm and the height of the usable crown is 6.5–7.5 cm, the donor area can provide 28×7 cm=196 cm^2/0.125=1500 grafts, if removed in totality. In practice, however, only a half or third of this area can be removed. When removing strips to obtain micrografts, it is also possible to estimate the number of grafts obtainable by calculating the hair density at the donor area and its surface area.

Quality of Hair

Assessment of the quality of hair in the donor area is as important as assessment of its capacity. Alt has defined seven intrinsic factors essential to obtaining a good cosmetic result [1]:

- The extent of the safe donor area: the donor area must be the region of the scalp where the definitive hairs are of sufficient density to allow the taking of grafts. This area is bounded by a line drawn vertically from the external auditory meatuses and a lower horizontal line drawn between the external meatus and the median line of the occiput, the upper border being determined by a horizontal line drawn 7 cm from the lower limit (see under "Classification" for the reasons for this lower line), which corresponds to a useful surface area of about 200 cm^2 (Fig. 1). Respect for these limits of the donor area will prevent scars that were previously concealed by the hair becoming visible, even if the balding process continues.
- The potential extent of the recipient bald area.
- The scalp laxity of the bald area is a third determining factor in the indication for scalp reduction.

The other four factors relate to the donor area:

- The hair density per square centimetre
- The diameter of the hair shafts
- Whether the hair is curly or wavy
- Hair colour

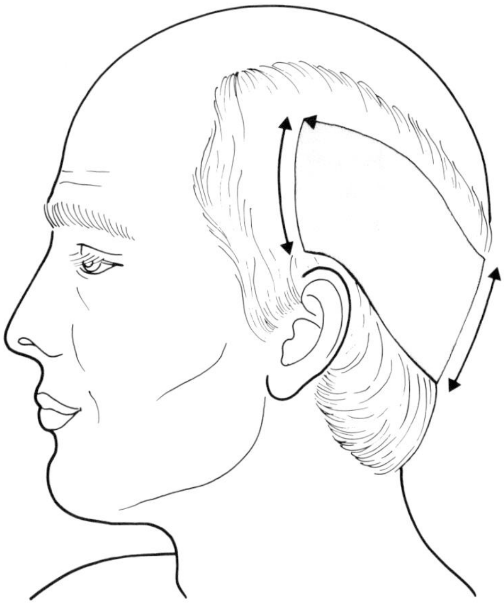

Fig. 1. Outlines of the harvesting area of autografts for male baldness

Hair Density (Photo 1)

The number of hairs per square centimetre is probably the most important intrinsic factor. The density varies considerably from one zone to another and from one individual to another. Thus the occipital zone is denser than the supra-auricular zone. The density may vary from 100 to 400 hairs per cm^2, so that a graft of 4 mm diameter (12.5 mm^2) may contain 12–50 hairs. The mid-occipital region is the best donor area because it is the densest.

A simple method of assessment consists in designing circles of 4 mm in diameter with a punch dipped in gentian violet. The hairs emerging within these circles are counted. According to Alt, if the density in the supra-auricular region is low, it is best to take the grafts before performing the session(s) for reduction of the vertex. In contrast, if the density is high, the reduction procedure may precede taking the grafts [1]. In practice, this problem ceases to exist once the grafts are considered in terms of their density and not of their diameter, as has been noted.

Diameter of Hair Shafts (Photos 2, 3)

The diameter of the hair shafts is an important factor. The hairs of greatest calibre are more rigid and therefore give a cosmetic aspect with more "body" to the hair. Thus, a graft which contains only eight to ten hairs may have its cosmetic efficiency compensated by the thickness and frizzy or wavy nature of the hair.

Conversely, fine hairs in blond or red-headed subjects are more supple and do not allow this possibility of giving body to the hair-style. On the other hand, these fine hairs have the undeniable advantage of creating a more natural anterior frontal line. Thus, in patients with thick hair it is recommended to choose the grafts intended for reconstruction of

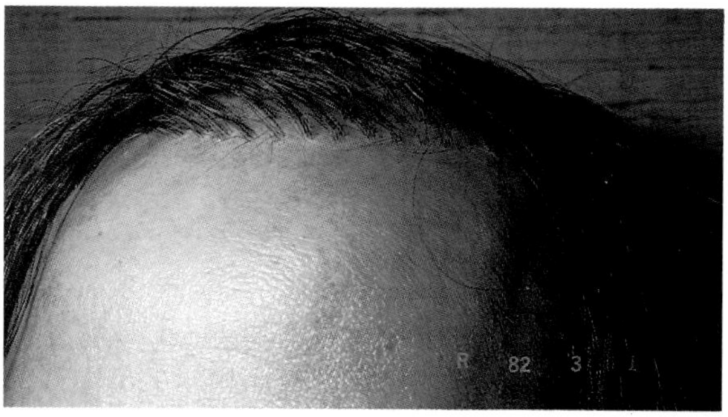

Photo 2. Poor indication: hairs stiff, black and thick (Asiatic)

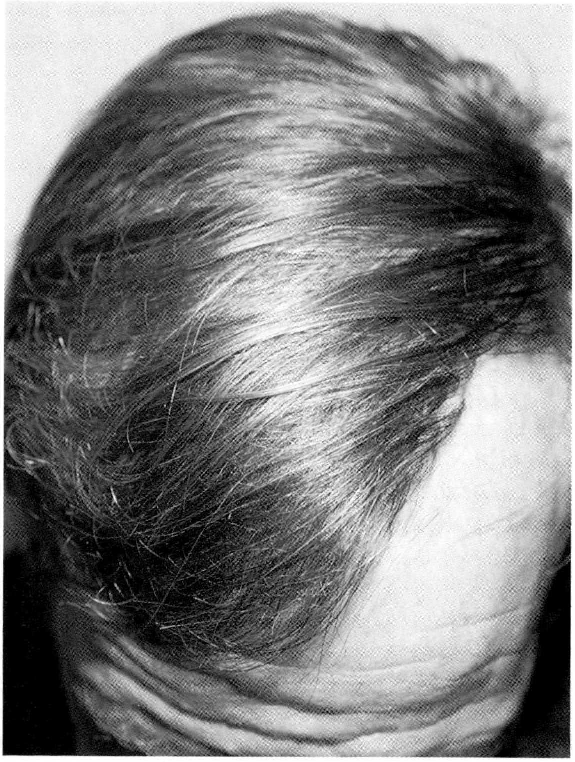

Photo 3. Hairs stiff but fine: good result after three sessions of 60 grafts

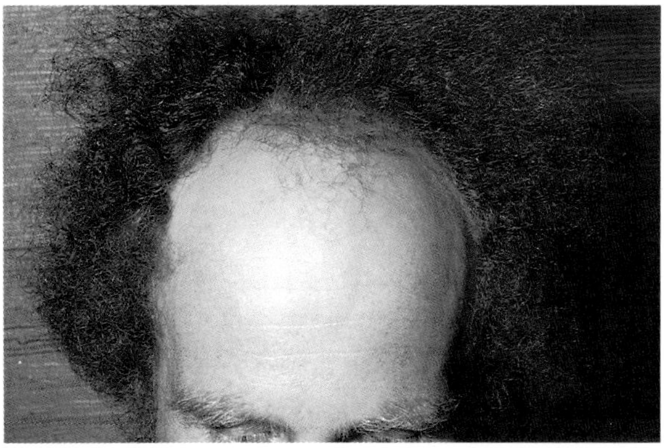

a

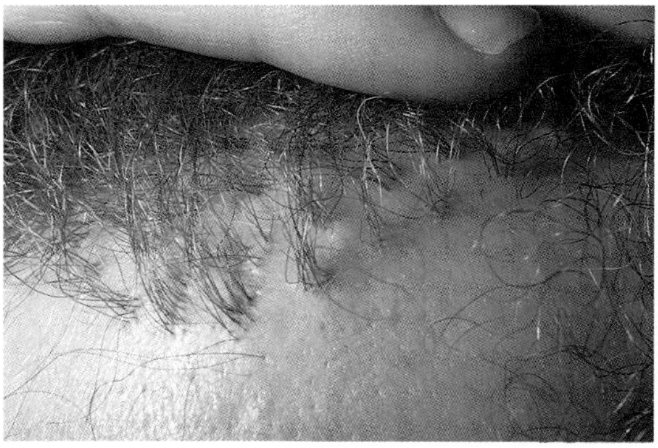

c

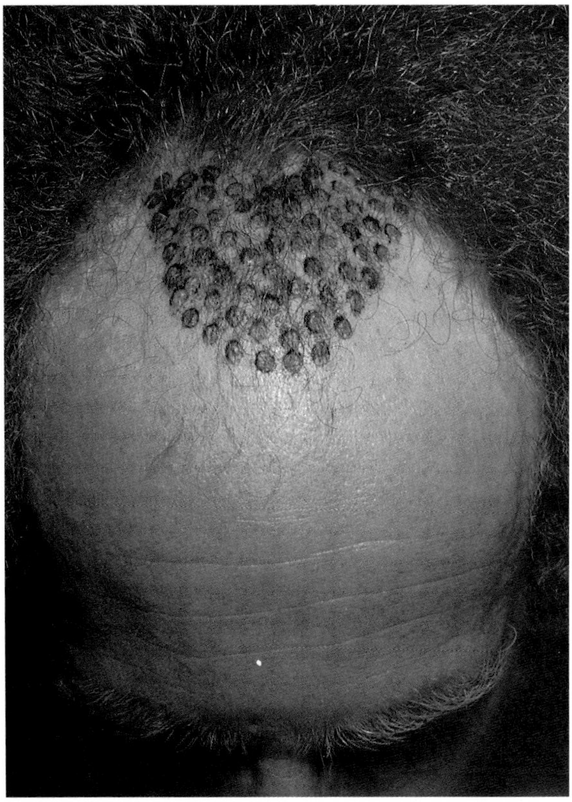

b

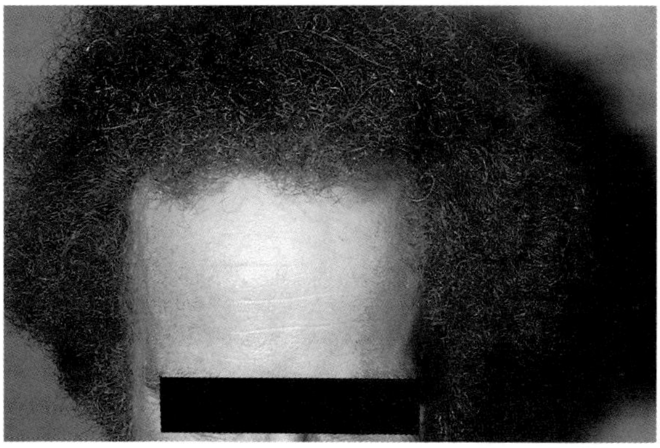

d

Photo 4. a Frontal alopecia in patient with frizzy hair. **b** Result 15 days after one transplantation session (60 grafts). **c** Result 6 months after a single session (patient voluntarily dishevelled). **d** Same patient with hair styled

the anterior line from a region where the hair has the least diameter. The resolution of this problem is one of the main reasons for the success of the micrograft.

Frizzy and Wavy Hair (Photo 4a–d)

Frizzy and wavy hair has the cosmetic advantage of giving "body" to the hair. The most confirmatory example is that of black subjects, in whom the density of the donor area can be less than that of the norm without impairing the cosmetic aspect. We may note the difficulty sometimes experienced in making an incision parallel to the hair bulbs in patients with crinkly hair. The penetration of the punch must be almost perpendicular to the plane of the scalp, unlike the obliquity classical for the removal of stiff or wavy hair.

Hair Colour (Photo 5)

Hair colour is an important factor insofar there may exist a contrast with the colour of the skin itself. In blond, red-headed or white-haired Caucasians, the nature of the hair is ideal because of the poor con-

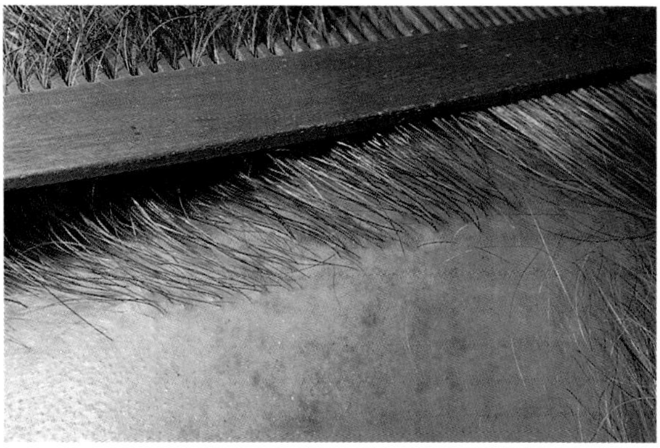

Photo 5. Frontal line of near-natural appearance after transplantation of grafts with light fine hairs

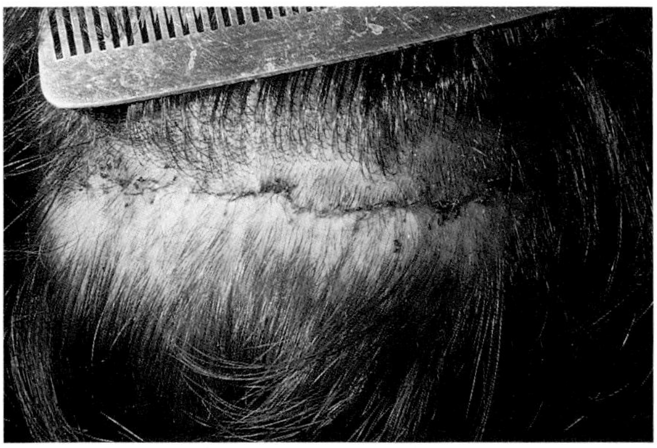

Photo 6. Camouflage of donor site by combing the hair above over it. Note that the grafts have been taken by the old method of separate orifices; above, running suture of a recent strip removal

trast with the underlying skin. Thus, fewer hairs are necessary to give a satisfactory appearance. Conversely, dark hairs give an unattractive appearance if their insuffcent density or calibre only incompletely camouflages the light underlying skin (Photo 2). The best candidate for hair transplantation is the subject with dense, thick, frizzy or wavy blond or grey hair.

Camouflage of Donor Area (Photo 6)

Postoperatively, camouflage of the donor area is as important as that of the receptor area. When the grafts are removed with a punch, a scattering of hairless circular scars 2–4 mm in diameter persists, usually well enough concealed when the patient's hair is properly styled, but evident when he or she is

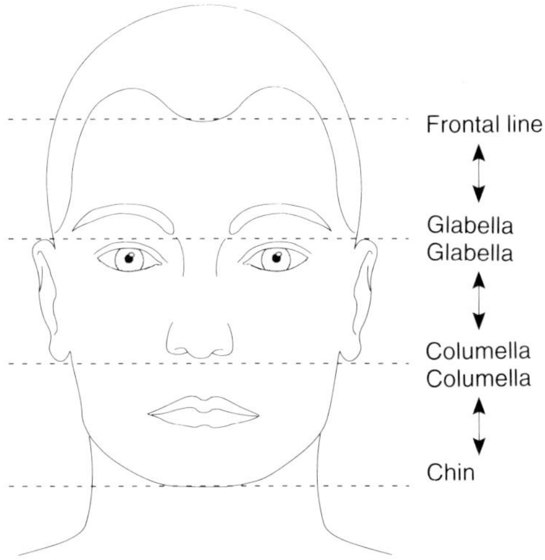

Fig. 2. Design and localisation of anterior frontal line

dishevelled, the hair is wet or when the donor area becomes too sparse and its hair too fine.

The removal of strips gives scars of better quality, provided these are transverse (see chapter on "Surgical Techniques", p. 64f). These are always hardly visible, even when only moderate in quality. Furthermore, this technique allows very numerous graft-taking sessions, using a different zone each time.

Recipient Area

Anterior Frontal Line (Fig. 2)

The design and localisation of the anterior frontal line (AFL) are among the most important factors [6]. Apart from good practical experience and an aesthetic sense adapted to each individual, certain factors are involved such as the age of the patient, the extent of the existing alopecia (see "Classification" and "Indications"), assessment of the progressive nature of the alopecia, the density, colour and shape of the hair and, finally, the personal cosmetic wishes of the patient [18].

1. The AFL must not be positioned too low down, for several reasons:
   - It is easier to correct an AFL by adding grafts to lower it than vice versa.
   - If the AFL does not have a sufficiently natural appearance, it is easier to conceal it with the remaining hair while awaiting the finishing touches (see "Micrografts").
   - Because of the forward orientation of the hairs, a very densely haired aspect may be obtained

without the AFL being too low, and the anterior line may also come to seem lower than was previously intended.
2. The AFL must never be straight or angulated, but form curved lines to make a more or less symmetrical oval depending on the patient's physiognomy.
3. The median point of the AFL must be situated at least two fingerbreadths above the highest median frontal crease (this approximate point depending on the breadth of the surgeon's fingers). This point can also be determined by using the rule of three equivalent distances: chin to base of nose, base of nose to root of nose, root of nose to AFL.
4. The design of this frontal line is shown to the patient, informing him of the impossibility of bringing the AFL too low down and of completely filling the two areas of fronto-temporal recession.

Transplantation to the Vertex

Transplantation to the vertex (Fig. 3, Photos 7a–c) is performed only after having confirmed or verified the absence of any indication for vertical reduction or for flaps intended for the vertex and frontal region (see "Indications").

The grafts are inserted at an oblique angulation identical with that of the down and of the existing hair and following a "wheel-spoke" pattern starting from a point situated in the lower quadrant and contralateral in relation to the parieto-frontal hair-parting. Forage of the receptor sites near this "centre" must allow sufficient spacing to prevent any unintended connection of the receptor pits. The grafts of the anterior part of the crown should have the same orientation as those of the vertex.

Complications Common to All Graft Types

Complications Resolving Spontaneously

Complications resolving spontaneously include normal and unpredictable developments:

- Postoperative oedema will distend the frontal region during the 3 following days and disappear spontaneously in 2–3 days as it diffuses toward the eyelids and root of the nose. It can be reduced in a quarter of the cases by the preoperative intramuscular injection of corticoids and the application of an ice-pack to the forehead postoperatively.
- Persistent anaesthesia or hypoaesthesia after section of the nerve-endings is spontaneously corrected in the following 6–18 months.
- Modifications of the aspect of the grafted hairs are uncommon, not very embarrassing and often resolve spontaneously during the following 6 months to 3 years. They may regrow darker, thicker or frizzier than at their original site. We should note the occasional difficulty in achieving

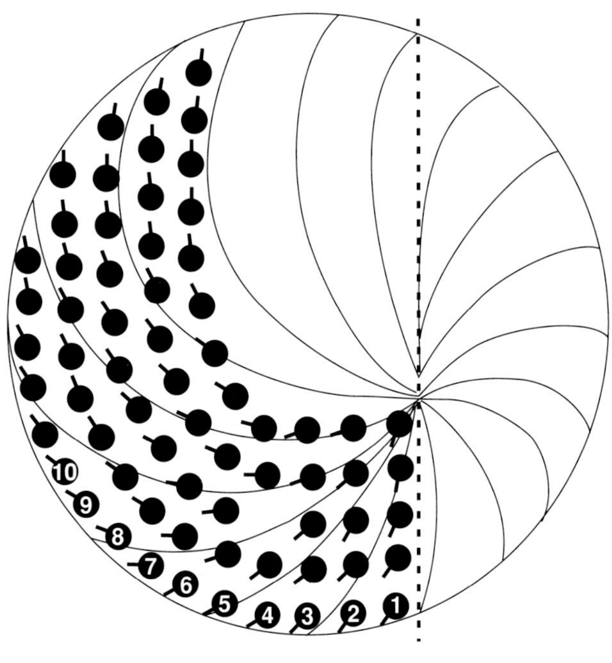

Fig. 3. Distribution and orientation of grafts transplanted to vertex baldness

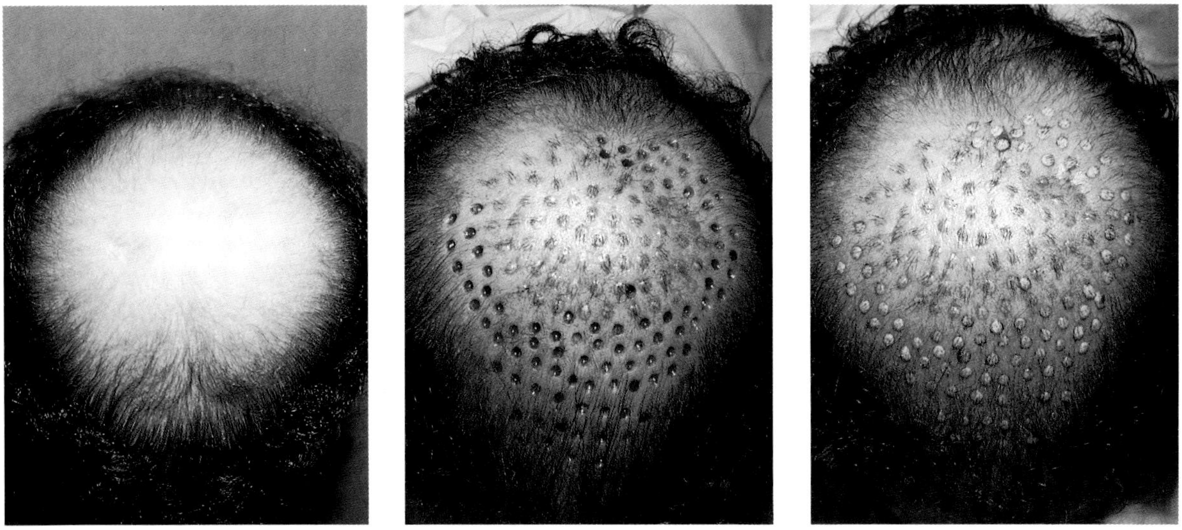

a b,c

Photo 7a–c. Distribution of two successive sessions with perioperative views of transplantation of punch grafts to vertex baldness

decolouration throughout the length of the hair shaft; the first few millimetres are remarkably refractory.

Complications at the Anterior Frontal Line

Anterior Frontal Line Incorrectly Situated (Photo 8, Fig. 4a)

Usually, if the AFL is incorrectly situated, it is too low. It is essential to respect the rule of the three facial distances or of the minimum distance of two fingerbreadths above the highest median forehead crease.

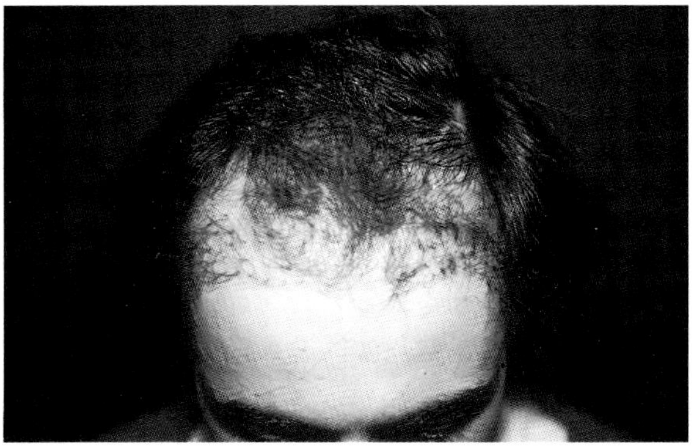

Photo 8. Frontal line too low and filling of frontal recession unaesthetic

Anterior Frontal Line Incorrectly Designed (Photo 9)

The oval of the design of the AFL must be more open or closed according to the breadth of the forehead (Fig. 4b). The oval design, more or less asymmetric depending on the physiognomy, must never be straight (Fig. 4c), arabesque, angular (Mephistophelian; Fig. 4d) or cover the fronto-temporal recession completely (Fig. 4e, Photo 10a,b).

Poor Angulation of Grafts (Photo 11)

Grafts inserted too vertically give an uncosmetic or "doll's hair" aspect. Grafts placed very transversely have a natural covering effect and cosmetic aspect, but the filling of the spaces between the grafts becomes trickier and the density is less.

Poor Orientation of Grafts (Photo 12)

Poor orientation of grafts, a common error, gives a particularly unpleasing appearance at the AFL, with grafts going in all directions in an anarchic, disorderly fashion.

Poor Optimisation of the Covering Effect

A higher concentration of grafts is necessary at the AFL and on the side of the parting.

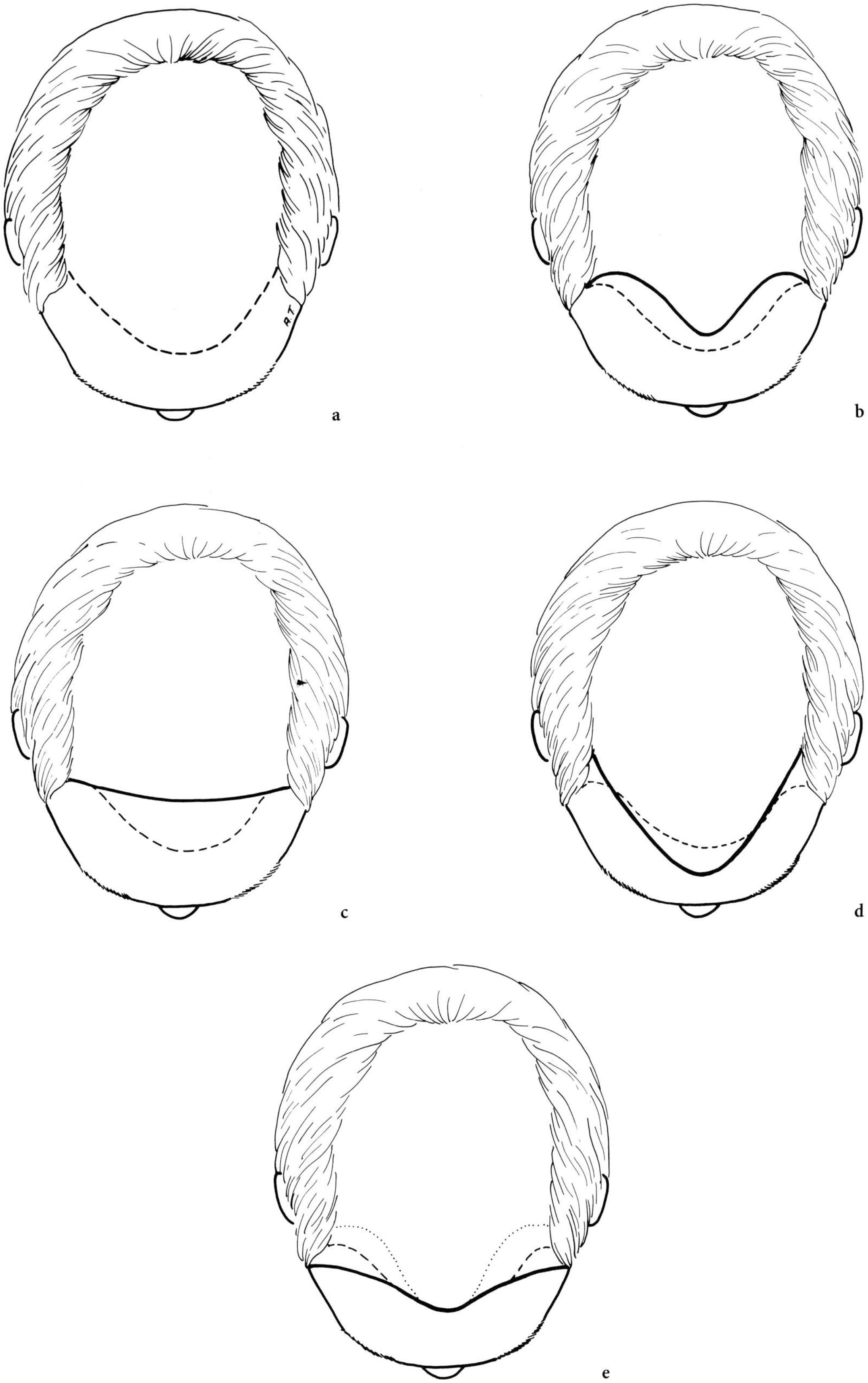

Fig. 4. **a** Ideal normal anterior frontal line. **b** Incorrect frontal line ("arabesque"). **c** Frontal line too straight. **d** Frontal line too pointed ("Mephistophelian"). **e** Filling of frontal recession is unaesthetic

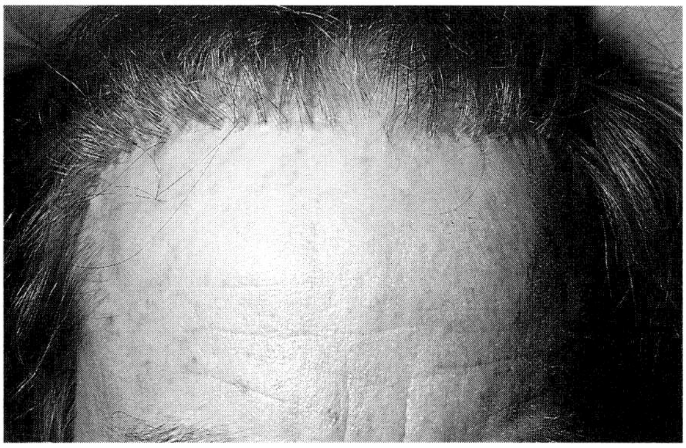

Photo 9. Frontal line too straight and too high

a

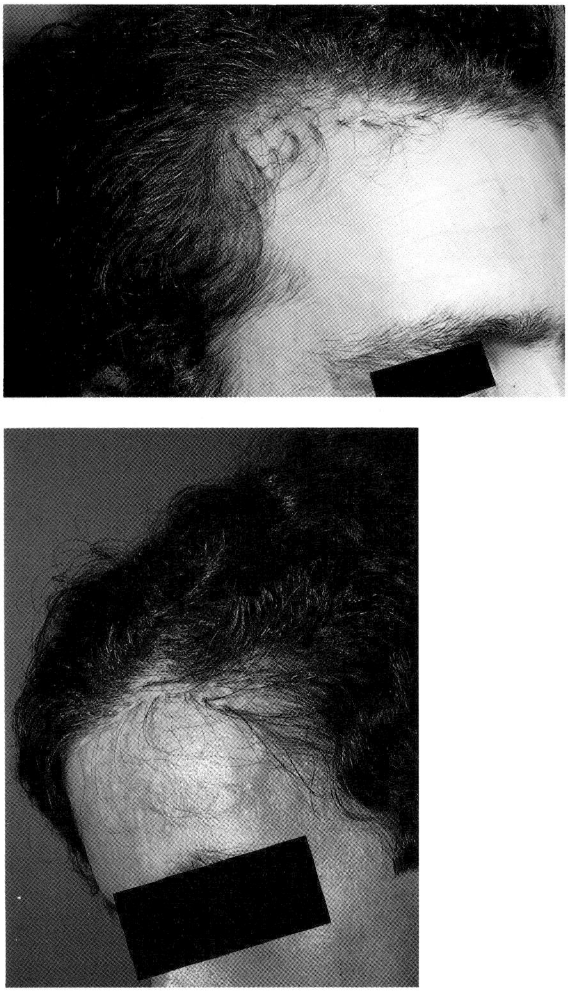

b

Photo 10. **a** Inappropriate transplantation of frontal recession. **b** Inappropriate transplantation of anterior temporal line

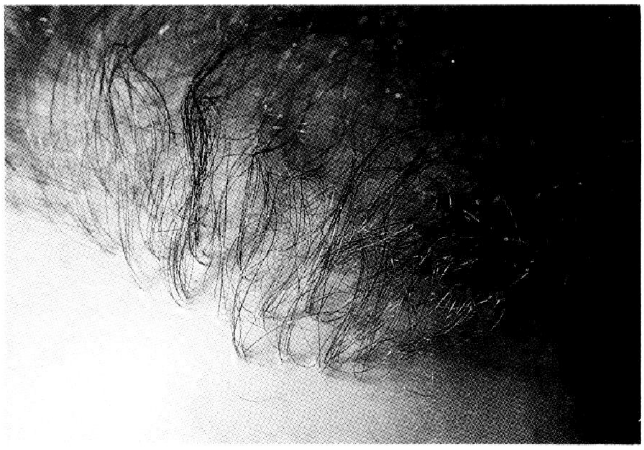

Photo 11. Poor angulation of grafts transplanted too vertically

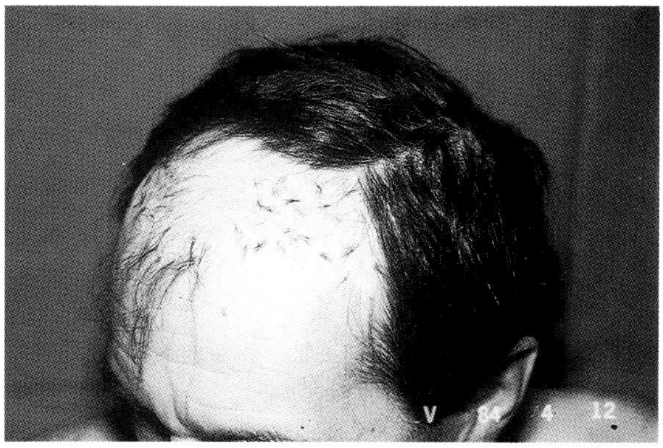

Photo 12. Disorderly transplantation at frontal region of cylindrical grafts, hairs going in all directions

Description of the Technique

Preparation of the Patient

An antiseptic shampoo is prescribed for the previous evening and on the actual day of the operation. The hairs of the donor area are cut to 1–2 mm above their emergence with scissors or an electric razor.

Local Anaesthesia

Adrenalinised 1% Xylocaine diluted by half with normal saline is infiltrated intradermally 20 min before the procedure. This preparation gives adequate haemostasis at the donor and receptor sites such that there is no need to resort to the use of a scalp haemostat (compressive helmet). Infiltration of the donor area with normal saline considerably reduces the distortion of the supple skin. However, the saline must be infiltrated in adequate amounts into small areas so as to rigidify the skin during the short period when the grafts are being taken. This infiltration of the donor site also promotes resistance of the subcutaneous tissues to compression and thus prevents crushing of the hair roots just before penetration of the punch or the scalpel blade.

Removal and Placement of Grafts

The removal and placement of grafts is related to the type of graft employed. The graft, held by very fine Adson forceps by its epidermal portion, is inserted into the orifice of the receptor site along an appropriate axis, properly orientated (specific orientations in terms of topography, nature of the hair etc.) and to a depth sufficient to prevent any protrusion. It may be that some rotation is required to give it the correct orientation. The assistant exerts brief, gentle compression on the graft (or for longer if bleeding has been caused).

In the event of persistent protrusion of the graft, one must either change it for a thinner one, cautiously reduce the deep hypodermal portion, deepen the forage or modify the axis on penetration to make it more oblique.

Siting of the Grafts

The grafts of best quality must always have priority of insertion at the alopecic zones, where they can ensure the best cover, making allowances for the type of coiffure. In the majority of cases, this particularly involves concentrating the grafts at the AFL on the side of the parting and in arranging them all in the same direction. The parting must not be placed in the midst of the grafted hairs. This lateral concentration of the grafts of the best quality may also be recommended for the regions of the vertex.

Angulation and Orientation of Grafts (Photo 13)

The angulation and orientation of the grafts are two fundamental elements, determined by the sum of the factors discussed above. As a rule, the angulation and orientation should follow that of the existing or previously existing down and hair, seeking to achieve maximal covering effect rather than extreme density. Nevertheless, in certain circumstances or at certain sites, it will be necessary to reduce the angle and change the orientation very slightly and gradually, particularly during construction of the AFL or during transplantation to receptor sites of lesser thickness. In some patients, because of the magnitude of the alopecia or the poverty of the donor area, grafts are placed at the AFL but orientated backward. Fine, clear hairs, stiff or wavy, emerging from grafts of a diameter less than 4 mm, will give a covering aspect without providing a dense hair cover. The interval between two transplantation sessions should be at least a month if the operation is not in the same region. However, the minimum interval should be 3–4 months in the case of transplantation to an already treated zone in order to fill in the spaces between the grafts. The surgeon may then assess the hair density of each graft previously inserted and carry out replacement of those which have not sprouted. Moreover, he can obtain perfect angulation and orientation by referring to the hairs emerging from the grafts already in place.

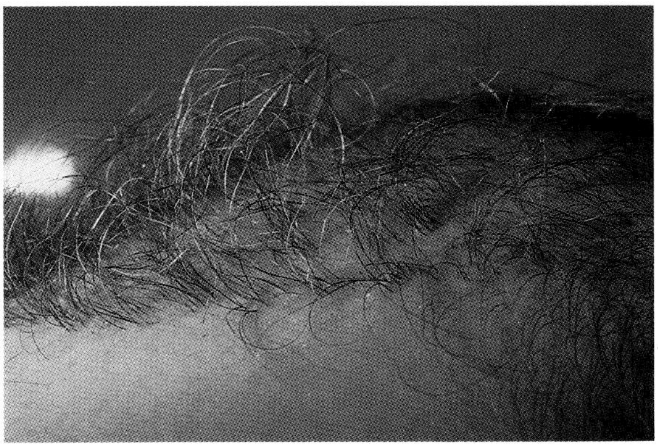

Photo 13. Angulation and orientation of grafts at anterior frontal line 4 months after single session

The sequence of the transplantation sessions can be reversed relating to the choice of the initial receptor site. Thus the first session is followed by one at the vertex and two at the frontal region. This sequence allows the patient to avoid the transient appearance of scabs by covering them with the previously grafted hairs.

Dressing

Inspection, cleansing with normal saline and observation of the receptor and donor areas for 10 min to detect any bleeding are followed by application of the dressing, but this is not routine.

Each surgeon will have his own technique of bandaging. At the donor and receptor areas we apply tulle gras or non-stick pads, covered with pads fixed with a classical Velpeau bandage and gathered under the chin to secure the best compression of the receptor area. Although this type of bandage may be judged too conspicuous by the patient, it is advised by some authors for its efficacy. It can be removed after 12–18 h.

Postoperative Management

A disinfectant shampoo is applied cautiously 24–48 h after operation. Some authors recommend the use of tulle gras and the application of antibiotic ointments covered with Telfa; in such cases the cleansing of the hair is less effective.

During the days following the operation, each graft assumes a pink color [9] and becomes covered by a scab of varying thickness. The dark and thick nature of this scab seems to be proportional to the degree of damage to the graft. During the following 3–4 weeks the scabs become detached spontaneously and fall off, taking the grafted hairs with them. Hair regrowth occurs towards the third or fourth month [9] (Photos 14a–d).

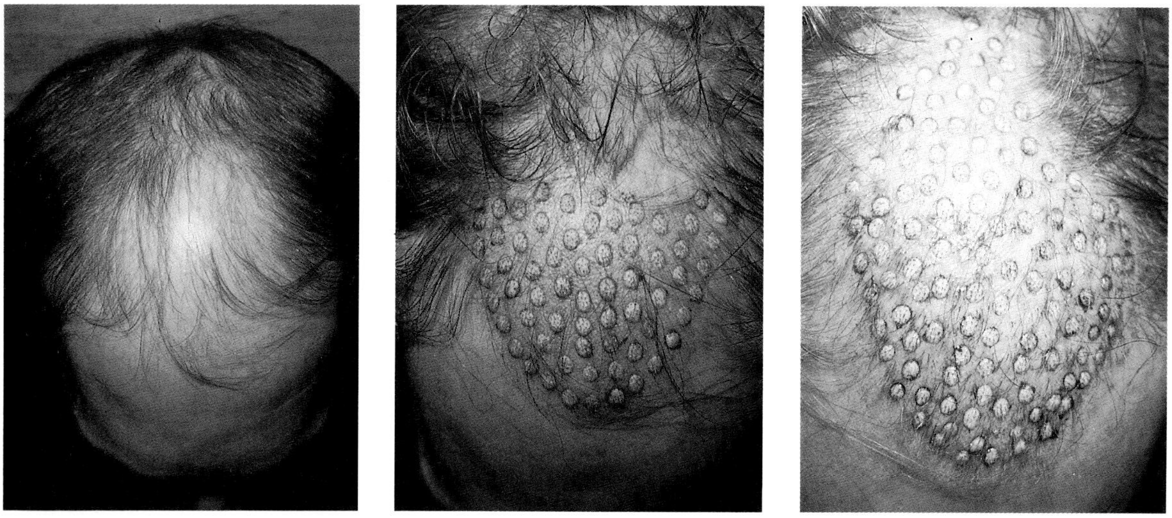

a b, c

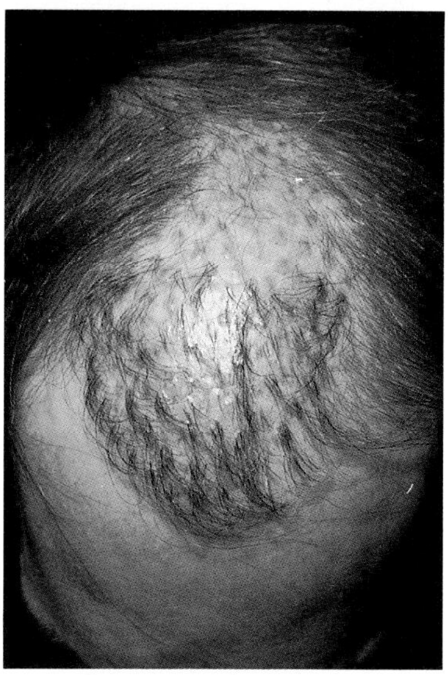

d

Photo 14a–d. Sequence of two transplantation sessions. **a** Patient before transplantation. **b** Perioperative aspect after first graft session. **c** Perioperative aspect after second graft session. **d** Aspect 4 months after first session and 1 month after second session

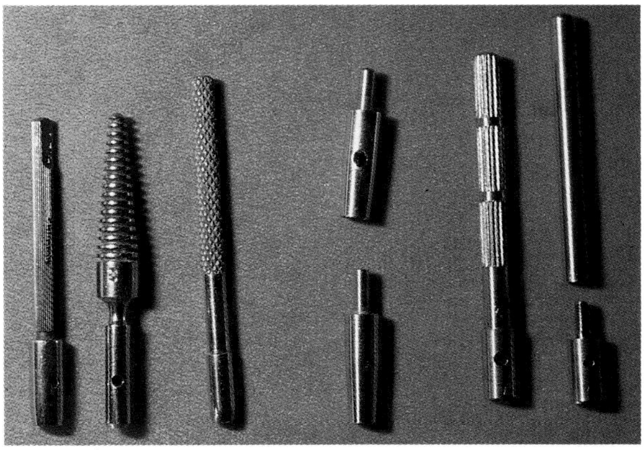

Photo 15. Various types of hand punch

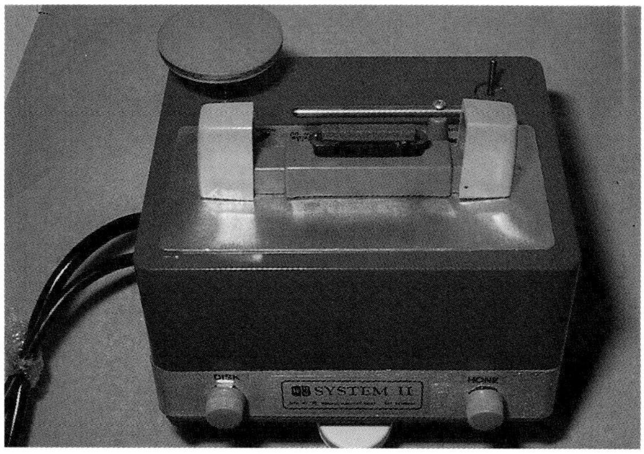

Photo 16. Motor for sharpening punch

Different Types of Graft

Cylindrical Grafts

Instrumentation

Each procedure for the transplantation of scalp autografts requires the appropriate instrumentation, the choice and care of which are discussed here.

Choice of Punch (Photo 15)

The essential instrument is the manually or motor-operated punch. Its choice is guided by various factors. The walls of the cylinder must be fine, and made of an alloy, such as carbon steel [29], resistant enough to retain its sharpness after the removal of a hundred or so grafts and to allow regular autoclave sterilisation. The handle of the manual punch can be diamonded or longitudinally grooved [33]. The latter is easier to clean and offers an adequate grip for easy penetration if the shaft has been properly sharpened.

Maintenance of the Punch (Photo 16)

Sharpening is done very cautiously after each transplantation session by applying the interior and exterior of the cylinder tangentially against a conical mandrel of metal or Arkansas stone activated by a rotary motor [12]. An agent facilitating the sharpening is applied beforehand, and a lens allows better monitoring of the procedure. The quality of the cutting edge can be assessed by testing for easy shaving of the hairs on a small area of the forearm. The punch is then cleaned with hot water and alcohol, dried in the drier, wrapped and placed in the autoclave.

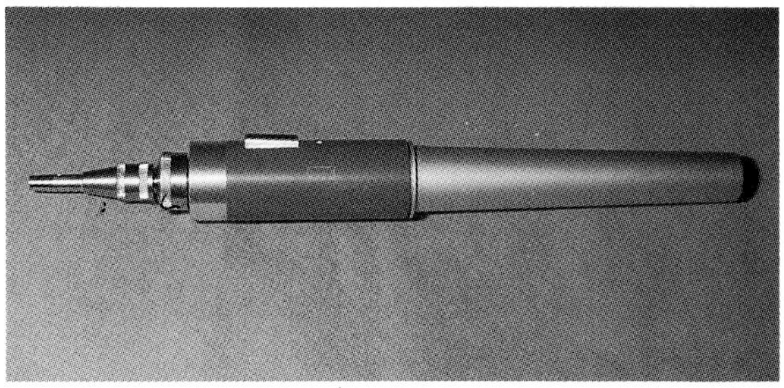

Photo 17. Battery-operated tool for graft removal by power punch

Power Punches

The use of power punches greatly facilitates taking the grafts. They should possess a speed control and especially a control permitting instant cessation of rotation when the contact is broken (Photo 17).

Techniques of Graft Removal

The cylindrical graft should have a diameter of between 3 and 4.5 mm. Below 3 mm it is difficult to obtain a good-quality graft. Above 4.5 mm, the reliability of regrowth is more uncertain. The Europeans, Australians and Scandinavians tend to choose a diameter of 4.5 mm. The Americans as a rule prefer a diameter of 4 mm.

Infiltration of the donor area with normal saline [42] allows firming-up and rigidifying of the skin and thus avoids distortion during penetration of the

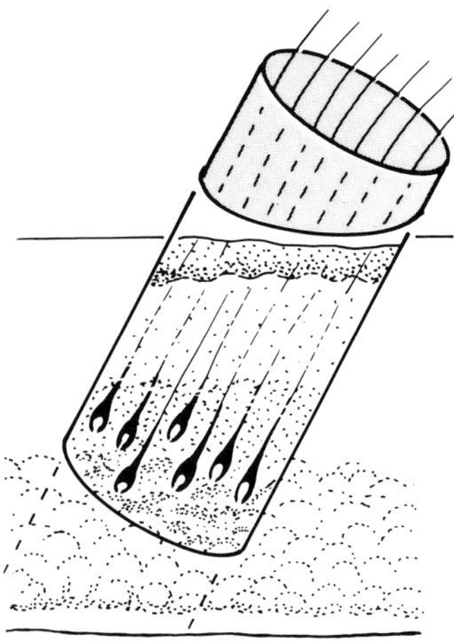
5

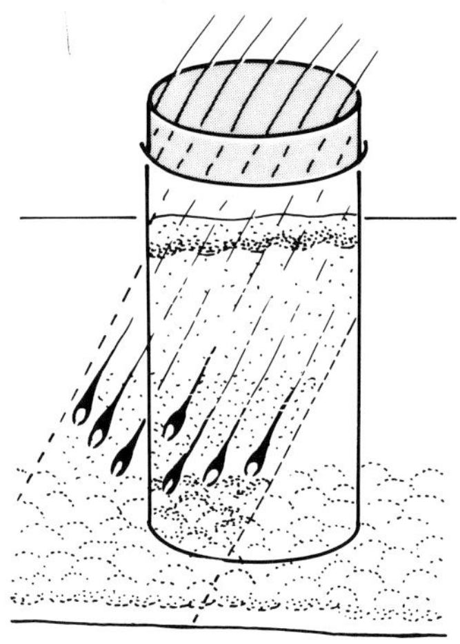
6a

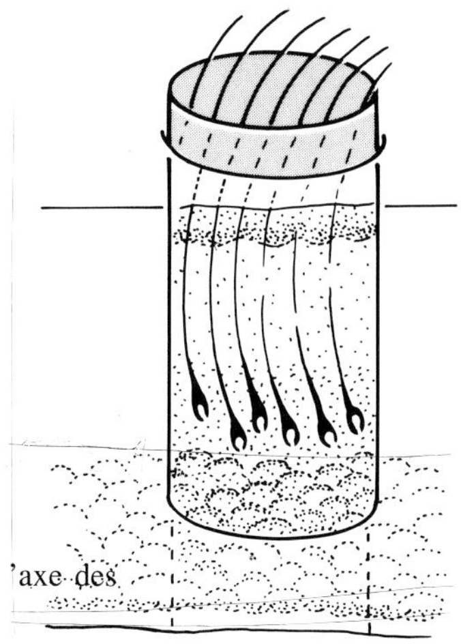

6b

Fig. 5. Penetration of punch parallel to axes of follicles

Fig. 6. **a** Incorrect penetration of punch. **b** Vertical penetration parallel to axes of follicles in subjects with crinkly hair

punch, so that the grafts are of much better quality [2].

A second series of so-called extrinsic factors [2] has an important effect of the quality of a transplant. These are:

- Most importantly, penetration of the punch strictly parallel to the axis of the hair bulbs (Fig. 5)
- Fineness of the cutting edge of the punch
- Speed of rotation of the blade
- Firmness of the donor area
- Rapid penetration of the punch
- Position of the head and trunk

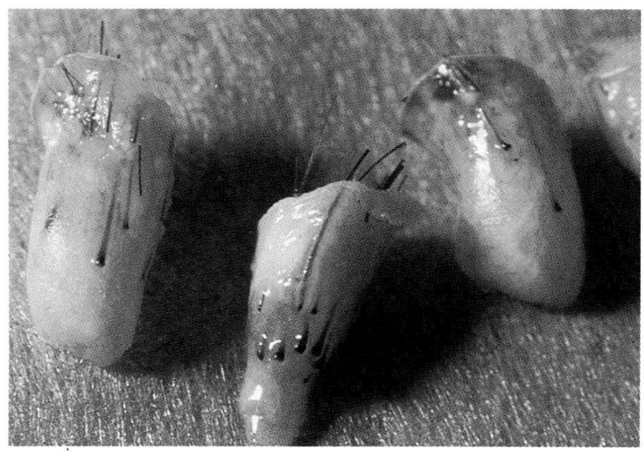

Photo 18. Punch grafts of poor quality

Distortion

Distortion of the skin during the taking of the graft is the main cause of poor quality of a graft (Fig. 6). This may be due to:

- Blunt punches
- Use of a manually operated punch
- Too supple a skin
- Rapid penetration of the punch
- Position of the head and trunk

It is obvious that a blunt punch will, during its rotation, produce a distortion which will destroy or impair the viability of the hair roots. This phenomenon will be greater when the hairs at the donor area are fine and of low density (Photo 18). The use of a well-sharpened punch activated by a motor plus rigidification of the donor area by normal saline allows the cutting out of a graft without transection of the bulbs and without torsion of the subcutaneous tissue (Photo 19).

The second cause of distortion is compression. When the punch is blunt, the surgeon exerts pressure on the skin of the donor area so as to stretch it better. The follicles are then compressed and the roots situated at the periphery of the graft are sectioned; this manoeuvre will also produce conical grafts with a subcutaneous apex. Compression thus produces skin distortion creating an oval with an epidermal beak at each end.

Preparation and Cleaning of Grafts

The grafts are aligned in a sterile Petri dish containing Ringer's solution with lactate, a solution which is more physiologic than normal saline. An assistant checks each graft to complete its preparation by cleaning it, removing the excess hypodermis to 1 mm below the roots and discarding the roots whose stems have been cut. The grafts are then arranged in order of decreasing quality.

Some authors [2] prefer to drill the receptor site before performing removal of the grafts at the donor site for two reasons: firstly, so that all bleeding has stopped at the time of insertion of the grafts, and secondly, so that only the necessary number of grafts is transplanted.

Suture of the Donor Area (Fig. 6, Photos 20, 21)

Suture of the donor area has been the subject of much discussion. Until 1978, most authors did not suture the donor area, leaving each orifice to heal spontaneously and thus producing rows of hypopigmented scars. Since then, routine suture of the graft orifices has been made by continuous suture with monofilament 3-O or an absorbable suture. This procedure has allowed considerable reduction of postoperative bleeding, pain and scabbing [3]. Any tension on the suture must be avoided to prevent ischaemia of the inter-orificial skin bridges and thus any permanent scar alopecia.

In 1979 Pierce proposed continuous suture by sectioning the inter-orificial bridges and meshing them together. In 1980, Alt suggested simple suture passing as a bridge above the margins of the donor zone, the suture traversing the epidermis from place to place at a distance from the margins [1]. Morrison proposed eliminating the inter-orificial bridges after removal of the grafts at two or three rows with well-sharpened steel or carbon-steel punches [25]. The indented margins thus created are brought together (see "Technique of Pierce"). This procedure allows the removal of grafts in great quantity, but not always of good quality [39]. The scalp bridges excised can be used for the transplantation of mini- or micrografts. We prefer Pierce's technique for graft removal and suture [37], adjusted to the laxity of the donor area: three rows if there is adequate laxity and one or two rows if the scalp lacks elasticity.

Currently, we no longer remove any grafts with a rotary instrument, whether manually or mechanically operated. We prefer to excise and segment scalp fragments of variable size using a scalpel blade.

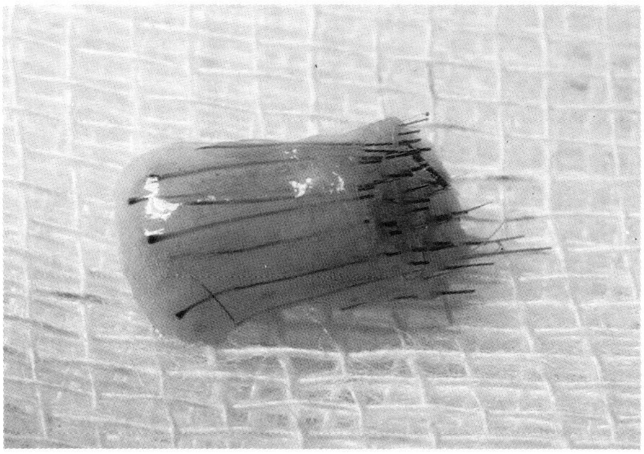

Photo 19. Punch graft of good quality

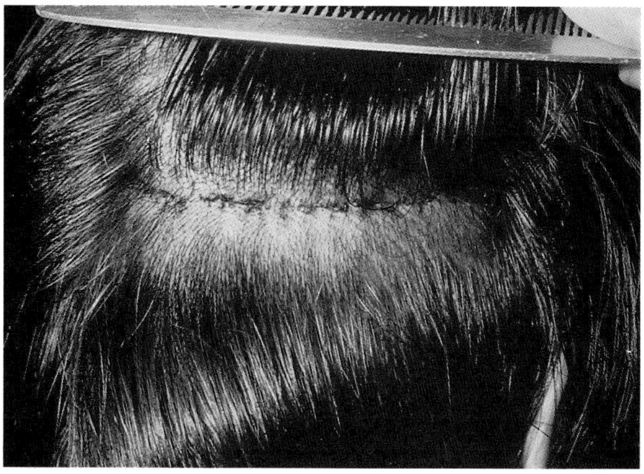

Photo 20. Running suture after removal of 70 punch grafts and excision of inter-orificial skin bridges (postoperative aspect)

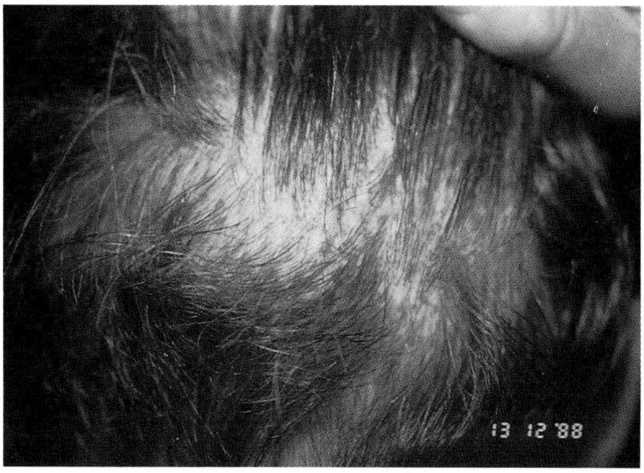

Photo 21. Healing without suture of donor zone after graft removal

Forage of the Recipient Site

Classically, punches are used whose diameter is 0.25–0.75 mm less than those used for taking the graft. The punch is embedded as deeply as possible, while avoiding contact with the bony cranial vault. If the scalp of the receptor area is not very thick, more extensive preliminary infiltration with normal saline is advisable.

The obliquity of the penetration of the punch must be absolutely parallel to the obliquity of the existing or previously existing hairs. If a manually activated punch is used, we adhere to a double obliquity of penetration. The axis is between 70° and 80° during passage through the epidermis and superficial dermis and is then changed to between 30° and 70° depending on the natural orientation of the hairs and the thickness of the smooth zone. If the punch is activated by a rotary electric motor, the sole axis of penetration is between 60° and 70° from the outset. We should note the risk during rotation of unfortunately catching adjacent hairs and of embedding the blade so deeply as to contact the bony vault. Each skin cylinder must then be cut with short, pointed, fine scissors at the deepest possible part of the hypodermis.

Distribution of Grafts

Frontal Area

Schematically, we distinguish between the classical distribution of the grafts to allow optimal coverage of the frontal region and a different distribution allowing satisfactory coverage using a lesser number of grafts.

Classical Distribution. Four successive sessions of transplantation of grafts of 4 mm are needed (see Fig. 7). At the fronto-temporal area and also at the region of the occipital crown, the mode of arranging the hair (e.g. from left to right) will encourage the use of a greater number of grafts (Fig. 8).

Two or three transplantation sessions are sufficient at the vertex and the lateral region opposite the side of the parting. The most prolific grafts are inserted at the lateral region of the parting. However, one should try not to become too dependent on the direction of styling the hair. In all, eight to ten sessions are needed to cover the entire bald area.

Minimal Distribution. The "quincunx" pattern of distribution of the grafts at the frontal region allows re-

7

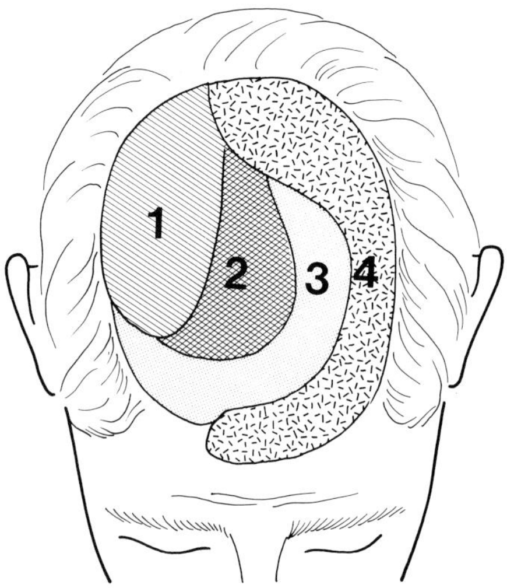

8

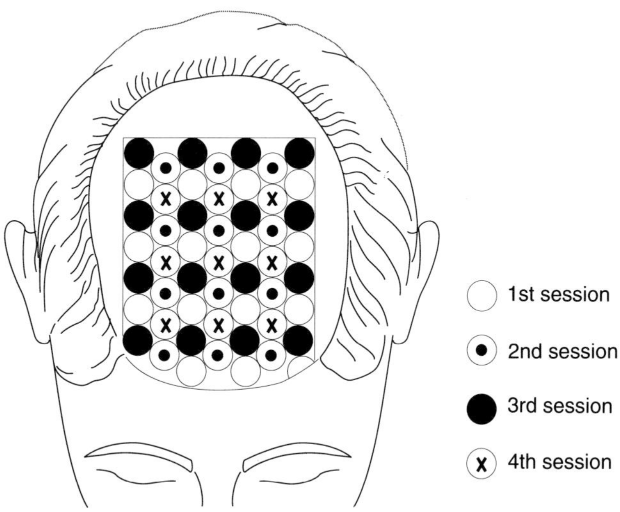

Fig. 7. Classical distribution of grafts: four successive sessions on the side of the parting (*4*), two to three sessions at the vertex (*2, 3*) and one session on the opposite side (*1*)

Fig. 8. Classical distribution of grafts transplanted at four sessions

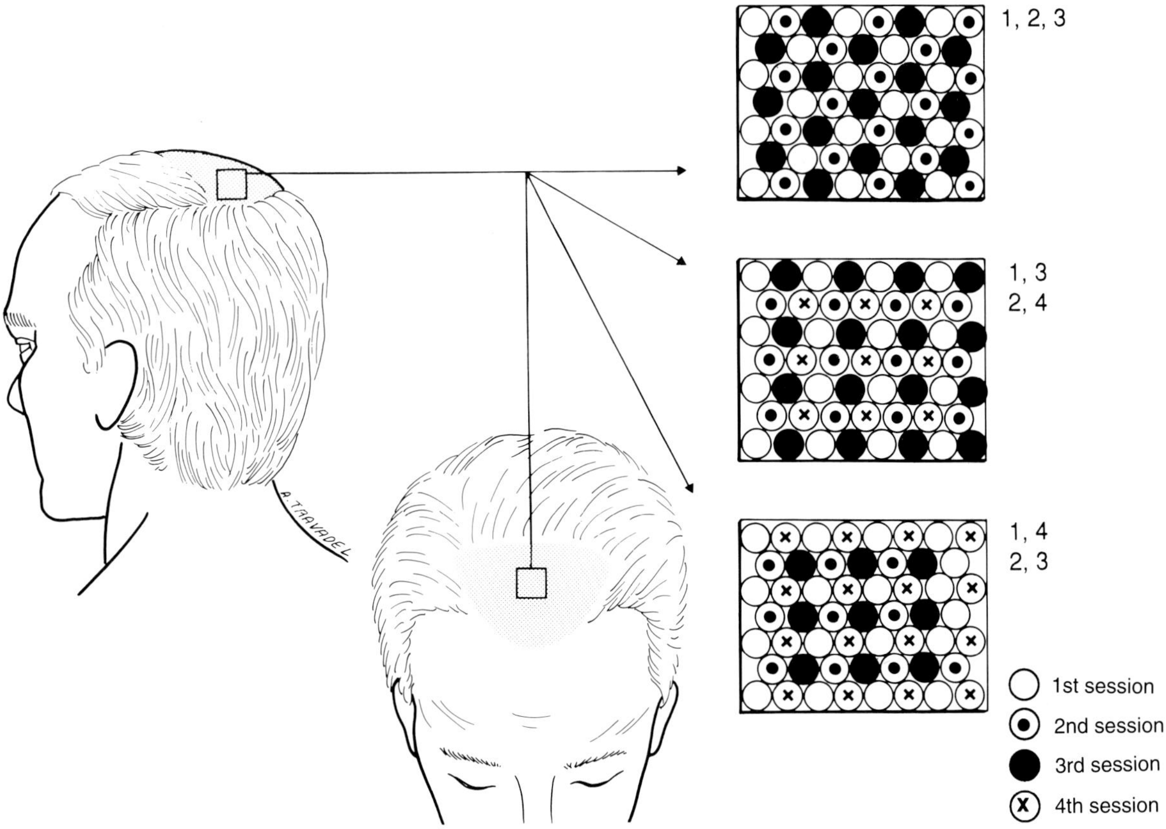

Fig. 9. Sequential localisation of grafts. The optimal use of four successive sessions may sometimes be reduced to three

duction of the number of sessions to two [2] (see Fig. 9). However, sometimes it is preferable not to transplant a very extensive bald area with a relatively reduced number of grafts. Then one must cover more restricted areas, but using an adequate density of grafts, thus avoiding having to resort to manipulation of the available hair. (NB: Insufficient donor areas make it necessary to use the less dense, but uniform distribution of mini- and micrografts) (Photo 14a–d).

Sequential Positioning of Grafts (Fig. 9). The grafts, separated by a space corresponding to the diameter of the punch, are positioned according to a precise pattern at each session. This optimal sequence for the performance of four sessions may be reduced to two or three sessions in some cases. For grafts situated at the two most anterior frontal lines, a slight overlapping may give a more continuous and aesthetic appearance.

Vertical Area

Here again, we may distinguish the classical distribution of grafts allowing optimal coverage of the vertex from a different distribution using a smaller number of grafts.

Classical Distribution [43] (Fig. 10). Four successive transplantation sessions of 4-mm grafts, which are distributed according to a precise sequential pattern and a spiral orientation (Photo 7a–c).

Minimal Distribution. According to Unger [20], two plans may be advised: either superimposed "U"s (Fig. 10a–d) or the procedure of successive waves (Fig. 11a–c).

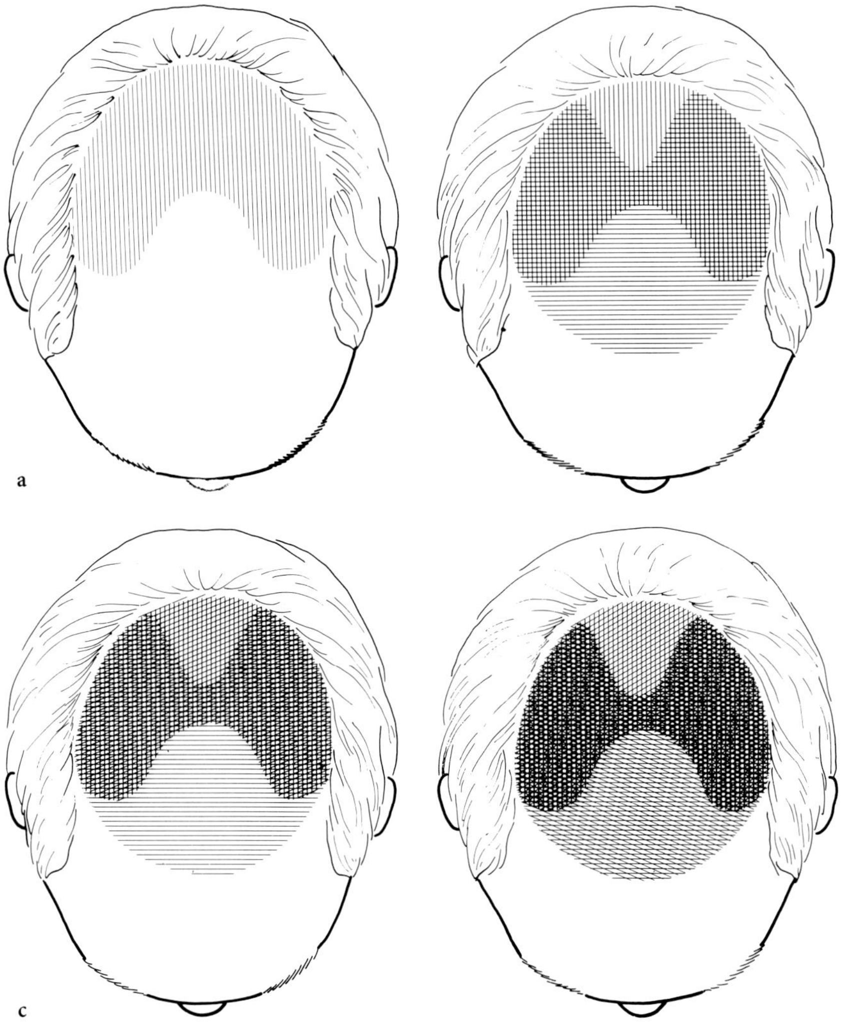

Fig. 10a–d. Superimposed "U" distribution of cylindrical grafts at vertex in four sessions (Unger)

Complications of Cylindrical Grafts

A good knowledge of the possible complications is fundamental if they are to be prevented or corrected. As a rule, a good technique, excellent equipment and the right indications will prevent most of the complications.

The prevention and treatment of syncope and vagal disorders are discussed in the section on "Anaesthesia" (p. 57ff).

As far as bleeding is concerned, an operative field at both donor and receptor sites with little or no haemorrhage can be secured by the following measures: assessment of coagulation status, avoidance of such medication as aspirin and the consumption of alcohol, detection of arterial hypertension, possible premedication with coagulants (vitamin K and dicynone), perfect relaxation of the patient with Atarax and Valium, by a calm atmosphere in the operating room and continuous dialogue with the surgeon, preliminary anaesthesia with adrenalinised 1% Xylocaine, nerve block (frontal, retro-auricular, occipital) and anaesthesia by intradermal injection (mesoflash) under pressure using a dermojet or with a 30-gauge needle. If there is major bleeding after drilling of one or more orifices, compression for a few seconds with a swab or the insertion of a cotton bud should stop haemorrhage from the small artery injured. A preliminary subcutaneous injection of normal saline will usually prevent section of these arteries, which travel under the hypodermis in an upper double fold of the galea. Exceptionally, we resort to simple or cruciform suture of the orifice.

Note the very exceptional rupture of an arteriovenous malformation, requiring ligature of the pedicles.

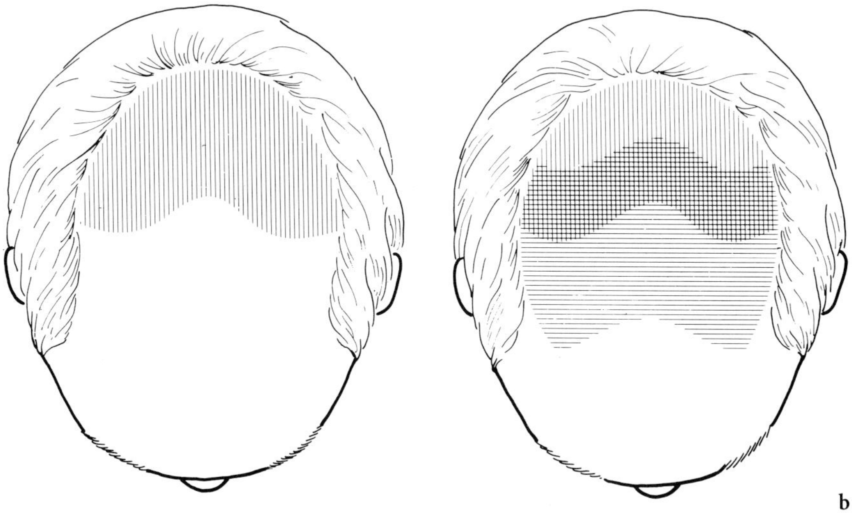

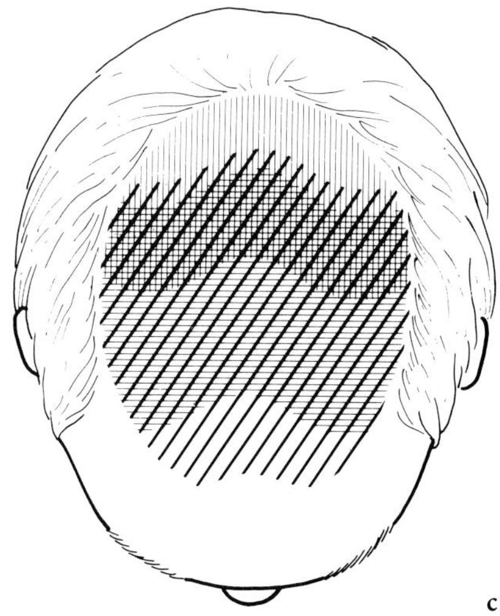

Fig. 11a–c. Distribution of cylindrical grafts in “successive waves” in three sessions (Unger). **a** First session. **b** Second session. **c** Third session

Complications at the Donor Site

Abnormal Clinical Course. The course taken is often relatively abnormal and need not necessarily be regarded as a complication:

- The formation of. scabs is greater at unsutured donor sites. They may be detached at an early stage by applying moist compresses for 30 min one to three times a day.
- Hypoaesthesia or anaesthesia is bound to occur above the zone of graft-taking in 100% of cases, but this disappears spontaneously in 1–6 months, rarely longer.
- Aseptic abscess or foreign body reaction is apparently a reaction to the suture material, especially if this is absorbable, and always regresses after removal of the sutures.
- Occasional pruritus is treated by the application of cortisone lotions and coal-tar shampoos.

Real Complications. Any unforeseen course marked by transient or permanent disorders is to be regarded as a complication:

- Necrosis of the donor site may have two causes [29] (Photo 22): (1) taking a considerable number of grafts whose orifices are separated by very narrow skin bridges damages the circulation and leads to ischaemia and also to tissue necrosis [7–9]; (2) the second cause is probably excessive tension after suture of the donor area or major granulation of the donor site when it has been left unsutured or when the grafts have been taken too closely.
- Major residual scars (Photo 23): the essential cause is the drilling of orifices not separated by scalp bridges and closed by improper suture. Tissue necrosis after the drilling of several rows of orifices (four or more) and closure under tension is the second cause of large scars.

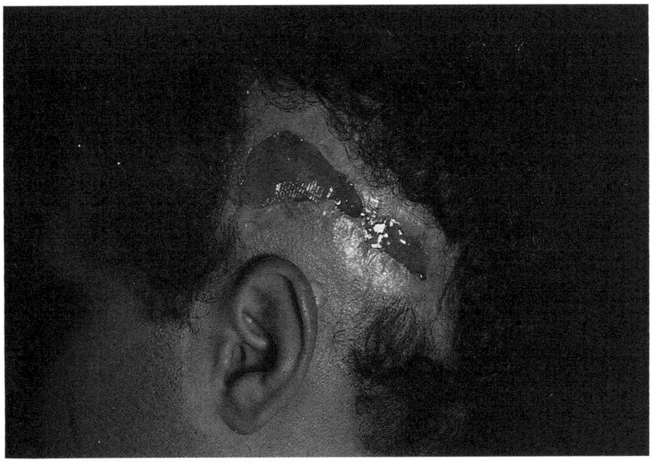

Photo 22. Rare appearance of necrosis of donor zone after excessive removal of punch grafts at one session

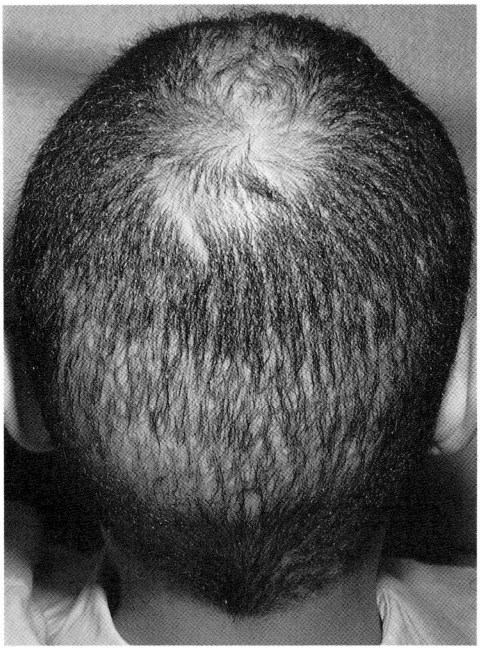

Photo 23. Major residual scars after removal of a large number of grafts in several rows

- Vascular malformations are unusual complications of this type of surgery and seem probably due to the failure to close the donor zone by suture. This arteriovenous fistula or pseudo-aneurysm is evidenced by a pulsatile and often painful swelling.
- Anagenic defluvium: during the days or weeks following operation, a sudden and sometimes massive loss of hair at the donor site may disquiet the patient and sometimes the inexperienced surgeon. The hairs have been precipitated toward a telogenic phase or a dystrophic anagenic phase [10]. This transient balding is followed by complete regrowth in the ensuing months [9]. This phenomenon is due to transient circulatory impairment.

Complications at the Recipient Area

Absent or Inadequate Regrowth of Hair on the Grafts. Inadequate regrowth of hair on the grafts is a complication often encountered [17]. It is therefore fundamental to be aware of the various possible causes if they are to be avoided [2] (Photo 24):

- Poor taking of the graft, usually due to the use of defective equipment.
- Poor angulation of the drilling or inadequate firming-up by the injection of the donor site with normal saline.
- Inadequate spacing of the grafts, hindering their vascularisation.
- Transplantation sessions too close together in time at the same receptor site (the interval should be no less than 3 months).
- Insufficient vascularisation of the posterior grafts due to repeated transplantations on an AFL, forming a circulatory barrier.
- Poor fitting of the graft in the recipient orifice. The graft protrudes in relation to the surrounding skin area and may undergo more or less complete desiccation. Deliberate pressure applied to secure better adjustment of the graft will incurve the follicles, giving rise to frizzy hairs.
- Insufficiently oblique insertion of the grafts in a very fine scalp.
- A hypertrophic scar (Photo 25); the graft assumes a bulging, erythematous glossy aspect and gives rise to a reduced number of hairs.

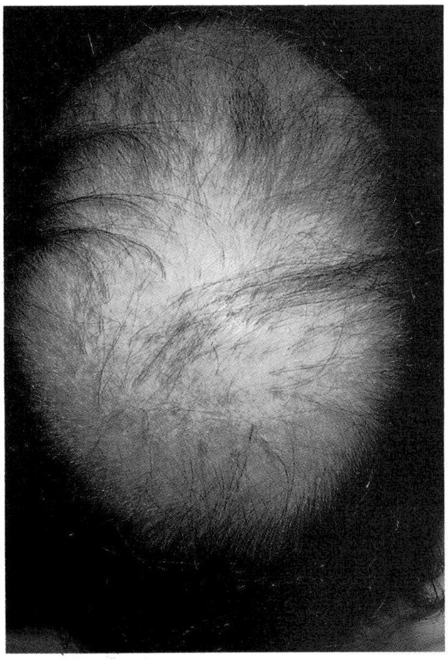

Photo 24. Near-total absence of regrowth after transplantation of 200 cylindrical grafts

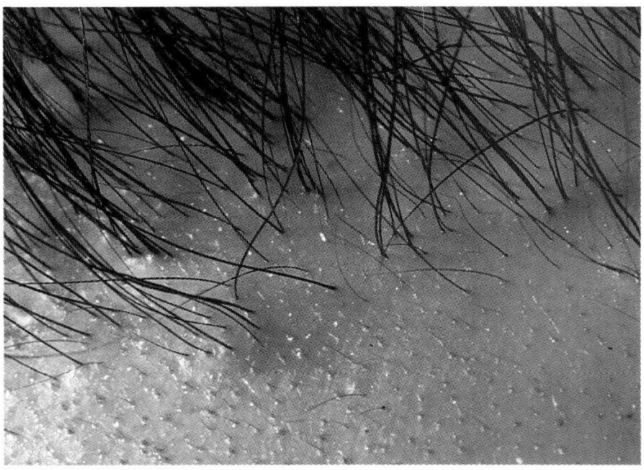

Photo 25. Hypertrophic scar giving bulging aspect to grafts

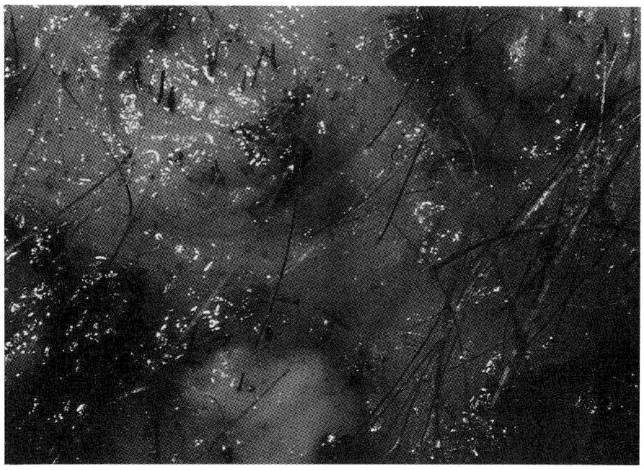

Photo 26. Pustular infection of two grafts

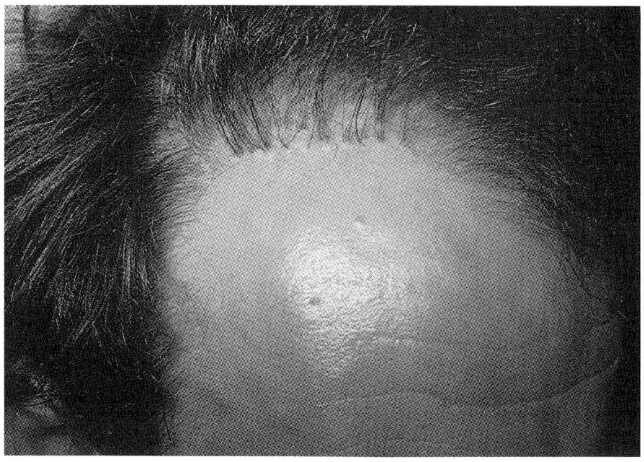

Photo 27. Grafts standing out to give an unaesthetic "cobblestone" aspect

- Central necrosis of the grafts: only the peripheral hairs of the grafts survive. This phenomenon is due to insufficient vascularisation following excessive vasoconstriction after the injection of adrenalinised Xylocaine. The scabs of these grafts are thicker and adhere longer than usual.
- Postoperative infection (Photo 26) of the scalp in general and the grafts in particular is uncommon because of the great vascularity of this region. It may consist of a pustule, with or without peripheral erythematous inflammatory reaction evident at the third to fifth day after the operation [9]. Wide-spectrum antibiotherapy can be adjusted in the light of the findings of bacteriological examination with an antibiogram. If graft infections occur repeatedly in successive patients, a check must be made of the quality of sterilisation of the equipment and the absence of cutaneous or ENT (ear, nose and throat) sepsis in the staff. A case of osteomyelitis after graft transplantation and vertical reduction has been reported [2].

"Cobblestone" Aspect (Photo 27). This unpleasing appearance is given by prominence of the grafts [42]. If this protrusion of the grafts persists, correction is necessary. To prevent this complication, the recipient orifices should be drilled sufficiently and well-cleansed grafts inserted without difficulty, with excision of excess hypodermis.

Other Complications. These include the following:

- Arteriovenous malformations may also develop at the receptor zone in the shape of a bulging, pulsatile swelling which increases progressively in size and then stabilises and gradually regresses in 2–3 months. In the event of rapid growth threatening rupture, the lesion should be excised by a plastic surgeon [29].
- Dermal cysts [29] are due to the unfortunate insertion of two successive grafts in the same orifice, resulting from over-deep drilling after the subcutaneous injection of normal saline. Excision of this painless, non-pulsatile tumour liberates caseous matter with hair bulbs and hair.

Correction of Complications and Poor Results

Unaesthetic Frontal Lines

Incorrectly Placed Anterior Frontal Line. This is the essential cause of unaesthetic results, sources of dissatisfaction. The design of the AFL may have been awkwardly placed: too high or too far forward, too pointed or too wide, too straight or over-ornate ("arabesque"). Correction is made by:

- Excision of any malpositioned grafts (Photo 28a,b)
- Insertion of supplementary mini- and micrografts (Photo 29a,b)
- Use of one or two vertical flaps (Photo 30a–c)

If the disappointed patient declines a further operation, electrical depilation of the grafts may be done or in some cases a frontal lifting (see "Indications").

Grafts of Poor Quality or Badly Inserted. Unsatisfactory regrowth of hair on the grafts may be due to different causes [42] (see "Complications"). Correction may be made by supplementing or exchanging these grafts with supplementary grafts of good quality and appropriate size, inserted at the proper angle and with the right orientation.

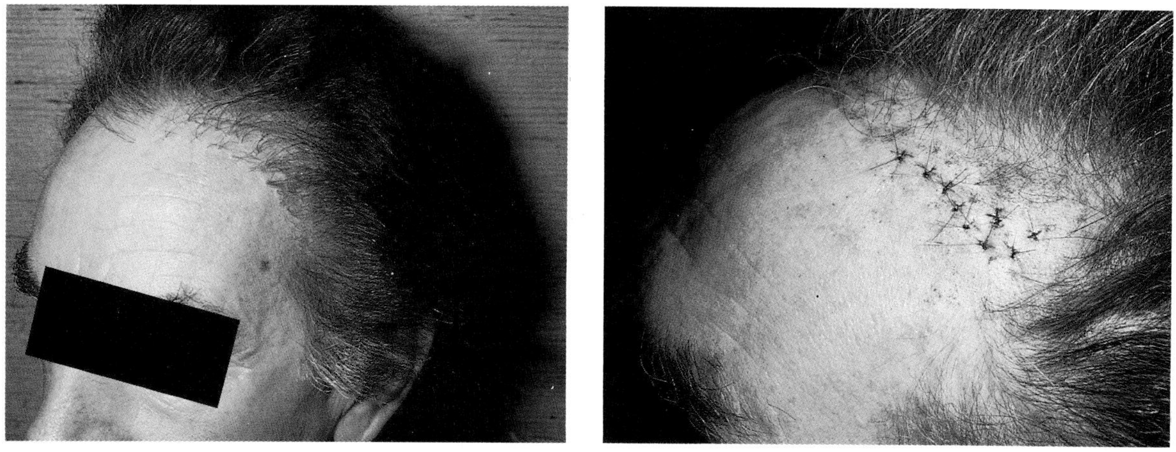

a b

Photo 28. **a** Punch grafts placed incorrectly at the frontal recession. **b** Excision and suture of each malplaced graft

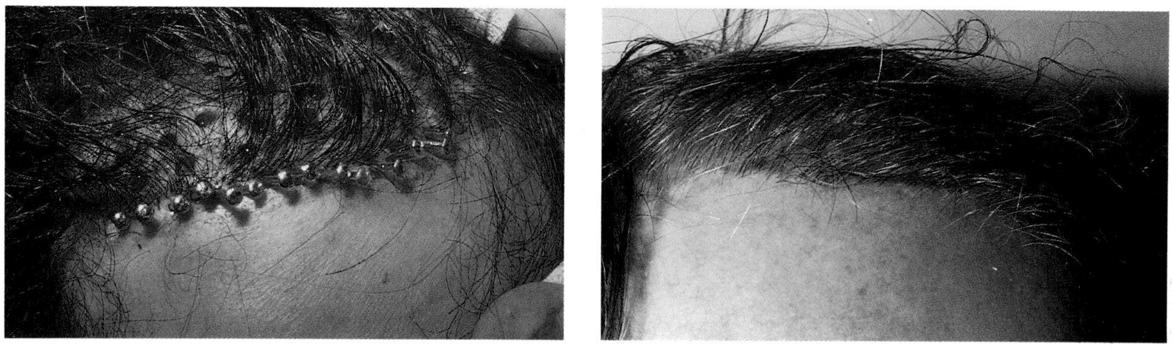

a b

Photo 29a,b. Correction of unaesthetic line of punch grafts by transplantation of mini- and micrografts

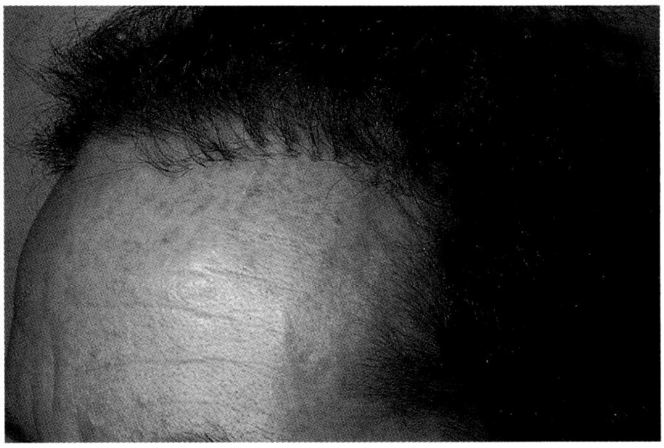

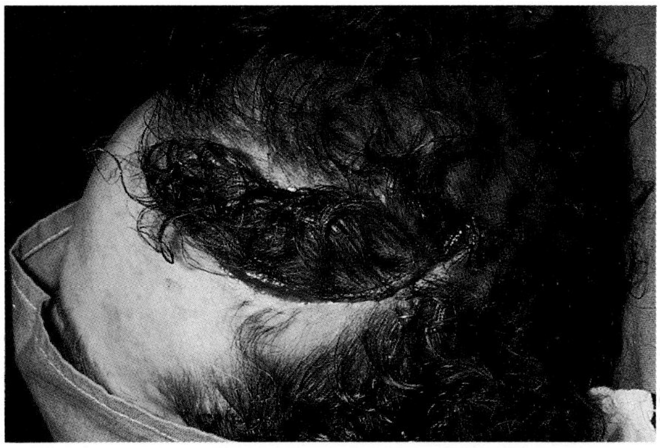

b

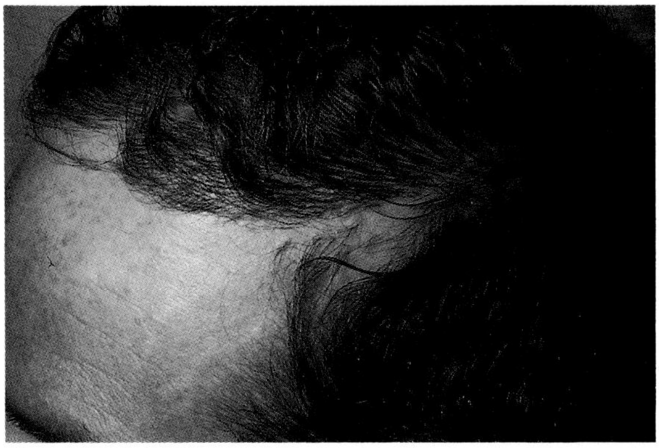

c

Photo 30. **a** Unaesthetic frontal line after transplantation of punch grafts. **b** Perioperative aspect after correction by flap. **c** Aspect 1 month after transposition of flap

"Doll's Hair" Aspect (Photo 31). This unaesthetic appearance of the AFL is the chief defect of this technique [5, 6]. Actually, this result is due essentially to the too vertical insertion of grafts of large diameter or of thick black hairs in a light skin. To prevent this, the technique should simply be replaced by a technique employing mini- and micrografts. To correct this aspect, the inter-graft spaces should be filled with mini- and micrografts (Photo 28), or a more anterior AFL may be constructed with fusiform grafts or micrografts.

Grafts arranged with an incorrect angle or orientation may be corrected by:

- Cutting them out with a punch of the same diameter and retransplanting them with the proper angle and orientation
- Inserting two fusiform grafts or transposing two vertical flaps

Grafts with a Hypertrophic Scar. These are unpredictable and may result in a poorer quality of regrowth and one whose appearance is delayed. To avoid this reaction, the graft must be perfectly cleansed and all hypodermal debris excised before insertion into a receptor pit of adequate breadth and depth. To correct bulging of this scar, we advise diathermy at the apex of the dome and daily application of a cortisone cream for 5–7 days. Postoperative intradermal injections of cortisone seem to have no significant preventive effect [29].

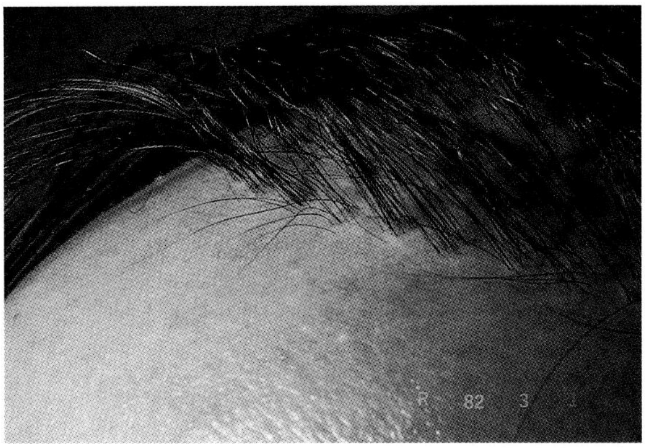

Photo 31. "Doll's hair" aspect after too vertical a transplantation of punch grafts, hair too dark and too thick (Asiatic type)

To prevent possible infection of the grafts, the methods available are:

- Prophylactic antibiotherapy started on the evening before the operation and continued for 48 h subsequently (erythromycin, mynocyclin)

- Antibiotic treatment as indicated by the results of culture of the pus with an antibiogram

Minigrafts and Micrografts

Small fragments of the scalp were first used in 1943 by Tamura [40] for pubic transplantation. In 1953, Fujita [19] recommended such micrografts for reconstruction of the eyelids. In 1980, Maritt [24] suggested the use of micrografts for the final touches to the AFL, and the value of this was confirmed by Bouhanna in 1983 [8].

Principle

The principle of minigrafts and micrografts consists in cutting strips of scalp into small fragments, each fragment carrying either one to two hairs (micrografts) or three to four hairs (minigrafts) (Photo 32a–c).

Aims

This procedure aims to recreate the natural emergence of two to three hairs through each pilo-sebaceous orifice (pili bigemini or trigemini). It is employed for transplantation of bald areas of the scalp in order to give them a natural and cosmetic aspect (Photo 33a,b), to achieve gradual refilling of the bald areas (Photo 34a,b), to correct the unattractive appearance of the anterior scar-line of certain flaps (Photo 35a,b) and to conceal certain over-obvious post-lifting temporal scars (Photo 36a,b).

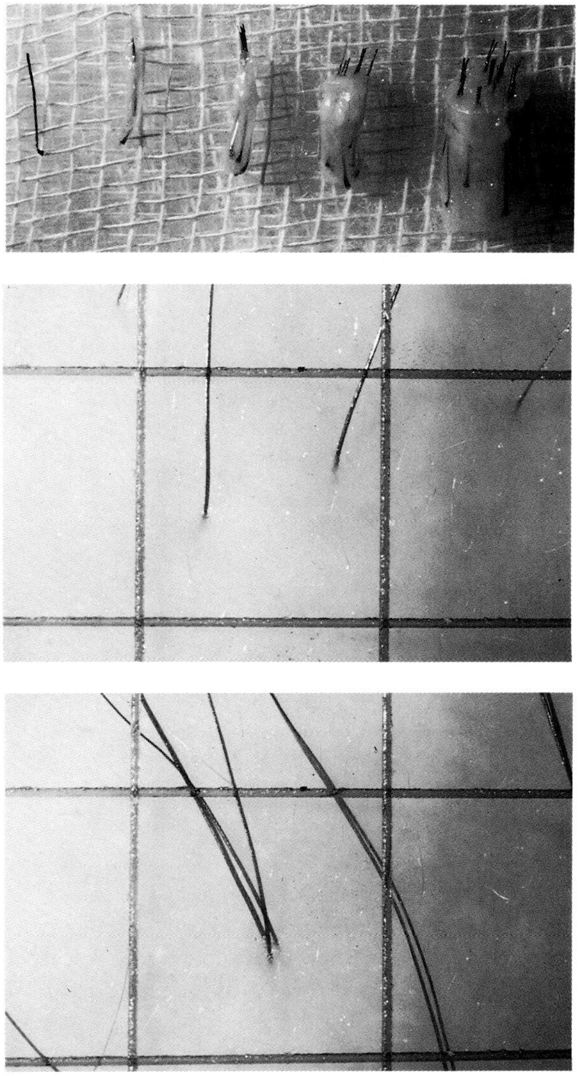

a b c

Photo 32. a Comparative aspects of punch graft, minigraft (three to four hairs) and micrograft (one to two hairs). **b** Macrophotographic aspect of transplanted micrograft. **c** Macrophotographic aspect of transplanted minigraft

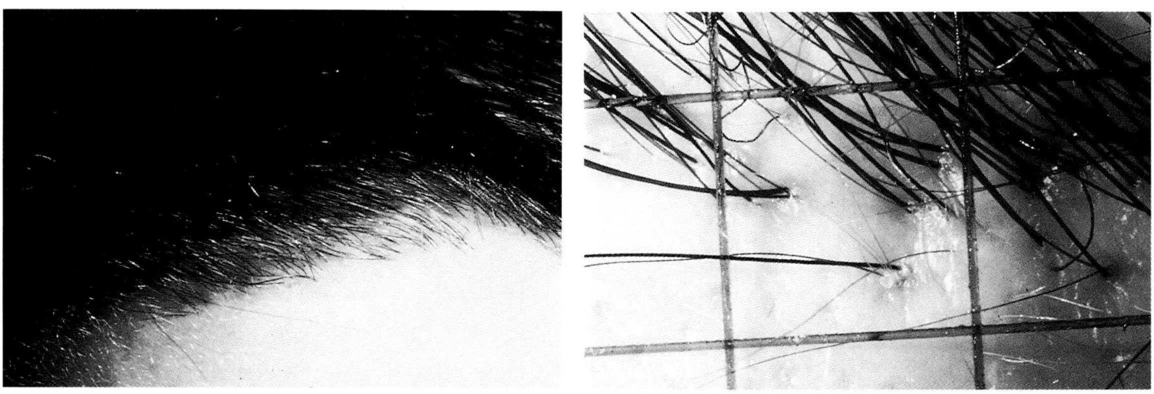

a b

Photo 33. a Anterior frontal line with minigrafts. **b** Macroscopic aspect of micro- and minigrafts a 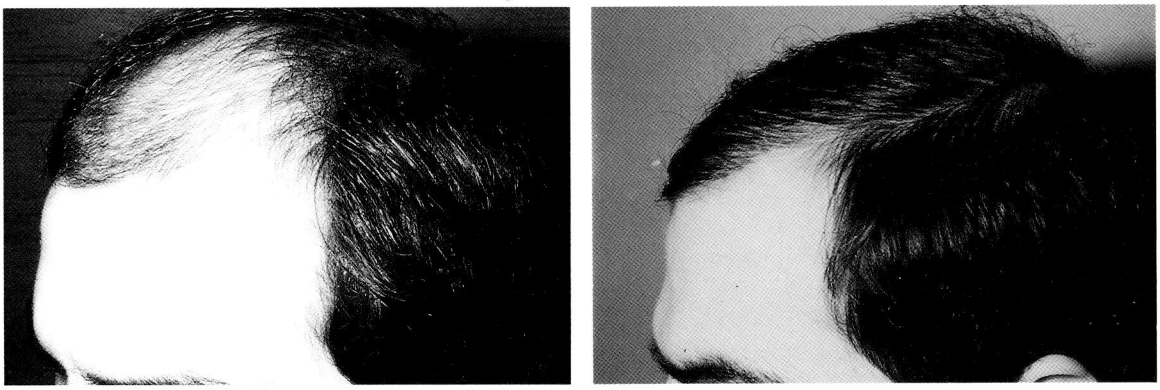 b

Photo 34a,b. Frontal baldness before and after "finishing touches" by minigrafts between grafts

a b c 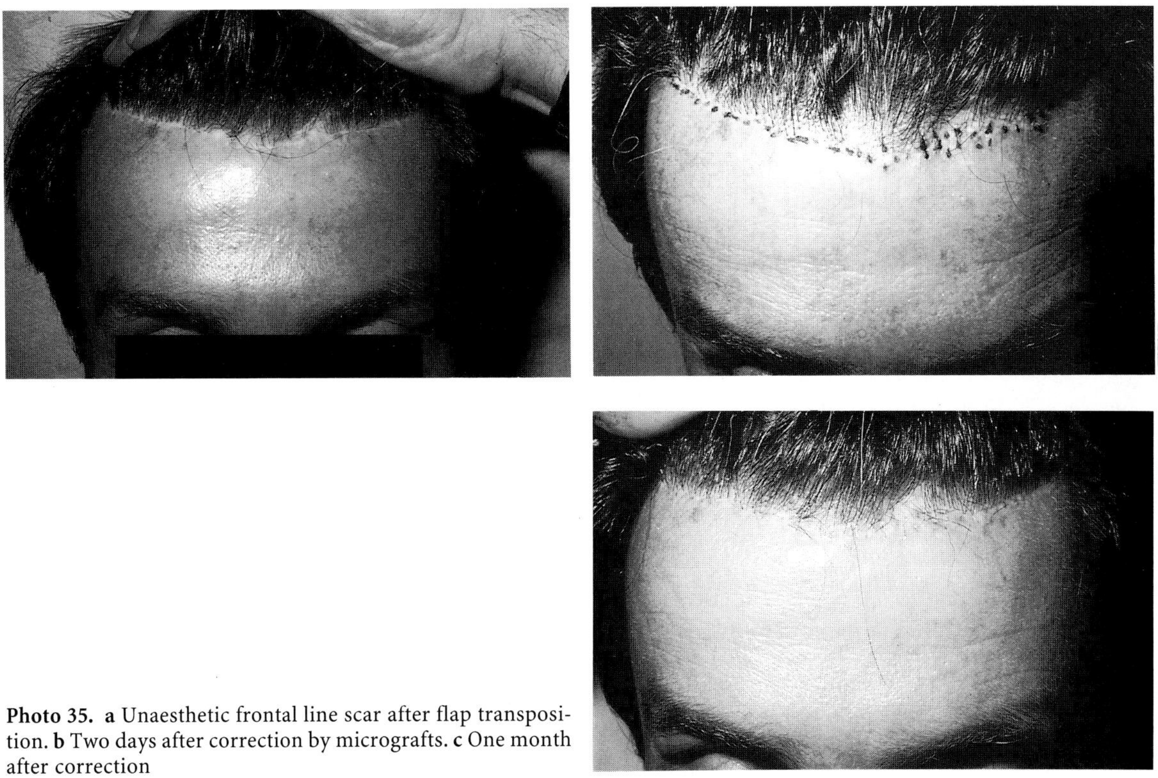

Photo 35. **a** Unaesthetic frontal line scar after flap transposition. **b** Two days after correction by micrografts. **c** One month after correction

Technique

The preparation, disinfection and anaesthesia of the donor and receptor areas resemble those performed for other types of grafts. Either the hairs are cut at their emergence with scissors or an electric razor or they are not cut at all [11].

Instrumentation

Taking the grafts at the donor area is done either with a scalpel with a no. 11 or 15 blade for removal of an elliptical strip (Photo 37) or with a scalpel bearing two, three or four no. 15 blades. These multiblade scalpels have undergone numerous modifica-

a
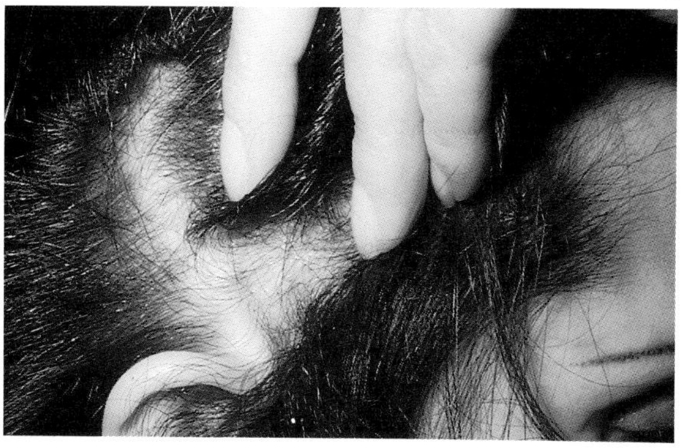

b
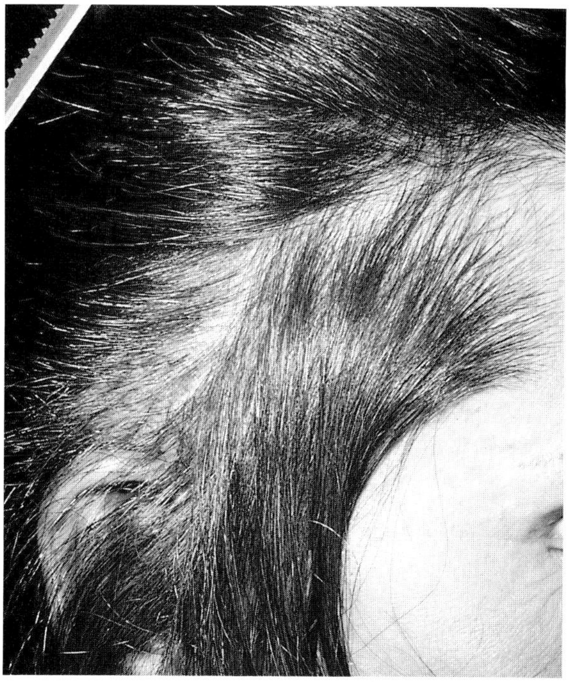

Photo 36. **a** Unaesthetic temporal scar after face-lifting. **b** After correction by minigrafts

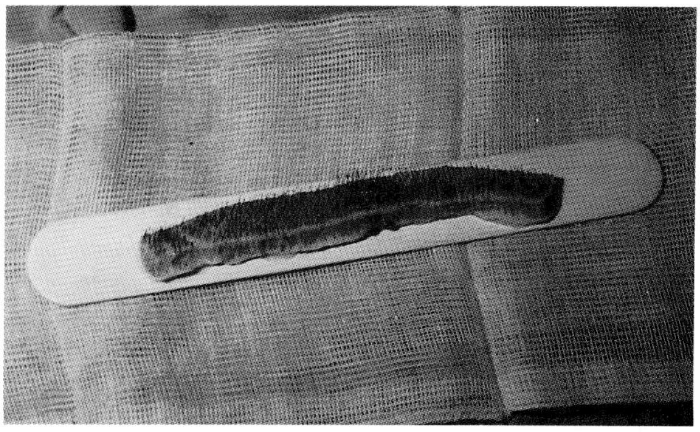

Photo 37. Scalp strip removed for cutting into mini- and micrografts

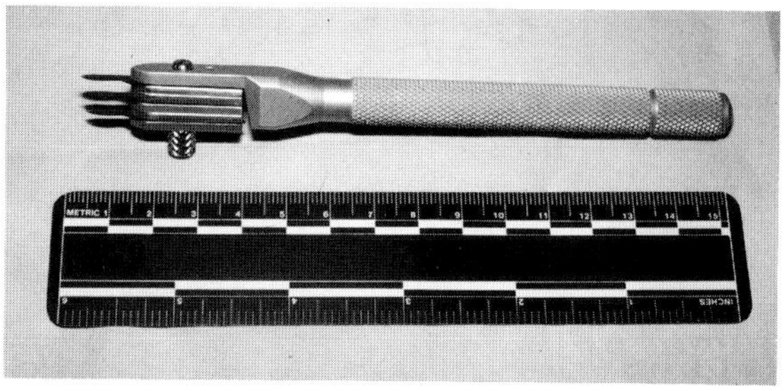

Photo 38. Multi-blade scalpel (van Sickle)

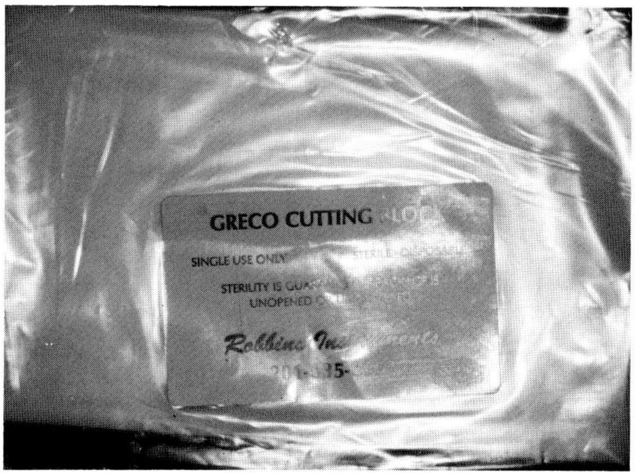

Photo 39. Greco acrylic cutting block (Robbins)

tions since the original description by Vallis (Photo 38).

Cutting out of individual grafts is made on a wooden base (tongue-depressor) or on a plastic base (Photo 39), using either no. 11 blades (the best results are with "feather" or "persona plus" blades), a no. 10 or 22 blade or the multi-blade scalpel mentioned above.

Preparation of the receptor zone can be done in various manners:

- Drilling with a hand- or motor-operated punch, giving grafts of a diameter of 1–2.5 mm
- Incision with a no. 11 or 15 blade, a 69 blade or a stitch-cutter (Fig. 12, Photo 40)
- Perforation with 16- or 18-gauge needles combined with the use of dilators (Fig. 13, Photos 41, 42)
- Perforation and incision with Nokor's 16- or 18-gauge lanceolate needles (Photo 43)

Each micro- or minigraft is inserted with a fine, untoothed, straight or curved forceps such as a jeweller's forceps or an iridectomy forceps (Photo 44).

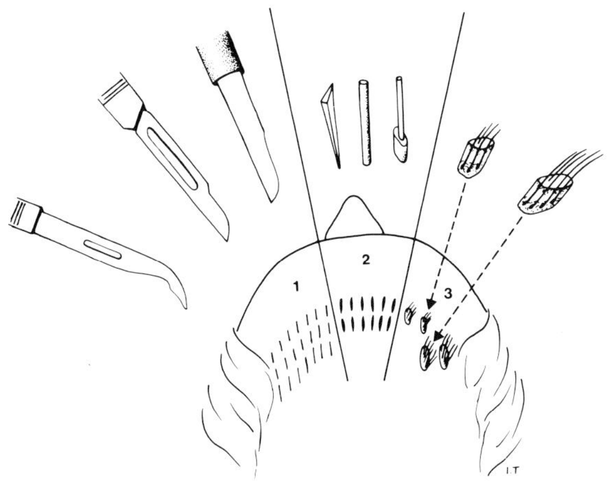

Fig. 12. Instrumentation for transplantation of minigrafts. *1*, Incisions with no. 12, 15 or 64 blade. *2*, Dilatation with wooden stem of cotton-bud, wooden gum massager, metal mini-dilator. *3*, Insertion of minigrafts

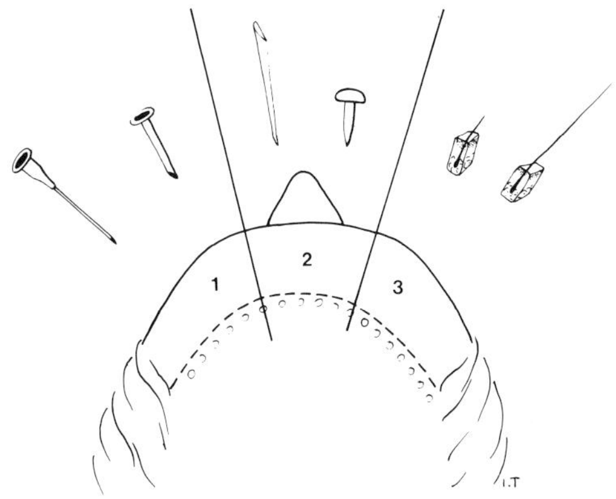

Fig. 13. Instrumentation for transplantation of micrografts. *1*, Perforation by 18-gauge needle or perforator–dilator. *2*, Dilatation by wooden or metal dilators. *3*, Insertion of micrografts

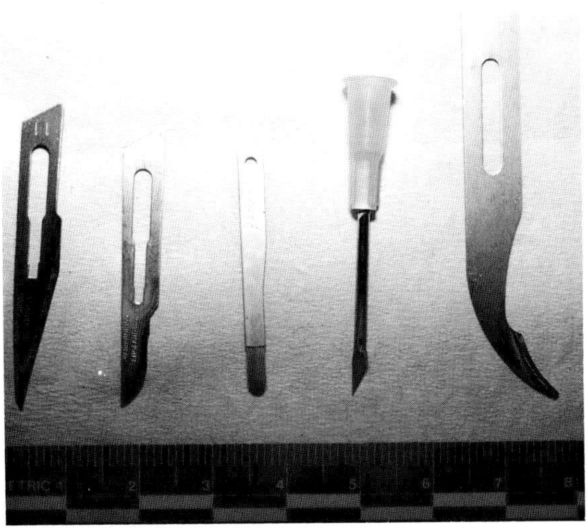

Photo 40. Instrumentation for incision: 11 blade, 15 blade, 69 blade, Nokor needle, stitch cutter blade (Beaver, Persona, Swann-Morton, Feather)

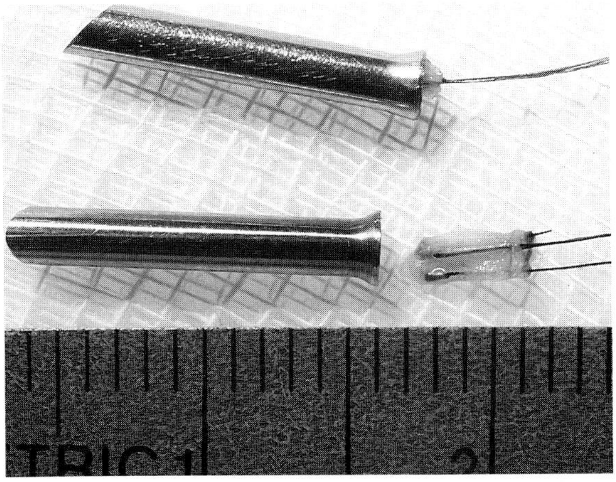

Photo 42. Macroscopic view of micrografts and Bouhanna perforator–insertors

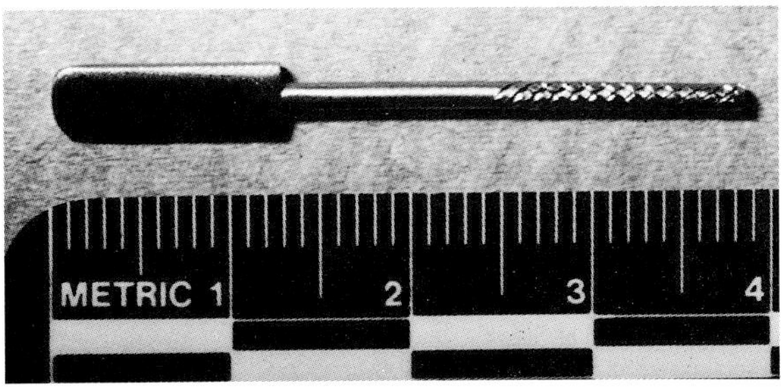

Photo 41. Lepaw's metal dilator

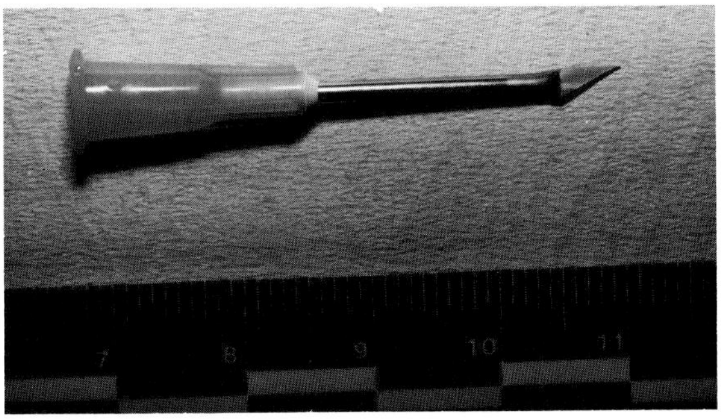

Photo 43. Nokor needle (16 or 18 gauges)

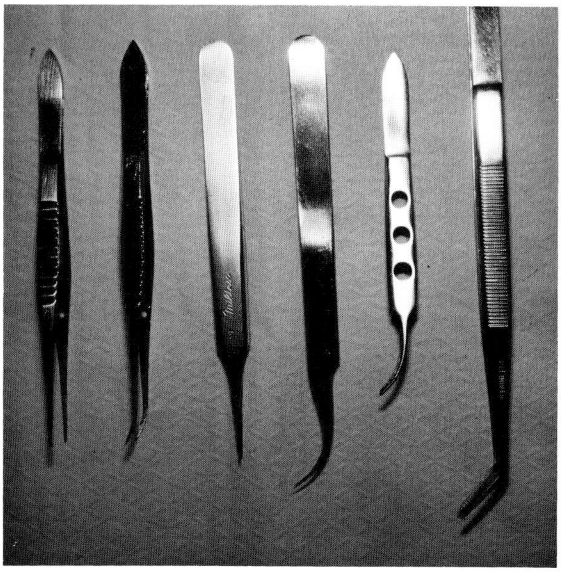

Photo 44. Instrumentation for implantation: untoothed straight or curved forceps such as jeweller's forceps, iridectomy forceps

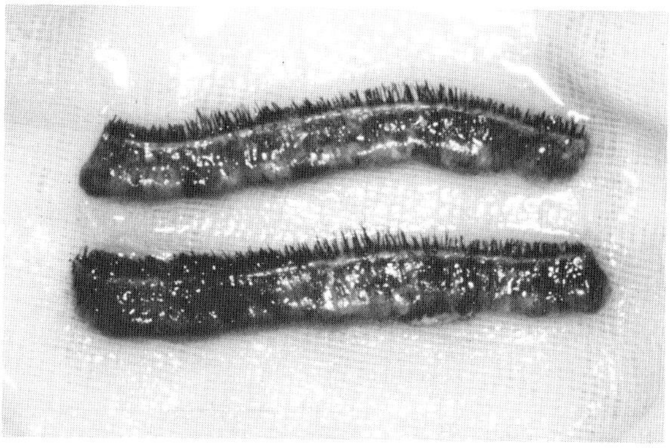

Photo 45. Two strips removed with the multi-blade scalpel

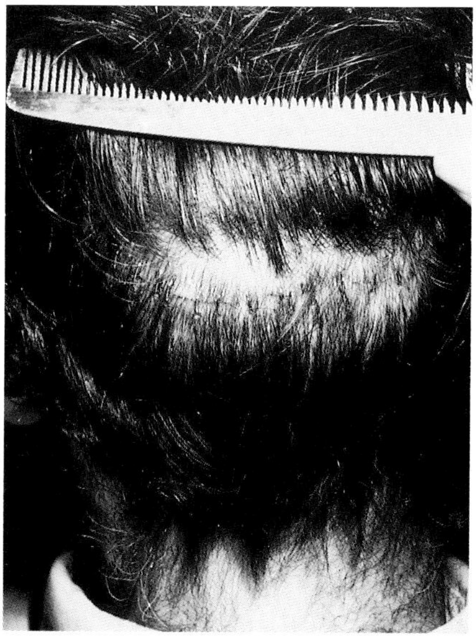

Photo 46. Two superimposed scars from graft removal. The staples are removed at the tenth day

Preparation of Micro- and Minigrafts

Micro- and minigrafts are removed at the donor occipital region by one of two methods:

- By excision with an 11- or 15-blade scalpel of a strip 10–20 cm long and 0.5–2 cm wide, the size depending on the number of micro- or minigrafts desired
- By removal of two, three or four strips with the multi-bladed scalpel originally described by Vallis [42] (Photo 45)

Closure of the margins of the donor zone is made with a continuous suture of 3/0 monofil, an adsorbable intradermal running suture or with skin staples (Photo 46).

The excised strip is set out on a swab in a Petri dish containing normal saline and is then segmented at the surgeon's convenience, either by cutting the fragments on a wooden tongue-depressor using a no. 11 blade, each graft being freed of all excess hypodermis, or by using very sharp straight iridectomy scissors (Photo 47a–c). The fragments are arranged in the four compartments of a Petri dish according to the number of hairs borne by each fragment. Preliminary de-epithelialisation of the micrografts is still advised by some authors.

Preparation of the Receptor Area

While the excised scalp strips are being cut into mini- and micrografts by one or two assistants wearing magnifying spectacles under good illumination, the surgeon will prepare the anaesthetised receptor zone by making perforations and incisions, possibly followed by dilatation. It is essential to infiltrate the receptor zone liberally with normal saline. A preliminary design with a skin pencil marks out the area to be transplanted (Photo 48).

Perforation and Incision

The perforation and incision stage varies with different authors. Most perforate the skin covering with a 16- or 18-gauge needle, Nokor's lanceolate needle

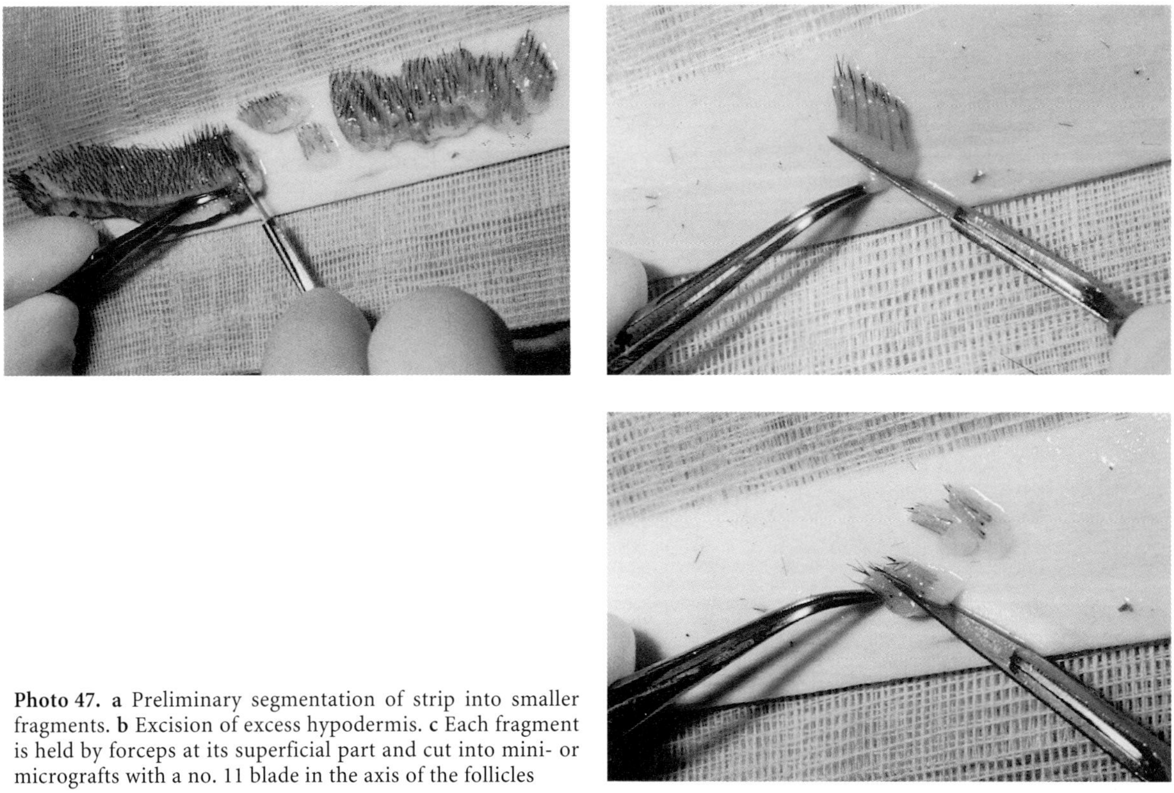

a b c

Photo 47. **a** Preliminary segmentation of strip into smaller fragments. **b** Excision of excess hypodermis. **c** Each fragment is held by forceps at its superficial part and cut into mini- or micrografts with a no. 11 blade in the axis of the follicles

being the most suitable. Others prefer to make incisions with a 15-blade scalpel or a no. 69 blade mounted on a round-handled scalpel. In practice, needle perforation is usually preferred for the implantation of micrografts and scalpel incision for that of mini- and micrografts (Photo 49).

Dilatation

The dilatation stage is not routinely essential. Some workers perform preliminary dilatation of the orifices or incisions with dilators of various shapes and materials before implantation (Photo 50). Some are wooden and very improvised, such as the stems of cotton-buds; others are of wood with a pyramidal point (Wooden-Udent) and are normally used for gum massage in the treatment of parodentitis. Others are metallic and of various shapes, e.g. the minidilators of Marritt or Lepaw. Those of Bouhanna are nail-shaped, with a diameter of 1–1.5 or 2 mm and a length of 15 mm. The pointed tip allows better penetration through the original needle perforation, while the rounded head at the other end facilitates its manipulation.

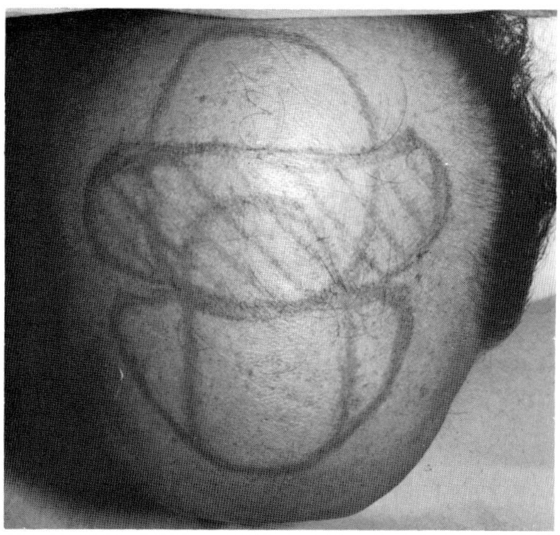

Photo 48. Design with a skin pencil of the bald area to be transplanted

However, we have abandoned the use of the perforator-insertor that we developed earlier. Each micrograft was placed in one of these cylindrical instruments; its pointed end perforated the skin and the micrograft was then pushed into the orifice while withdrawing the instrument.

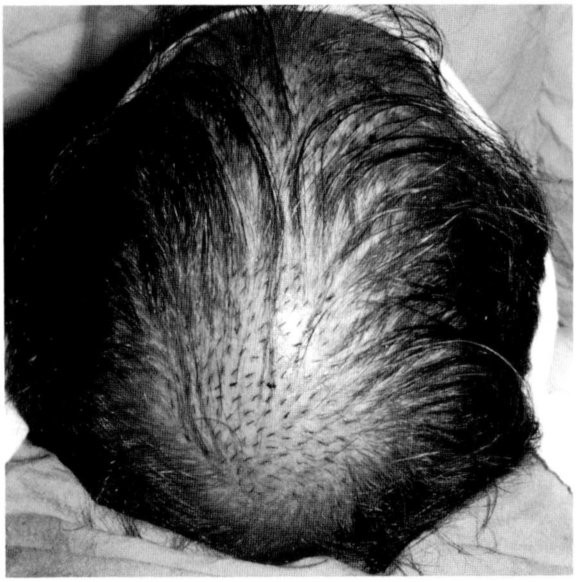

Photo 49. Bald area after incisions with 15 blade, 69 blade and Nokor needle

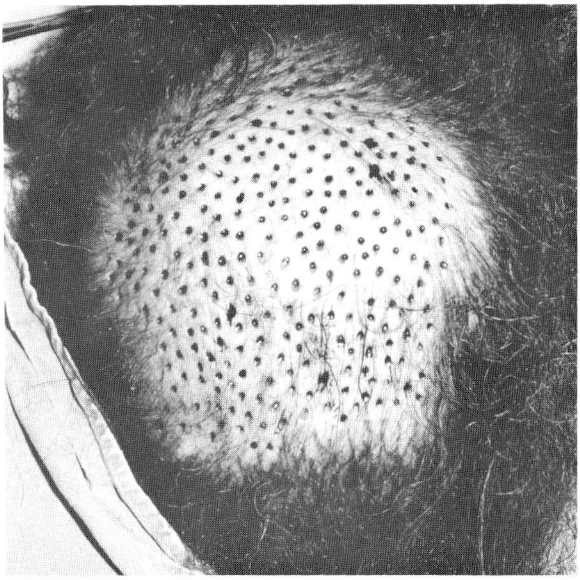

Photo 51. Bald area after drilling with micro-punches (1, 1.25 and 1.5 mm)

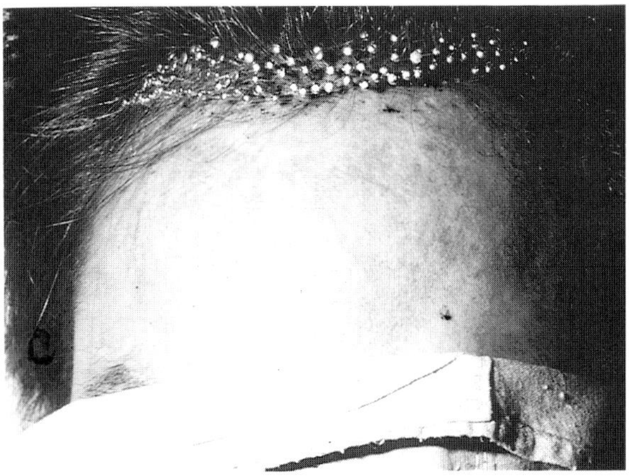

Photo 50. Immediate aspect after use of Bouhanna perforator-dilators and before insertion of micrografts

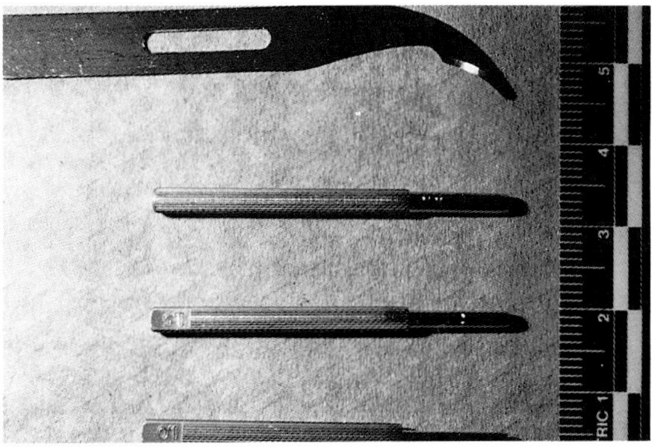

Photo 52. 1- to 1.5-mm punch and stitch-cutter used for transplantation of mini- and micrografts

Cylindrical Orifices

Drilling of the receptor area with a punch of 1–1.25–1.5 mm is widely used for macrografts and a diameter of 1.75–2.25 mm for minigrafts (Photos 51, 52).

Implantation

As graft-cutting proceeds, the mini- and micrografts are placed in a Petri dish containing normal saline. Each fragment is chosen and then inserted through a perforation or incision after checking its quality and cleaning it of hypodermal or keratin debris. If dilators have been used, they are removed as the implantation proceeds (Photo 53a,b). Most authors grasp the fragments with very fine, untoothed forceps (jeweller's type) or with curved ends (Photo 54). Each mini- or micrograft is held delicately along its entire extent with the forceps and threaded through the previously perforated or incised skin cover. Some auhors insert the micrograft in the orifice with the point of a needle, transfixing the deep hypodermal part of the graft. The mini- or micrograft sometimes tends to be extruded just after its insertion. This embarrassing incident is due to several factors: a taut skin, over-proximity of the perforations, frag-

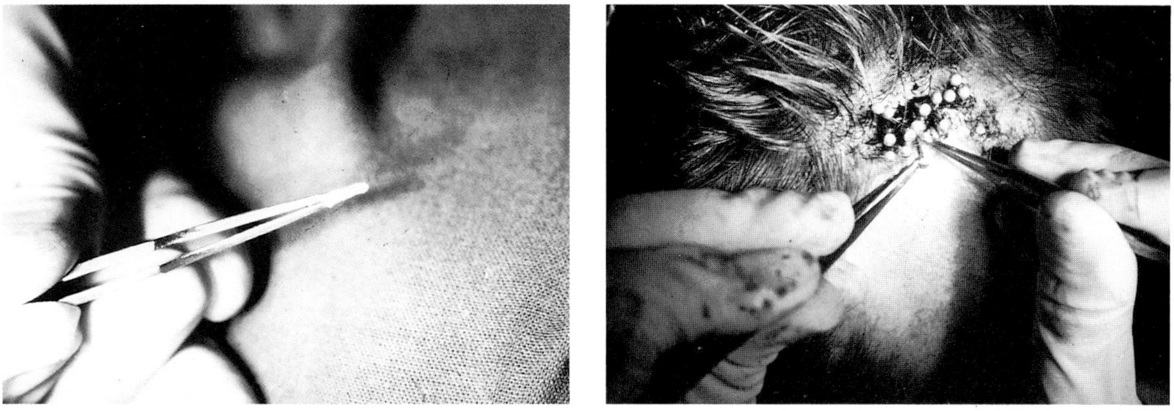

a b

Photo 53. **a** Grasping of micrograft with jeweller's forceps. **b** Insertion of micrograft into an orifice from which the perforator-dilator has just been withdrawn

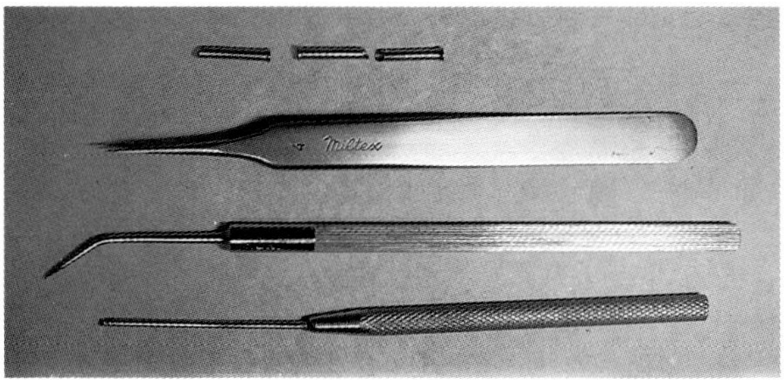

Photo 54. Instruments for insertion of micrografts

ments which are too small or too large in relation to the orifices and small haemorrhages at the base of the incision. Because of this, preliminary dilatation with the instruments described above permits not only easier penetration, but also better retention of the transplant. To avoid this snag, Bouhanna has developed a different procedure (see the section on "Immediate Long-haired Autografts", p. 106ff.).

The technique consists in a first stage of preliminary oblique penetration with an Orentreich manual punch, whose diameter (1–2.5 mm) depends on the size of the fragments (Fig. 14). This stage is identical with that advised for the transplantation of cylindrical grafts. The fragments of smooth skin cut are excised. At a second stage, using the cutting instrument employed for suture removal (the Swann-Morton stitch-cutter), we incise each orifice to debride it. The point of the instrument should first penetrate vertically into the anterior wall of the orifice and is then rotated backward in the depth of the dermo-hypodermis. At the end of this movement the blade also produces a slight nick in the superficial posterior part of the orifice.

This initial procedure has the following advantages:

- Insertion of the micro- or minigraft is easy.
- The deep bed is easily stretched and so prevents rejection of the transplant.
- The superficial incision allows deformation of the initial circle and therefore adaptation to the geometric shape of the graft without being cylindrical.
- Drilling with the punch allows the excision of multiple smooth areas and thus reduction of the bald area.

It is therefore possible to manage without the use of dilators.

It is currently possible, during a single session, to transplant several hundred mini- and micrografts. Rassman, Uebel and Pravitz have exceeded a thousand implanted micrografts in one session. During reconstruction of a bald frontal region, the fragments chosen to construct the AFL will be those with two to three hairs (1 mm) in the first row, three to four hairs (1.5 mm) in the second row and finally five to seven hairs (2 mm) (Fig. 15).

At the end of the session, gentle compression is applied for 3 min with swabs soaked in normal saline or hydrogen peroxide. Using an operating microscope, we check all of the grafts to confirm their proper insertion and good orientation (Photos 55a,b, 56).

The patient remains supine for 3 h, and a further check is made at the end of this rest period. Depending on the preference of the surgeon, a dressing may or may not be applied for 24 h. A foaming antiseptic shampoo is applied from the next morning. The minuscule scabs which form over the micro- and minigrafts fall off spontaneously in the following 10

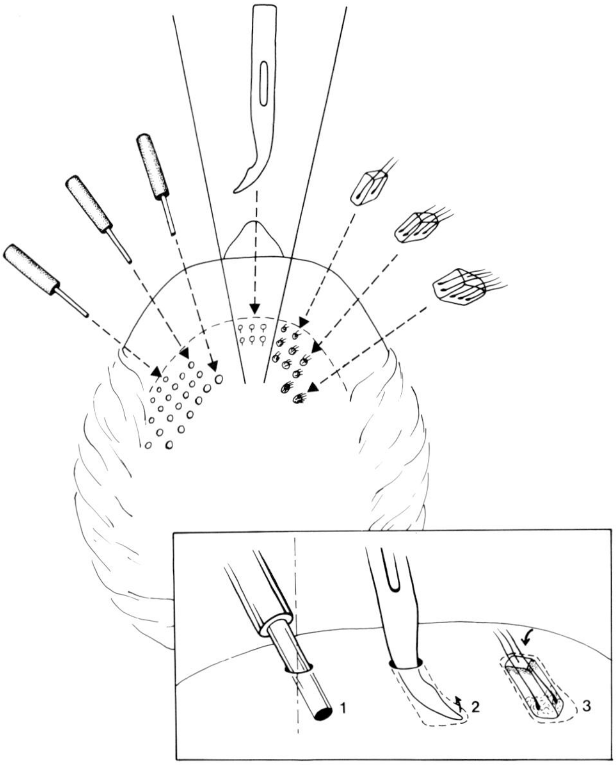

Fig. 14. Instrumentation for insertion of mini- and micrografts (Bouhanna). *1*, Oblique forage with 1.5 to 2-mm punch. *2*, Intra-orificial incision with "stitch-cutter". *3*, Insertion of mini- and micrografts

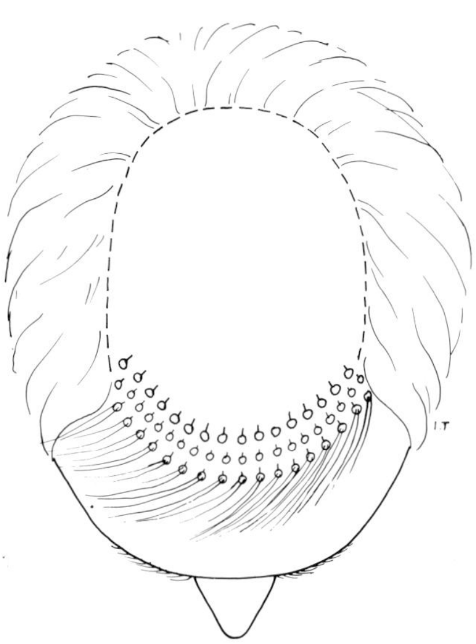

Fig. 15. Distribution of grafts at anterior frontal line: micrografts at first row and minigrafts at following rows (possibly with long hairs)

days. The hairs may fall out 15–20 days later and regrow after 3 months on average.

Technical Features in Women

The transplantation of minigrafts is the procedure most used to correct female alopecia. Because of the diffuse nature of the hair loss, removal of the strips can be performed only at the mid-occipital region, and subsequent grafts are always taken from the same scar (Fig. 16). Depending on the topography and extent of the baldness, the minigrafts are transplanted in one to three sessions in the frontal and vertical regions (Fig. 17, Photo 57a,c).

Complications

The complications that occur with mini- and micrografts resemble in incidence those of classical grafts, but are naturally reduced in extent by virtue of the small size of the fragments. On the other hand, we have to report that two complications have become more common with these new procedures:

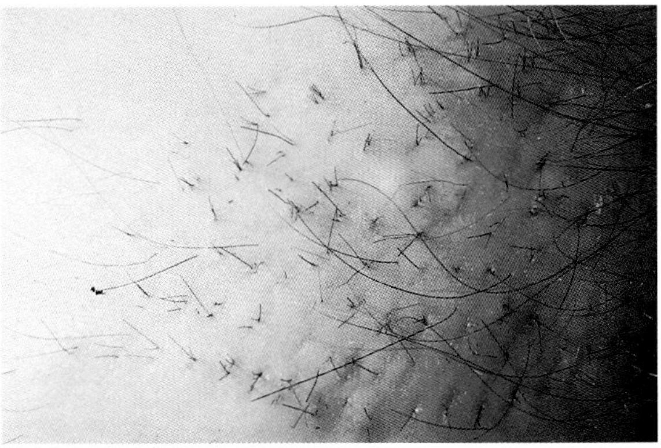

55a

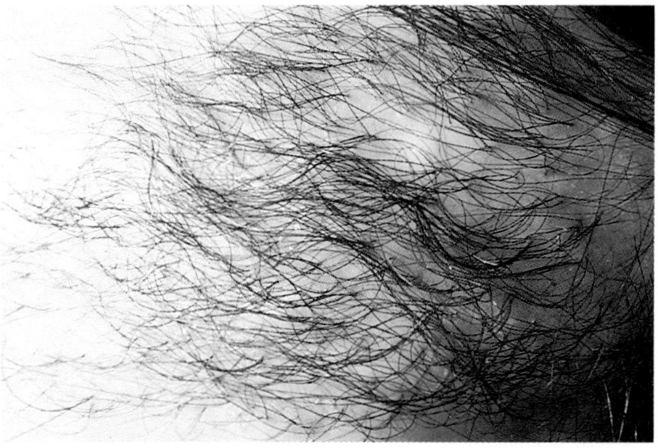

55b

Photo 55. a One month after transplantation of minigrafts to a bald area and pre- and postoperative application of minoxidil. **b** Aspect of grafted hairs 3 months after transplantation

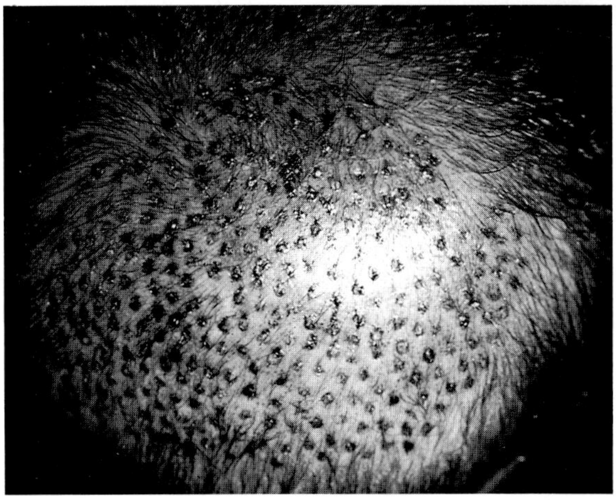

56

Photo 56. Vertex baldness immediately after transplantation of 300 minigrafts

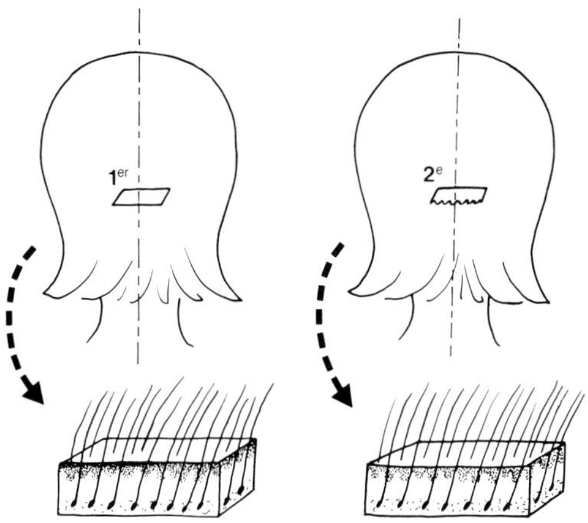

Fig. 16. Single or repeated removal of mid-occipital scalp strip before segmentation into minigrafts

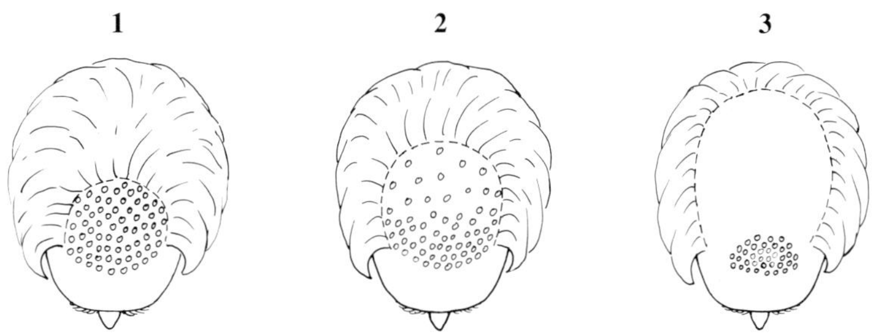

Fig. 17. Three sites of transplantation of minigrafts in women, depending on extent of baldness. *1*, 100–200 minigrafts in one session. *2*, 200–300 minigrafts in two sessions. *3*, 100 minigrafts in one session shafts

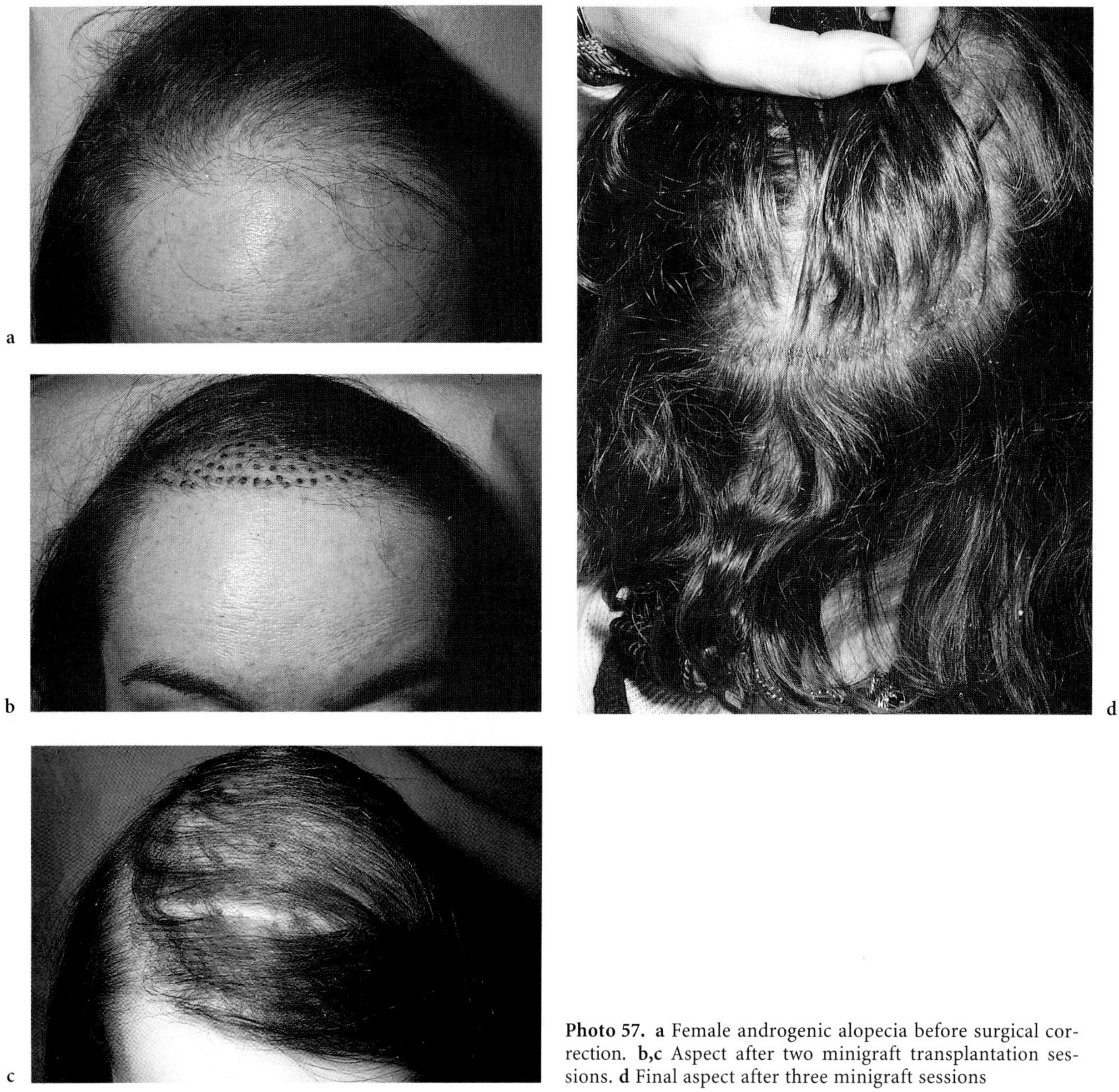

Photo 57. **a** Female androgenic alopecia before surgical correction. **b,c** Aspect after two minigraft transplantation sessions. **d** Final aspect after three minigraft sessions

- Cysts of the scalp after the inclusion of cutaneous or keratinous debris in the hole (Photo 58a,b). In the months after transplantation a cyst resembling a wen of the scalp may develop and remain quiescent. Sometimes, it may follow the same course as the cysts of acne with inflammation and discharge on the skin surface. During the inflammatory suppurative episode the lesion should be incised and evacuated after instituting antibiotherapy. If the cyst is not inflamed, incision and evacuation are just as for an epidermoid cyst, though there is no actual capsule. The material obtained is sebum agglomerated with hairs that have continued to grow.
- Ingrowing implanted hair. Hair growth directed inward is due to poor orientation of the transplant; the hairs continue to grow rolled up on themselves. Treatment consists of teasing out and uncoiling the hairs with the point of a needle or forceps (Photo 59).

Conclusion

Transplantation of mini- and micrografts has afforded considerable progress in the surgical management of male or female alopecia [37]. This technique allows for harmonious, uniform and

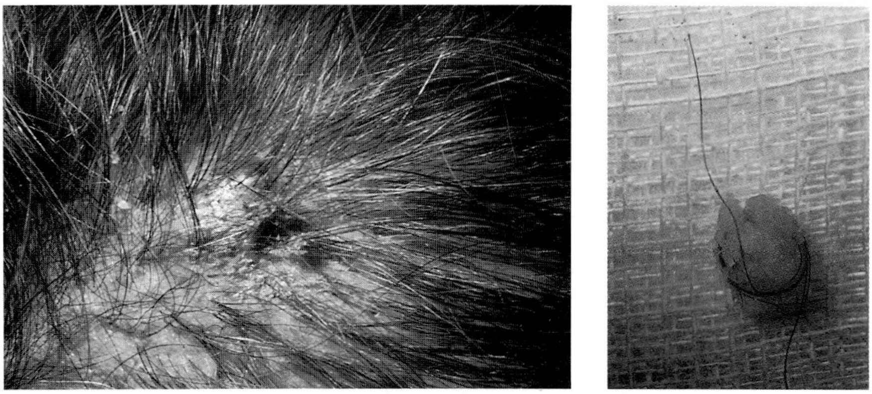

a b

Photo 58. **a** Superficial suppurative skin lesion due to epidermal cyst. **b** Epidermal cyst evacuated after incision: sebaceous material and hair

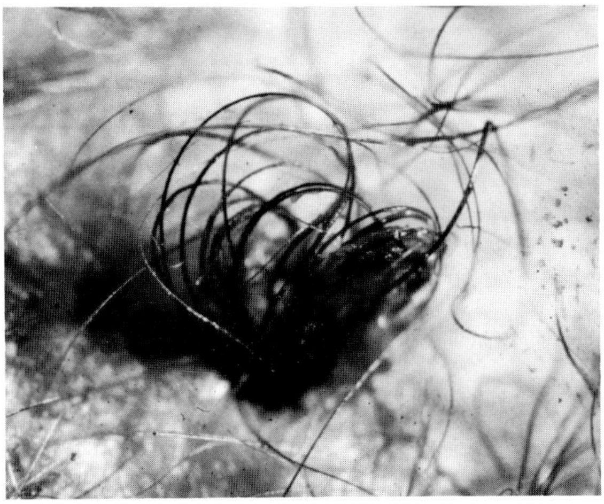

Photo 59. Ingrowing implanted hair due to poor orientation of the minigraft; hairs continue to grow rolled up on themselves; hairs need to be teased out with the point of a needle

cosmetic reconstruction between the bald and hairy donor areas. It also facilitates the correction of unaesthetic complications of previous scalp procedures.

Fusiform Grafts

Strips of scalp were recommended in 1967 by Vallis [45] for the creation of a hairy anterior line (Photo 60). The single fragment removed transversely at the donor occipital zone could be 12–15 cm long and 6–8 mm wide. This strip was placed on the frontal region [46] after preliminary excision of the corresponding area of smooth skin, following the classical design of the frontal line (see section on "Autografts", p. 106ff.). This graft, extending from one temple to the other was fixed by multiple interrupted sutures [47].

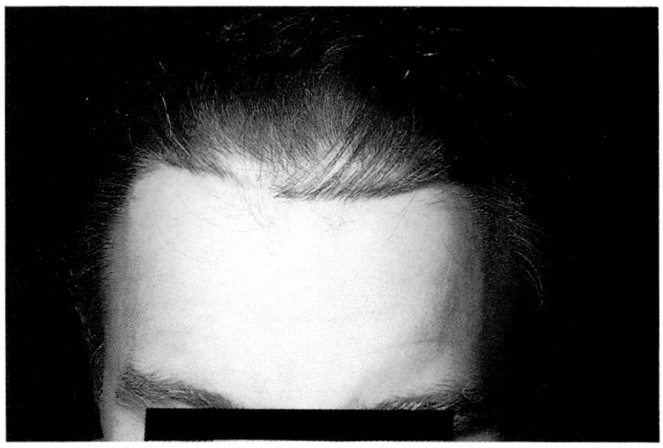

Photo 60. Aspect of anterior frontal line after transplantation of Vallis-type strip

In 1972, Nataf and Vissian [50] also suggested the transplantation of strips of a similar nature, but these so-called "fusiform" grafts had certain special features:

- They were removed vertically at the donor occipital region.
- They were smaller: 2–3 cm long and 4–5 mm wide.
- They were arranged like a necklace on the AFL.
- They were inserted in incisions without excision at the receptor frontal region.
- They were sutured at the four cardinal points.
- They were held in place by one or more acrylic strips whose perforations allowed discharge of any sero-sanguineous exudate.

In 1976, with Nataf et al. [5, 26], Bouhanna confirmed the cosmetic value of this procedure, while stressing that it was less reliable than cylindrical grafting. In 1988, Bouhanna [11, 13] standardised the procedure.

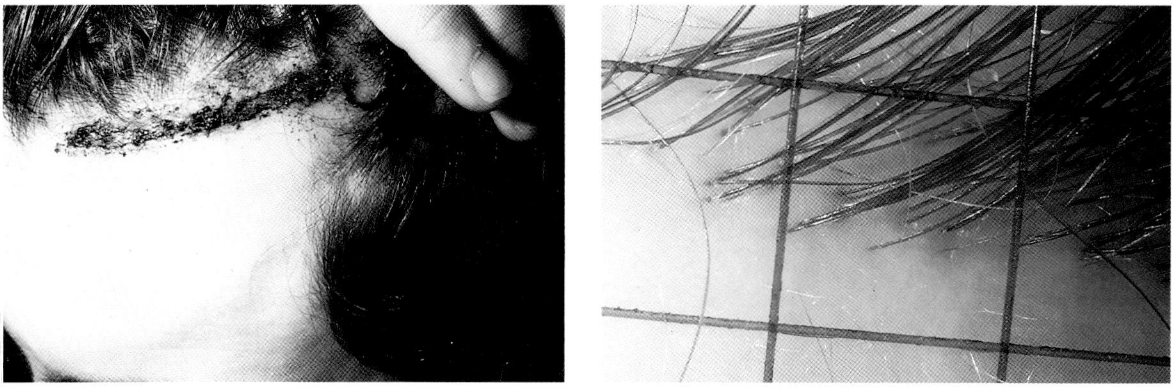

a b

Photo 61a,b. Transplantation of fusiform strip. **a** One week after transplantation. **b** Macrophotographic view of strip graft

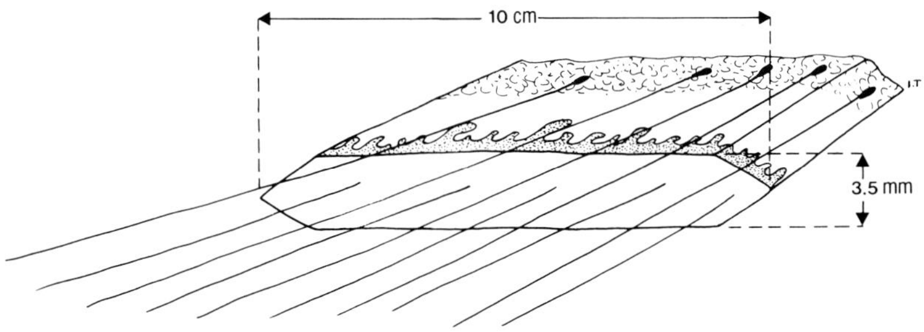

Fig. 18. Strip of scalp 10 cm long and 3.5 mm wide with an average of 300–350 hairs

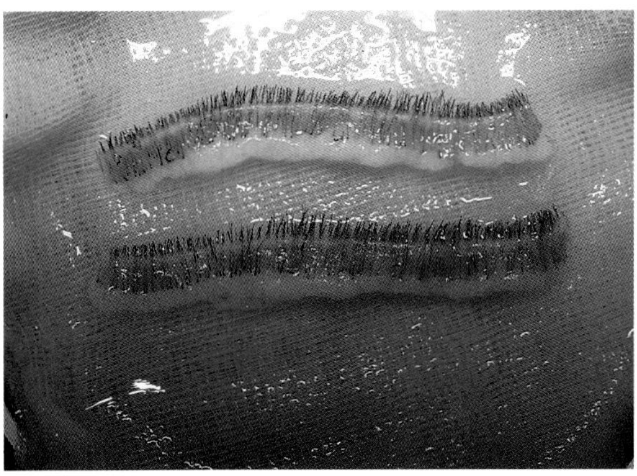

Photo 62. Strips removed and placed in normal saline

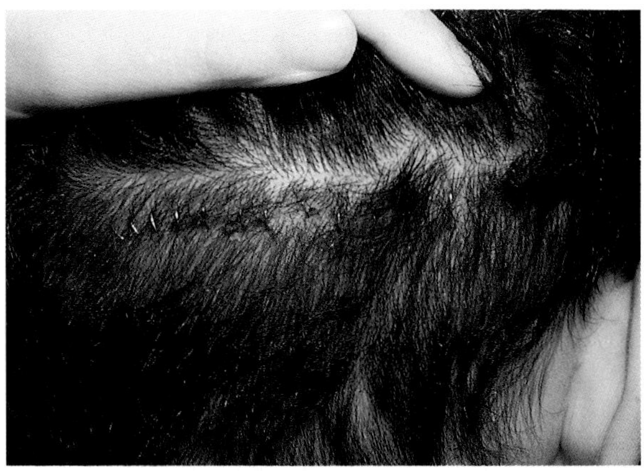

Photo 63. Aspect of donor area 8 days after staple closure

Aim

The aim of this procedure is to reconstruct a continuous AFL by transplanting a strip of occipital scalp to each frontal recession in a single session (Photo 61a,b).

Technique

Taking the Grafts

The technique of taking the grafts is similar to that used for micrografts. The strips are about 3.5–4 mm

Fig. 19. Filling of both frontal recessions by simultaneous transplantation of two Bouhanna-type strip grafts

Fig. 20. Bridge suture over both margins of strip graft. A 6/0 monofilament suture is recommended, to be removed at the fifth day

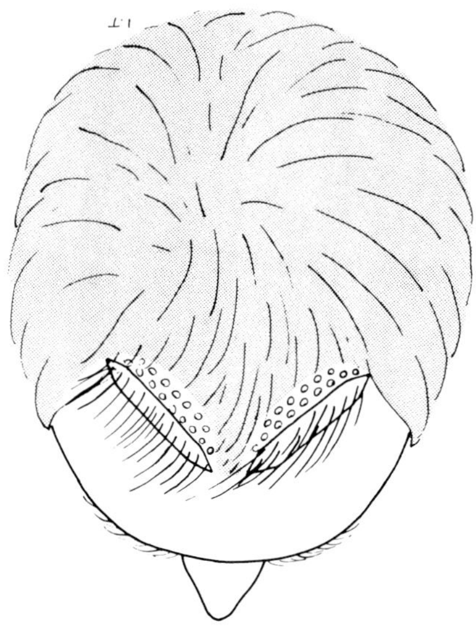

19

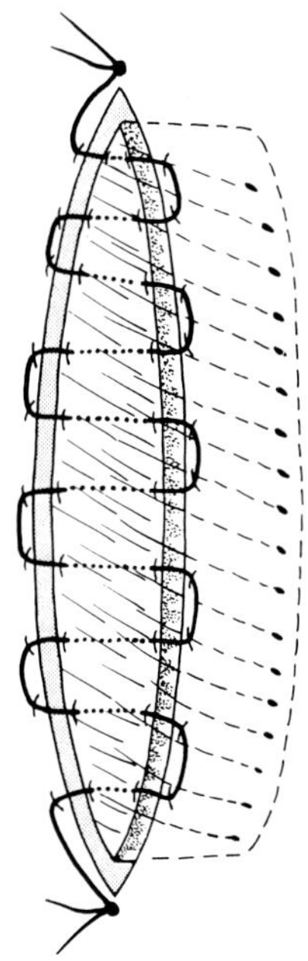

20

wide and 10 cm long and are taken horizontally (Fig. 18). The two strips are carefully cleansed from all epidermal fragments or hair stems; any excess aponeurotic or hypodermal tissue is excised (Photos 62, 63).

Transplantation of Strips

At the receptor frontal region the AFL designed using the classical criteria (see section on "Transplantation"). The scalp, firmed by previous injection of normal saline, is incised deeply down to the subgaleal layer over a length of 8–12 cm on each side, following the design of the planned frontal line. A simple incision is adequate, though sometimes an excision of 1–2 mm in width may be required (Fig. 19). After marginal haemostasis, the graft is carefully positioned and held in place by a continuous suture with monofil 5/0 passing as a bridge over it (Fig. 20). The strips are inserted so as to allow forward orientation of the hairs (Photo 64). Telfa and compresses are applied for 24 h by a slightly compressive bandage over the donor and receptor zones. This dressing is stripped off very cautiously. Shampooing is carried out on the second day. The sutures bridging the grafts are removed at the fifth day and the continuous suture of the donor area at the 12th day.

The programming for the strip graft is based on that observed after transplantation of cylindrical grafts (see sections on "Transplantation", "Grafts", "Minoxidil" and "Immediate Long-Haired Autografts").

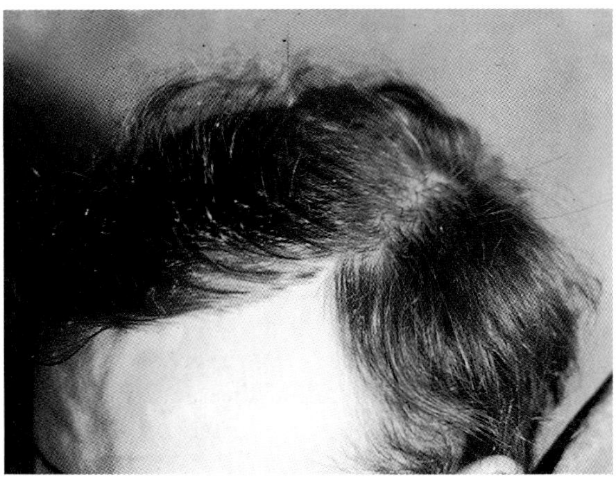

Photo 64. Aspect of a strip graft 6 months after transplantation to left frontal recession

Complications

The main complications are identical with those observed during the transplantation of cylindrical grafts:

- Impairment of central hair regrowth is due to poor vascularisation of the graft, amounting even to necrosis (excess of adrenaline, subjacent haematoma) (Photo 65).

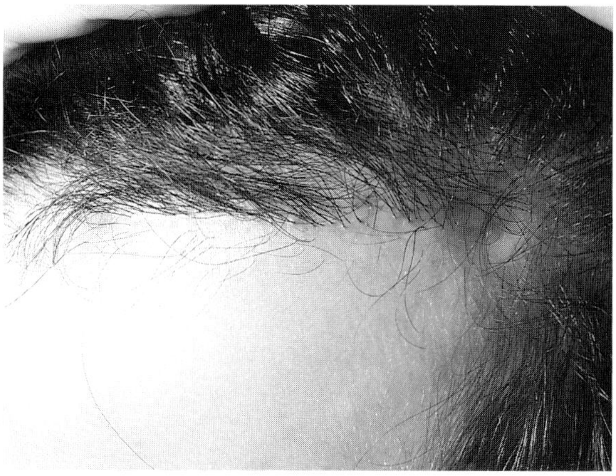

Photo 65. Partial regrowth defect of strip and whitish aspect of scar due to premature sun exposure

a 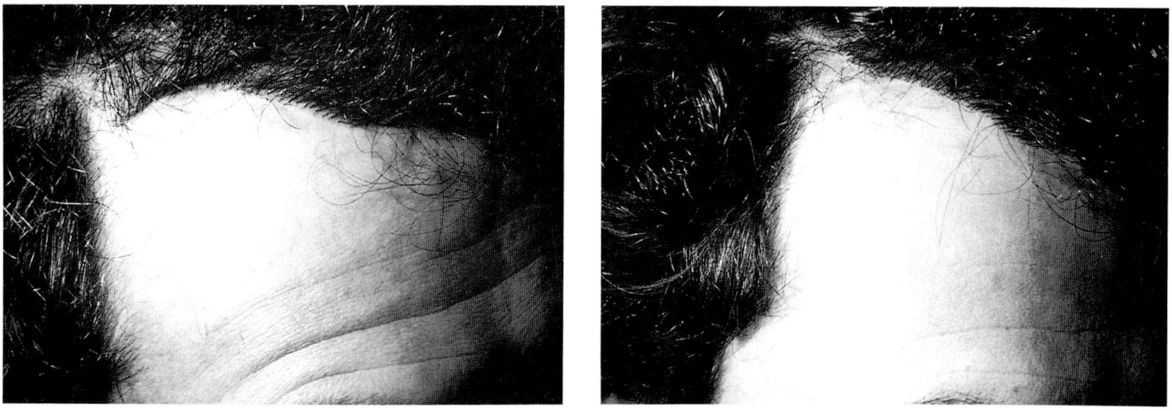 b

Photo 66. **a** Poor design of strip transplantation. **b** Aspect 6 months after correct reposition of proximal part of strip

- Impairment of peripheral hair regrowth is mainly due to improper section of the roots, the line of section not having been adequately parallel to the follicles.
- A fine but visible scar at the AFL is due to too early exposure to the sun (before 3 months). A session of micrografting can be advised to conceal any persistent scar.
- If the strip has been placed in poor position, it is easy to carry out reposition of all or part of the graft (Photo 66).
- If the hair density at the donor site is considerable, there is a risk that the strip may be too obvious.

Conclusion

Transplantation by strips may take its place among the different procedures capable of reconstructing an AFL of natural and cosmetic aspect. Its indication may be simply for the filling-in of slight recession of the frontal line, or it may be combined with other surgical techniques for the correction of more extensive alopecia.

Immediate Long-Haired Autografts of Bouhanna

Bouhanna's technique of immediate long-haired autografts allows the removal and transplantation of grafts of different shapes and sizes in which the hairs have not been shaved. The main value of this procedure is its ability to immediately conceal the operated region. The fate of these long hairs may follow two paths:

- They may fall out at the third week, regrowth occurring 3 months after the operation.
- All or some of these hairs continue to grow if a lotion based on 2% minoxidil has been prescribed before and after the operation (see section on "Minoxidil").

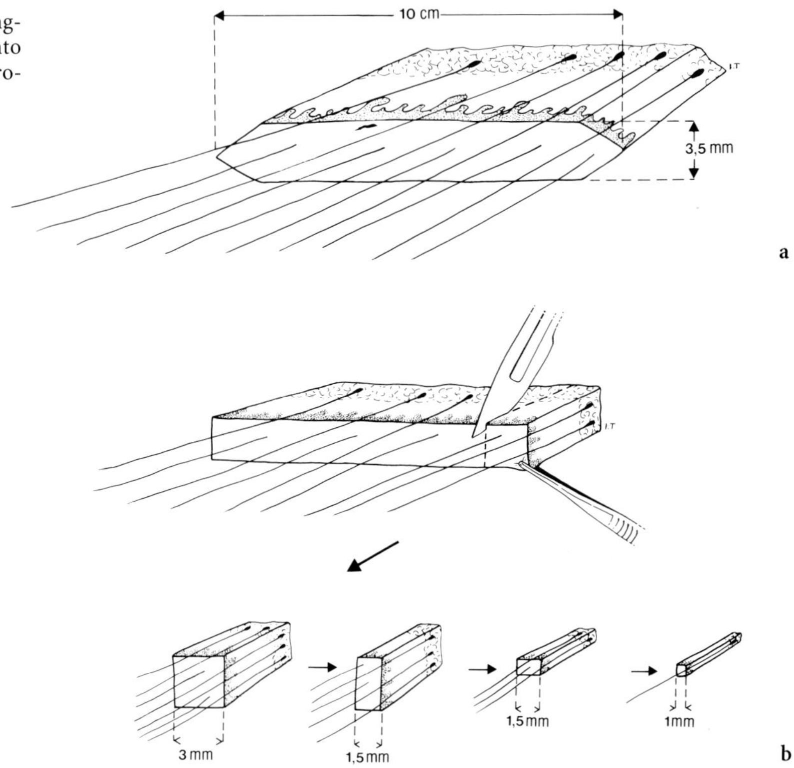

Fig. 21. a Usual size of fusiform long-haired graft. **b** Segmentation of strip into square or rectangular mini- or micro-grafts with long hairs

In every case involving the face, this procedure immediately provides the patient with an aspect that is sufficiently cosmetic for him to resume his family and professional activities after 24–48 h without embarrassment. In principle, three types of long-haired grafts can be used: fusiform grafts, micro- and minigrafts, and classical square grafts with sides of 2.5–3 mm. The indications for these different kinds of autografts are almost the same as those classically employed (see "Indications"). We estimate that this procedure is especially useful for coverage of completely bald areas. It is useless for the densification of sparsely haired regions.

Technique

Graft-Taking at the Occipital Region

One or two strips 10 cm long and 3.5 mm wide are marked out with a skin pencil. Depending on the type of grafts required, the density and calibre of the hairs and the scalp laxity, we prefer to remove a horizontal median occipital strip rather than a lateral vertical occipital one. The hairs are not shaved beforehand at the donor area (Fig. 21a,b).

Local anaesthesia of the donor and receptor areas is identical with that described above. The subcutaneous injection of 30–50 ml normal saline will firm up the surface sufficiently to allow an incision with a no. 11 blade perfectly parallel to the hair roots. The scalp strips are excised and the excess of hypodermis is carefully removed with scissors. The strips are then arranged in a Petri dish filled with normal saline. The margins of the excised regions are brought together in one layer without tension by means of clips or with a continuous 3/0 monofil suture (Photo 67).

Segmentation of the Scalp Strips

It is necessary to predict precisely the number, shape, size and density of the hairs on each fragment to be cut out (Fig. 22, Photo 68). For practical reasons, we suggest a classification of the different grafts (classification of Bouhanna):

- Strips, which are on average 10 cm long and 3.5 mm wide and may carry 250–350 long hairs
- Megagrafts, 3 mm^2 with more than eight hairs
- Macrografts, 2.5 mm long and 1.5 mm wide with five to seven hairs

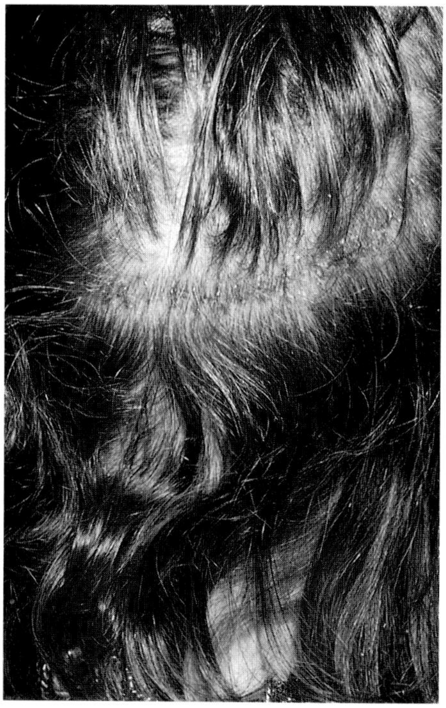

Photo 67. Removal of horizontal occipital scalp strip and closure by skin staples

- Minigrafts, 1.5 mm² with three to four hairs
- Micrografts, 1 mm² with one to two hairs

With the aid of magnifying spectacles and under good illumination, two assistants working simultaneously can cut out up to 500 fragments in a single session.

In the first stage, each strip deposited in a Petri dish containing normal saline is placed on a tongue-depressor kept permanently moist. With an 11-scalpel blade, an initial cutting-up of the strip, held with a fine forceps by its epidermis, parallel to the follicles, allows a first division into seven to ten fragments which are replaced in the normal saline. The fragments are then in turn placed on the tongue-depressor to be cut up according to the number, shape and size of grafts required. The scalpel blade must be changed regularly to ensure that the segmentation is of perfect quality (Photo 69). For reasons of comfort and reliability, the assistants who do the cutting and those who help with implantation at the orifices regularly change places. Each fragment cut is cleaned of all fragments of hair shaft or hypodermal debris before being placed in the container filled with normal saline.

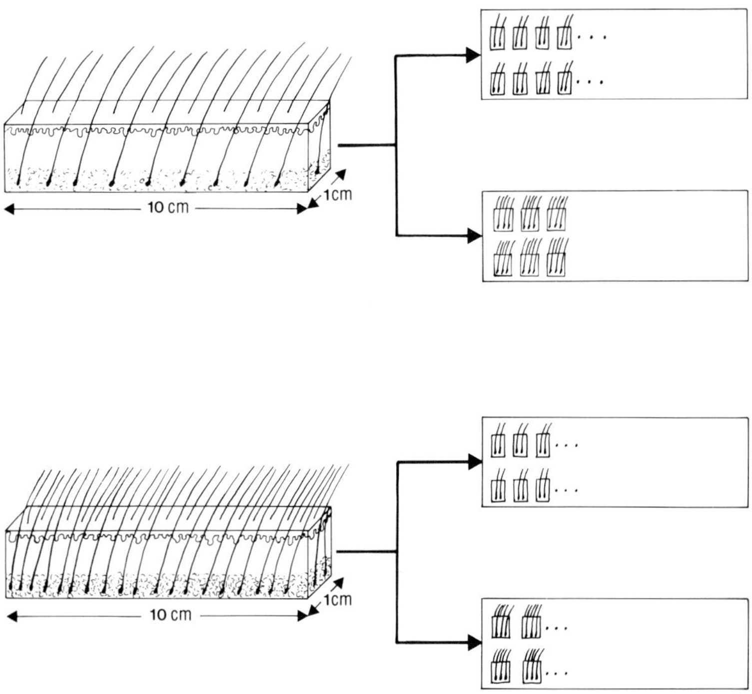

Fig. 22. Preliminary determination of size of strip for cutting up in relation to number, shape, size and density of each fragment

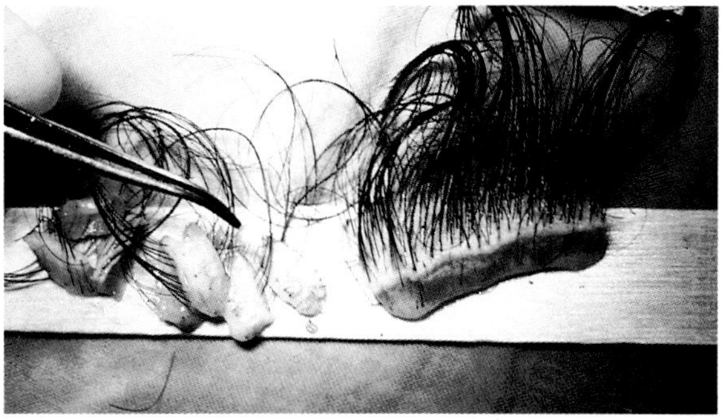

Photo 68. Scalp strip arranged on tongue-depressor and commencement of segmentation in axes of follicles

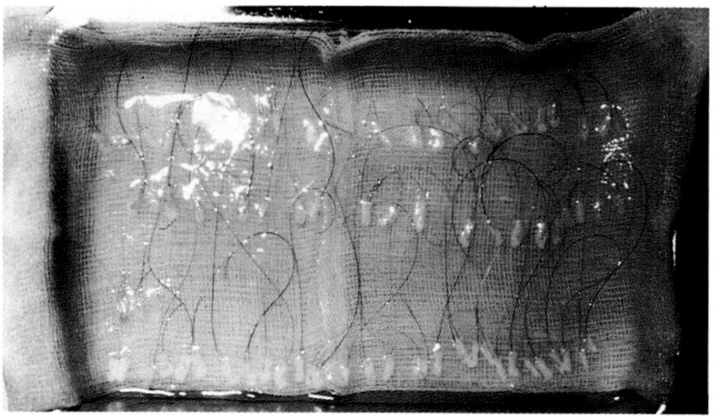

Photo 69. Long-haired micrografts placed in a dish containing normal saline

23

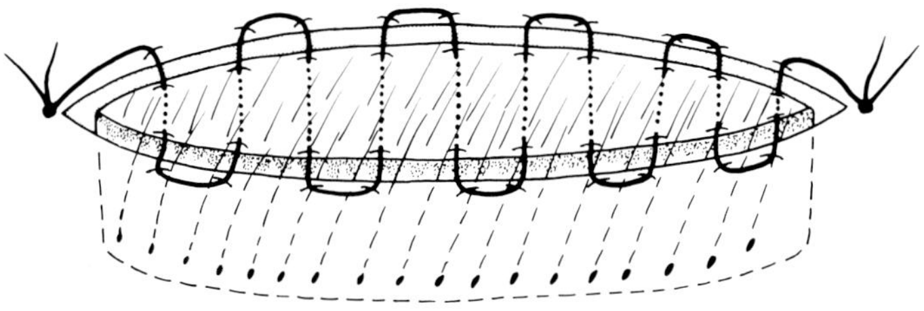

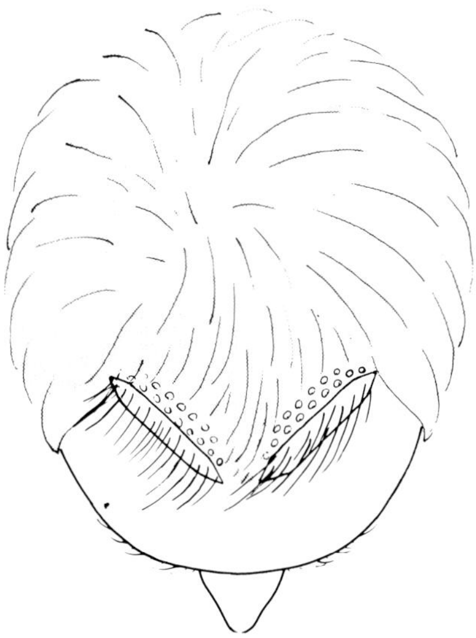

24

Fig. 23. Long-haired fusiform graft held in its bed by bridging running suture (Bouhanna)

Fig. 24. Long-haired fusiform graft at each frontal recession recreating anterior line and concealing the scabs of subsequent minigrafts

Preparation of the Receptor Region

The area to be grafted is demarcated with the skin pencil using the same criteria already mentioned for the transplantation of classical grafts. The areas corresponding to the choice of each type of graft must be determined and precisely designated. Only the transfer of fusiform strips is an isolated procedure. The other types of grafts can be combined during the same session.

Preparation of the graft-bed is guided by the size and shape of the grafts. The long-haired fusiform strip is inserted between the margins of an incision of the corresponding length. Little or no excision of the smooth area is necessary, but perfect haemostasis of the margins and the depth is essential. The fragment is held in place by a simple running 5/0 monofil suture bridging over the graft (Fig. 23). The long hairs are oriented forward, thus allowing immediate reconstruction of the frontal line. A strip may be placed in each frontal recession during the same session (Photo 70a–f, Fig. 24).

For all the other types of grafts cut out, preparation of the receptor site is uniform. In the first stage we perform drilling along an oblique axis of 45°–60° using an Orentreich type of manual punch. The diameter used depends on the size of the graft to be inserted into each orifice. The minimum space to be left between adjacent orifices must be equivalent to the diameter of the punch:

- A punch of 1 mm in diameter for micrografts
- A punch of 1.5 mm for minigrafts
- A 2-mm punch for macrografts
- A 2.5-mm punch for megagrafts

The scalp fragments cut out by the punch are withdrawn with fine-toothed forceps and iridectomy scissors (Fig. 16).

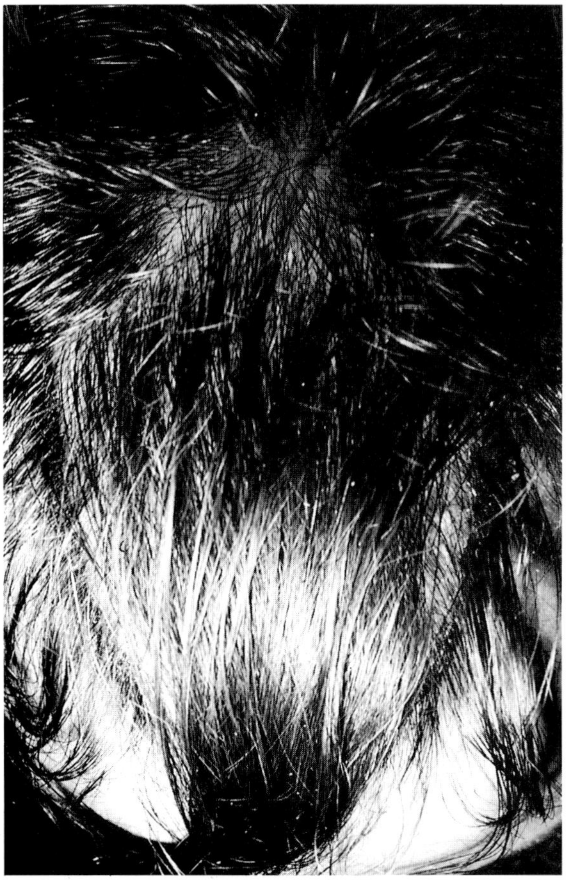
a

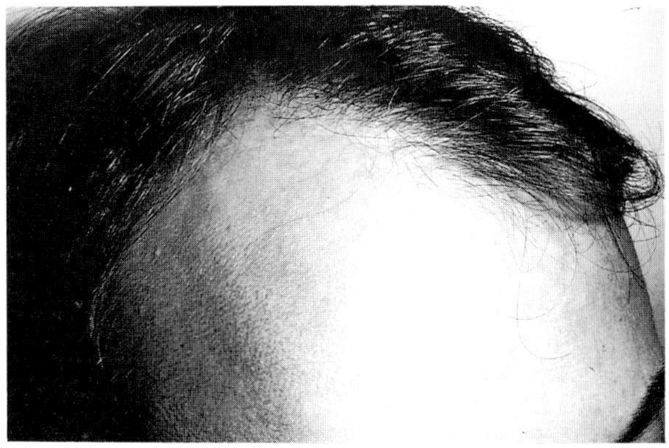
b

Photo 70. **a** Two long-haired fusiform grafts inserted at each frontal recession to reconstruct the first frontal hairline. **b** Aspect of right frontal recession before treatment. **c** Immediate postoperative aspect of long-haired fusiform graft held in place by continuous bridging suture. **d** Immediate postoperative aspect of long-haired fusiform graft at the right frontal recession. **e** Aspect of fusiform graft at seventh day with concealment of crusts by long hairs. **f** Aspect of right frontal recession at 4 months

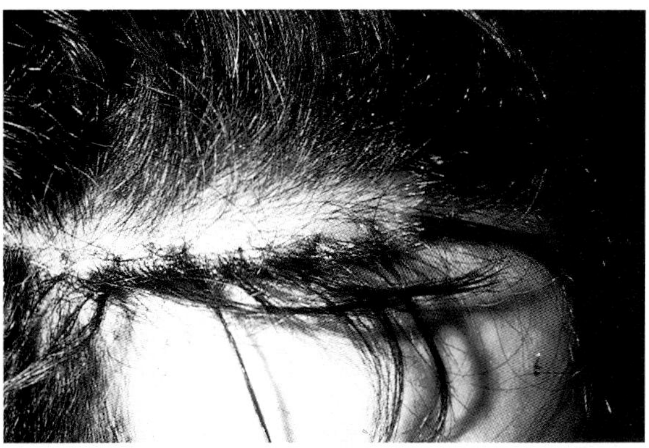
c

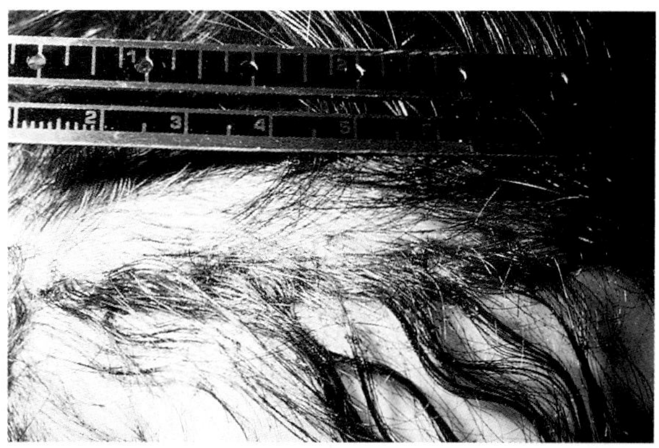
d

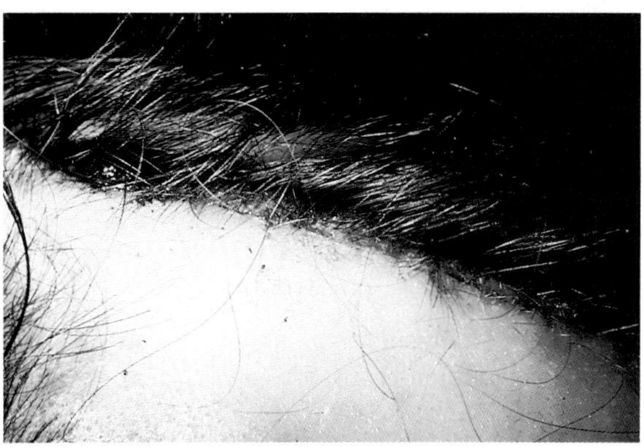
e

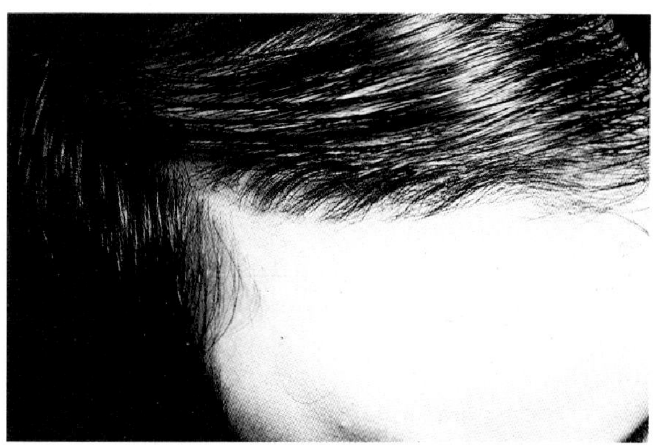
f

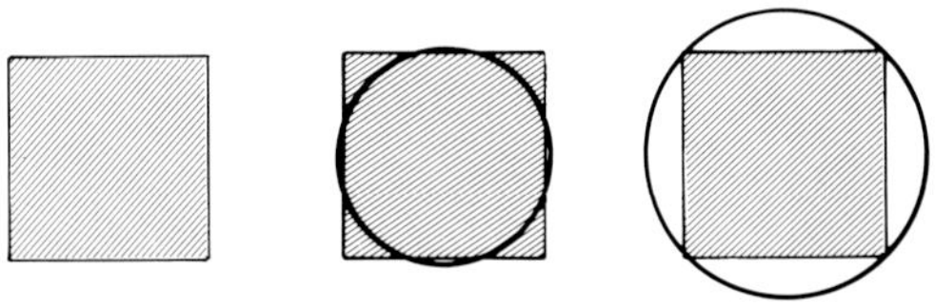

Fig. 25. Square grafts must be inserted in an orifice whose diameter is equal to the side of the square and not its diagonal

Before inserting the grafts in the corresponding orifices, a supplementary procedure is sometimes made wih a Swann-Morton stitch-cutter. The small curved tip of the blade is inserted from the front backwards, and the small cutting hook makes a slight incision at the posterior aspect of the orifice in its superficial part and a nick in the subjacent dermo-hypodermal structures. This simple manoeuvre allows each graft a bed suited to its size and so avoids its extrusion during the insertion of grafts into adjacent holes (Fig. 25).

After this last stage before implantation, it is important to check that no skin fragment remains in the orifices. Each long-haired graft is held in jeweller's forceps for insertion into its orifice. The micrografts are arranged in two rows at the level of the AFL. Behind this, and depending on the local conditions – fine AFL, hair colour (fair or dark) and shape (stiff or crinkly) – we choose between the three other types of grafts (minigrafts, macrografts or megagrafts). It is possible to transplant up to 400 grafts at one session.

Pre- and Postoperative Management

The grafted zone is manually compressed, first with swabs soaked in normal saline or hydrogen peroxide (10 volumes) and then with dry swabs for several minutes. No dressing is usually necessary and shampooing is performed after 48 h.

The strip technique may require a dressing for the first 24 h. To allow this to be removed more easily the following day, we apply Telfa directly. The whole is covered with pads and a slightly compressive bandage. Whatever procedure is chosen, the sutures and stitches are removed at the seventh to tenth day.

Course

Each graft, of whatever shape and size, follows the same stereotyped course as the cylindrical grafts (see "Grafts"). The scabs formed fall off between the second and fourth weeks. Complications are also very much the same. However, it should be noted that two complications are less frequent with long-haired mini- and micrografts:

- The secondary cyst associated with untoward insertion of a fragment in the same orifice where the skin fragment drilled by the punch remains in the depths.
- Ingrowing implanted hair: hair-growth directed inward is due to poor orientation of the graft.

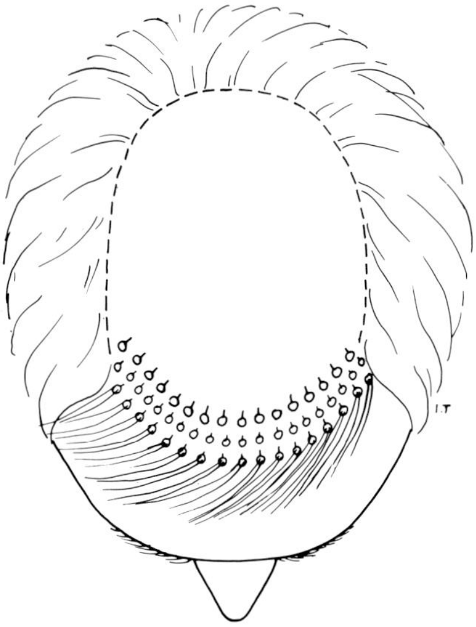

Fig. 26. The micrografts are inserted at the anterior frontal line and the minigrafts in the rows behind

Conclusion

This procedure of using grafts carrying long hairs provides the patient with a head of hair that looks natural immediately after the operation (Fig. 26, Photo 71a–d). Thus it is possible to avoid the cosmetic blemish due to scabbing and to over-prominent tufts of hair after the classical transplantation of cylindrical grafts or minigrafts. To promote continued growth of all or part of the transplanted hairs, the patient should apply a lotion based on 2% minoxidil to the recipient area 6 weeks before the transplantation. This local treatment is continued on the non-operated regions for 3 months following the procedure (see "Minoxidil") (Photo 72a,b).

Other advantages worthy of mention are the following:

- The different shapes and sizes of the grafts allow a choice suited to the cosmetic requirements of each individual.

a b

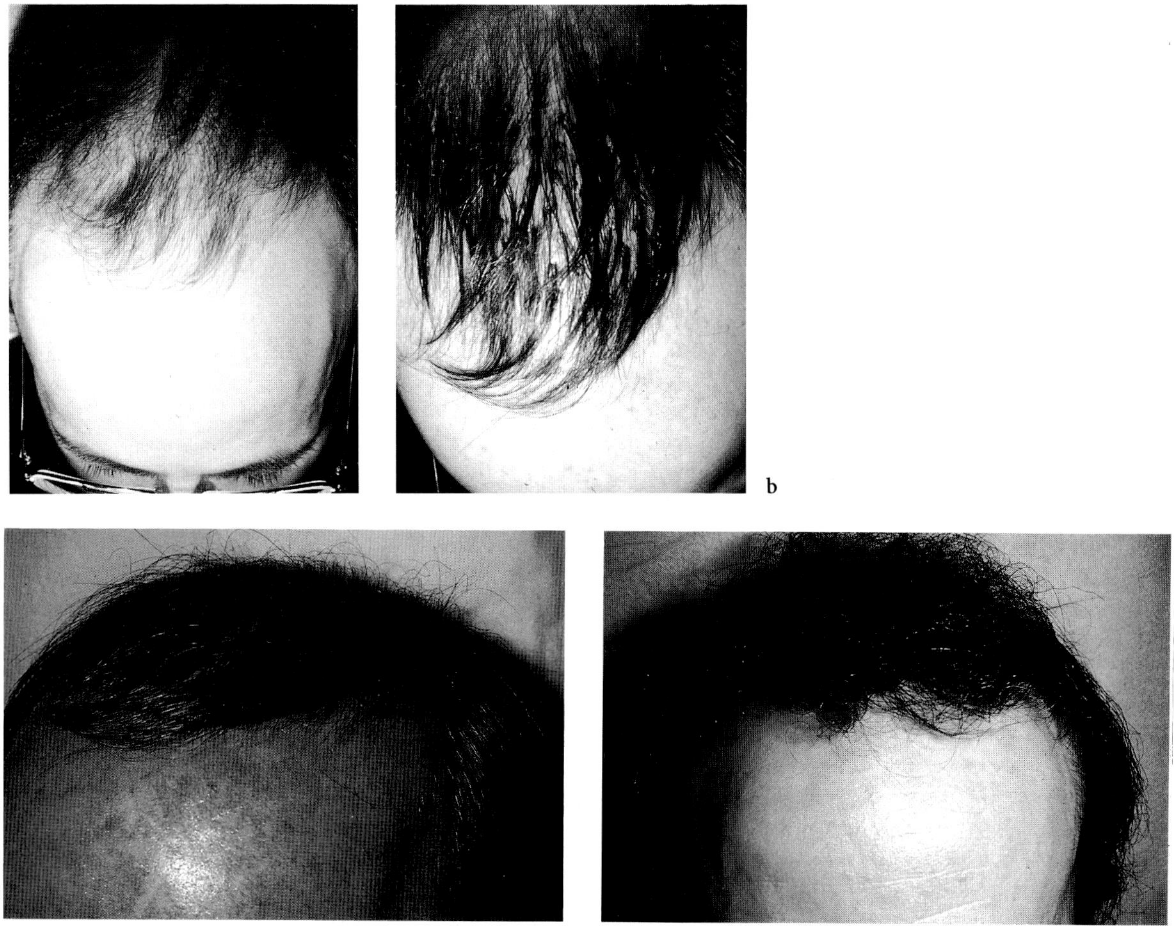

c d

Photo 71. **a** Male baldness before treatment. **b** Aspect 6 h after transplantation of long-haired grafts and application of swabs soaked in hydrogen peroxide. **c** Aspect of left frontal recession at eighth day; the long hairs mask the crusts. **d** Same patient after two transplantation sessions

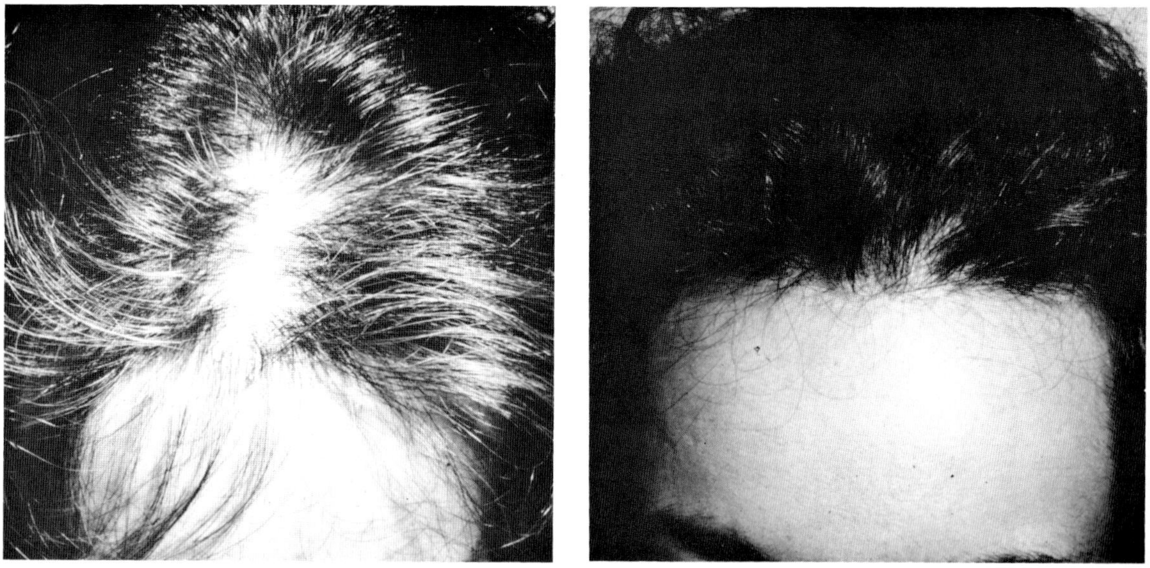

a b

Photo 72. **a** Frontal androgenic alopecia on a young woman before surgical correction. **b** After one session of mini- and micrografts

- The linear scar at the donor area is easily hidden by the hair.
- For the same number of grafts, the duration of the operation is much shorter than when grafts are taken with a motor-driven punch. On the other hand, this type of procedure calls for the aid of one or two assistants.
- Finally, even if some or all of the long-haired grafts should be rejected at the third or fourth week, the patient will nevertheless have benefited from temporary concealment of the operated zone during this period.

References

1. Alt TH (1984) Evaluation of donor harvesting techniques in hair transplantation. J Dermatol Surg Oncol 10: 799
2. Alt TH (1988) In: Unger WP, Nordstrom RE (eds) hair transplantation, 2nd edn. Dekker, New York, pp 145–209
3. Ayres S (1970) Hair transplantation. In : Epstein E (ed) Skin surgery. Thomas, Springfield, pp 453–508
4. Bouhanna P (1976) Le cuir chevelu. Les alopécies définitives et leurs traitements. Thesis, Paris
5. Bouhanna P, Nataf J (1976) À propos des transplantations de cuir chevelu. critiques et propositions. Rev Chir Esth 7(2): 17–23
6. Bouhanna P (1981) Considérations su le traitement chirurgical des alopécies masculines. J Méd Esth Chir Dermatol 29: 182–184
7. Bouhanna P (1982) The advantages of phototrichogram in hair surgery. The International Advanced Hair Replacement Symposium, Birmingham, February 3–4
8. Bouhanna P (1983)Study of the anterior frontal line in the surgical treatment of common male alopecia. The 4th International Congress on Dermatologic Surgery, Granada, October 2–5
9. Bouhanna P (1987) the phototrichogram: an objective technique used in hair replacement surgery evaluation. In: Unger WP, Nordstrom RE (eds) Hair transplantation, 2nd edn. Dekker, New York, pp 277–280
10. Bouhanna P (1989) Topical Minoxidil used before and after hair transplantation surgery. In: Vanneste D, Lachapelle JM, Antoine JL (eds) Trends in human hair growth and alopecia research. Kluwer, Boston, pp 257–263
11. Bouhanna P (1988) Grafts with immediate long hair (GILH). In: Transactions of the IX International Congress of Dermatologic Surgery, Edinburgh, September 25–28
12. Bouhanna P (1989) Topical Minoxidil used before and after hair transplantation surgery. J Dermatol Surg Oncol 15(1): 50–53
13. Bouhanna P (1989) Greffes à cheveux longs immediats. Nouv Dermatol 8(4): 418–420
14. Carrierao S, Lessa S (1978) New technic for closing punch graft donor sites. Plast Reconstr Surg 64: 455
15. Coiffmann P (1979) Use of square scalp grafts for male pattern baldness In: Unger WP (ed) Hair transplantation. Dekker, New York
16. Converse JM (1956) Vascularisation of skin autografts and monografts. Ann Surg 243: 306–315
17. Farber GA et al. (1972) Hair transplants for male pattern baldness. Long-term subjective evaluation. South Med J 65(11): 1380
18. Feit LJ (1969) Pathogenic classification of male pattern baldness. New innovation in surgical techniques. Int Surg 51(1): 58–67
19. Fujita K (1953) Reconstruction of eyebrow, Lepr Rev 22: 364
20. Goldman P (1985) Punch grafting the crown and vertex. J Dermatol Surg Oncol 11(2): 138–131
21. Hill TG (1980) Closure of the donor site in hair transplantation by a cluster technique. J Dermatol Surg Oncol 6(1): 190
22. Kassimir JJ (1987) Use of topical Minoxidil as a possible adjunct to hair transplant surgery. J Am Acad Dermatol 16: 685–687
23. Mac Leod N (1984) Sharpening method. In: Norwood OT Shiell RC (eds) Hair transplant surgery, 2nd edn. Thomas, Springfield
24. Mazzitt E (1984) Single hair transplantation for hairline refinement: a practical solution. J Dermatol Surg 10: 962–966
25. Morrison ID (1981) An improved method of suturing the donor site in hair transplant surgery. Plast Reconstr Surg 67: 378
26. Nataf J, Elbaz JS, Pollet J (1976) Étude critique des transplantations de cuir chevelu et proposition d'une optique. Ann Chir Plast 21(3): 199–206
27. Nataf J (1979) Special techniques of hair transplantation by fusiform grafts and flaps of many types. J Dermatol Surg Oncol 5(8): 620–624
28. Nataf J (1981) The flaps and navicular grafts in the surgical treatment of baldness. In: Orfanos CE, Montagna W, Stüttgen G (eds) Hair research. Springer, Heidelberg New York Berlin
29. Norwood OT, Shiell RC (1984) Hair transplant surgery, 2nd edn. Thomas, Springfield
30. Nordstrom RD (1981) Micrografts for improvements of the frontal hairline after transplantation. Aesthetic Plast Surg 5: 97–101
31. Okuda S (1939) Clinical and experimental studies of transplantation of living hairs. Jpn J Dermatol Urol 46: 135–138
32. Okuda S (1939) The study of clinical experiments and hair transplantation. Jpn J Dermatol 6/46: 135
33. Orentreich N (1959) Autografts in alopecia and other selected dermatological conditions. Ann NY Acad Sci 83: 463–479
34. Orentreich N (1971) Hair transplants: the punch grafts technique. Surg Clin North Am 51(2): 511–518
35. Orentreich N (1972) Hair transplants. NY State J Med 72(5): 78–82
36. Pierce HE (1973) Problems encountered with the strip graft hair transplant procedure. J Natl Med Assoc 65: 211
37. Rassman WR, Pomerantz MA (1993) The art and science of minigrafting. Int J Aesth Rest Surg 1: 27–36
38. Shiell RC, Norwood OT (1984) Micrografts and minigrafts in hair transplant surgery. Thomas, Springfield
39. Strum H (1984) The benefit of donor site closure in hair transplantation. J Dermatol Surg Oncol 10: 987
40. Tamura H (1943) Pubic hair transplantation. Jpn Dermatol 53: 76
41. Unger MG, Unger WP (1978) Management of alopecia of the scalp by a combination of excision and transplantation. J Dermatol Surg Oncol 4: 670–672
42. Unger WP (1979) Hair transplantation. Dekker, New York

43. Unger WP (1984) A new method of donor site harvesting. J Dermatol Surg Oncol 10: 524
44. Unger WP, Nordstrom R (1988) Hair transplantation. Dekker, New York
45. Vallis CP (1969) Surgical treatment of the receding hairline. Plast Reconst Surg 40(2): 138–146
46. Vallis CP (1969) Surgical treatment of the receding hairline. Plast Reconst Surg 44: 271–278
47. Vallis CP (1977) The strip graft method in hair transplantation. In: Epstein E (ed) Skin surgery. Thomas, Springfield, p 389
48. Vallis CP (1982) Hair transplant for the treatment of male pattern baldness. Thomas, Springfield
49. Villodres Ramos E (1986) Microinjerto de cabello. Piel 1(6): 19–22
50. Vissian L, Nataf J (1973) Advantages d'une technique d'implantation du cuir chevelu par greffons fusiformes. Bull Soc Fr Dermatol Syph 80(1): 65–67

Flaps

The surgery of flaps is a difficult technique requiring high technical skill from the surgeon and considerable experience in plastic surgery; errors are not forgiven and the penalty is often necrosis of the flap, However, the quality and rapidity of the result obtained by the flap technique when the indications are right, compared to those of graft cover, are such that the risks - minimal in expert hands - are amply compensated by the advantages.

After studying the principles of the technique, we shall consider the different type of flaps and their individual advantages and disadvantages. Of course, all the types of flaps described in plastic surgery can be used in the scalp, but in practice only long narrow flaps are of real value, especially when employed to cover frontal baldness, whereas alopecia of the vertex is more simply covered by reductions, which are often translation or rotation flaps, or by grafts.

In practice, since the grafts are raised in the temporo-parietal and occipital regions, they need to be long enough to cover the frontal region; also, as the elasticity of the scalp is reduced, they must be narrow to allow easy closure of the donor area [14].

General Principles of Flaps and Application to the Scalp

Definition

A skin flap is a unit comprising skin and subcutaneous tissues which can be transferred from a donor to a receptor site while preserving (for the time being or definitively) its vascular autonomy via its own pedicle.

Flaps of other types with different components are possible: purely muscular, musculo-cutaneous, fascio-cutaneous or compound (bone, cartilage etc.).

Classification

The different types of flaps can be classified in several ways:

1. In terms of their vascular anatomy [7]: this is the modern classification of McGregor and Morgan [43] into "conventional" or random flaps, and "axial" flaps. Conventional flaps, whose skin vascularisation is essentially ensured by the dermal and subdermal vascular plexuses, do not depend on a precise and macroscopically identifiable pedicle. The ratio of their length and breadth determines their viability.

   The so-called axial flaps include an arterial supply and venous drainage passing through a macroscopic vascular pedicle, the area of the flap being included in the autonomous vascular territory of its pedicle; these flaps may be used in the form of a peninsula, of islands and even as a free flap (Fig. 1).
2. In terms of whether their pedicle is permanent (the most usual case) or temporary (the nutrient pedicle being divided when the flap has acquired sufficient connexions with the receptor area).
3. In terms of their uni- or bipedicled nature (their migration being limited in the latter case).
4. In terms of whether or not they undergo preparation before transfer:
   - Flaps raised initially or in one stage (acute flap).
   - Flaps in several stages or delayed flaps, thanks to preliminary autonomisation by incisions of the margins and subsequent raising of the flap. Placement of an expansion prosthesis under the flap also constitutes the equivalent of autonomisation.
5. In terms of the movement they are subjected to:
   - The sliding or pure advancement flap (the "French" flap)
   - The rotation flap, stereotype of the Imre plasty [56]

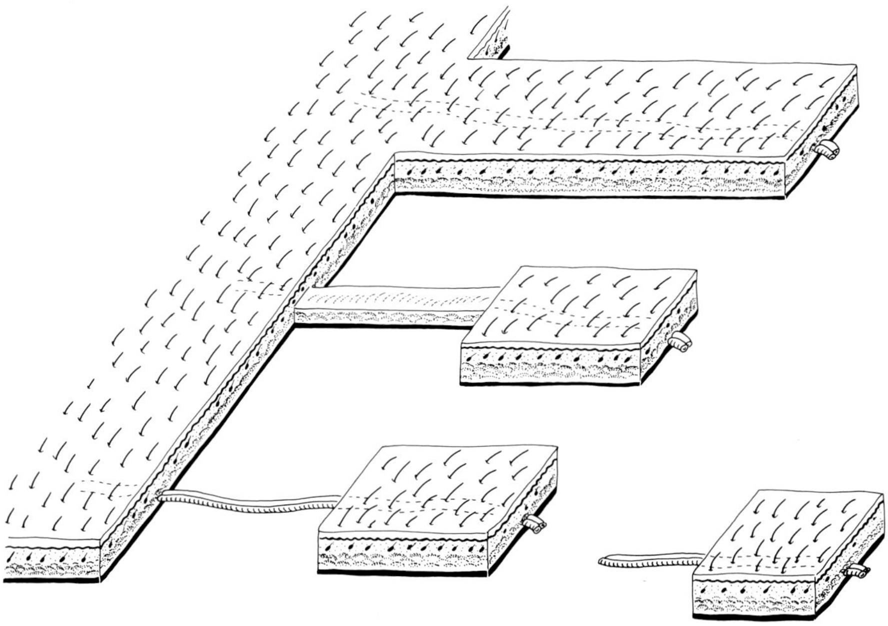

Fig. 1. Different types of flaps: peninsula, island, free flap

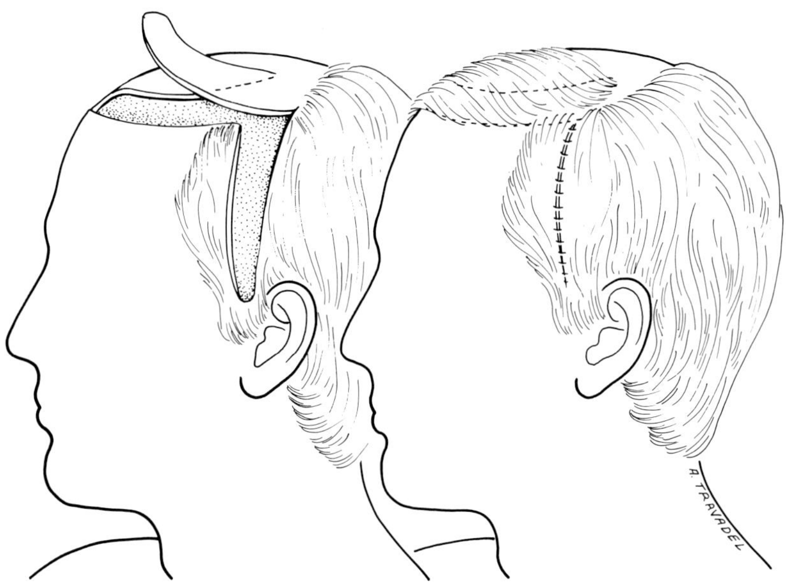

Fig. 2. Transposition flap

- Translation flaps, which are quadrilateral in shape (one of the sides being at the edge of the loss of substance) and which are tilted around their pedicle to create a narrow angle
- Transposition flaps, which resemble translation flaps, but their migration, instead of being adjacent to the loss of substance, straddles a portion of skin left in place. It will be seen that this type of flap is the one most used in the surgery of baldness (Fig. 2)
- Exchange flaps: Z plasty or the LLL plasty of Dufourmentel, which is actually a transposition flap using the excess of skin adjacent to the loss of substance. It is suitable for lozenge-shaped losses of substance.

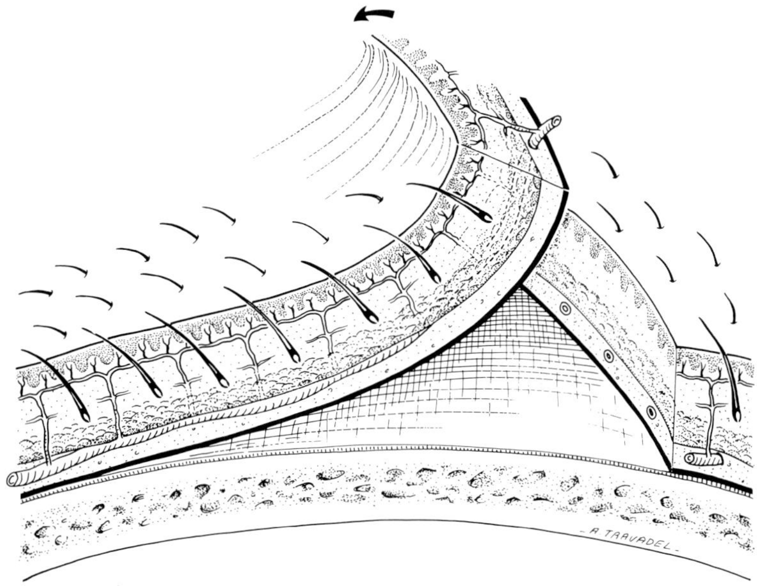

Fig. 3. Plane of stripping of scalp flap

Special Features and Application to Scalp Flaps

Scalp flaps usually have a useful skin island including the entire thickness of the skin (including the galea), so that their stripping is done in the subaponeurotic space of Merkel (Fig. 3). The particular anatomic and physiological features of the scalp produce certain constraints and some advantages in flap surgery [42].

Limitations

The poor elasticity of the scalp requires the use of flaps that are very extensive in relation to the zones to be covered, but their possibilities may be increased, either immediately, by slashing the galea to close the donor zone [25], or gradually, by insertion of a tissue expander, and these two procedures can be repeated. The particular shape of the skull often foreshadows possible deformation or reduced dimensions when the flap is mobilised, especially when it is intended for very convex regions such as the vertex.

Advantages

The vascular richness of the scalp allows the use not only of flaps based on the major pedicles (superficial temporal, occipital), but also of conventional flaps with considerable length to breadth ratios of up to 5:1 [4, 14, 23, 29]. Finally, the anatomic conditions (thick surface, firm support zone and strippable space of Merkel) are favourable to the placement of expansion prostheses.

Different Methods of Assessing Vascular Adequacy

The following methods of assessing vascular adequacy are available:

1. The simplest method of assessing vascular adequacy is to note the blanching at the extremity of the flap on digital pressure and the speed of capillary recolouration.
2. It is also possible to observe the extent of dermal bleeding at the end of the flap. This test is very valuable when positive, but is of no significance when negative because of the vasoconstrictor effect of the adrenalinised infiltration. However, these two methods are imprecise and give little information about the venous return.
3. The fluorescein test [39]. Dye is injected intravenously and after 20–30 min the tissues and vascular network are visualised under ultraviolet light. The method is precise and simple for assessing the circulation in the skin flaps at the time of injection of the medium.
4. Perfusion fluorometry [64]. The dose of dye is less with this method and the results can be read 2 min

after injection. Measurement of the tissue fluorescence is made with a luminous optical fibre, yielding an objective result in “fluorescence units”. This quantifiable method is more reliable and serial injections are possible.

5. Use of the laser Doppler to indicate blood-flow allows monitoring of the tissue blood-flow. This determines a value for the laser Doppler flow which indicates the number and speed of the erythrocytes and also a value for laser photometry by photoplethysmography [68]. The reading of the laser Doppler flow falls to a low level in response to arterial or venous occlusion. That of laser photometry does not change with arterial occlusion but decreases with venous occlusion, so that the two can be distinguished. This method is almost 100% reliable after 24 h.
6. Monitoring of the temperature is a simple method and very useful after digital re-implantations, but imprecise for assessing flap vitality.
7. Measurement of transcutaneous oxygen pressure (PO_2) [67] is a good test for assessing the adequacy of autonomisation procedures.
8. The vitality of the flaps can also be assessed by measuring the transcutaneous CO_2 pressure (pCO_2), the haematocrit and the blood pH.

Autonomised (Delayed) Flaps

Definition

Surgical interruption of part of the blood-supply of a flap during a preliminary stage of its transfer is called “preparation of the flap” (delayed flap). Its effect is to increase the possibility of survival of the flap (and therefore its length) and thus the chances of its successful transfer.

Mechanisms

The mechanisms are probably complex and debatable. It seems that they are involved in adaptation of the needs of the flap to the relative hypoxia created by the preparation, as well as the increase and orientation of the blood-supply of the prepared flap. There are several types of preparation of a flap:

- Simple incision of the margins of the flap: all sides at once (one-stage preparation) or at different times (e.g. incision of the two margins and then of the extremity, two operative stages)
- Combined with or followed by raising of the flap, which is replaced on its donor site with the possible interposition of a silastic sheet [47], which seems useful only when there are perforating vessels coming from the depth (scalp of the occipito-nuchal region; Fig. 4). However, it should be realised that preparatory raising of a flap has the disadvantage of increasing its thickness and reducing its laxity.

The stages necessary for preparation and severance of a flap depend very much on:

- The design and type of flap (delays are less useful for axial flaps)
- The localisation of the donor site (preparation more often needed for the lower limbs than at the face)
- The age of the patient (preparation more often necessary in elderly subjects)
- Assessment of the vitality of the flap
- Other factors, such as the presence of scars etc.

As for the time necessary for preparation, human clinical studies have shown that the maximum vascularisation is reached as a plateau at the end of the eighth day after preparation; from 2 weeks, return of the vascularisation of the flap develops with the onset of peripheral revascularisation, and at 3 weeks the vascular state is identical with that before preparation, with the same peripheral vascular connections.

Factors Influencing the Vitality of a Flap

Local Factors

Type and Site of Flap

Axial (vascular) flaps are more reliable provided their arteriovenous pedicle is respected and their territorial limits not transgressed [29–33], whereas so-called conventional flaps remain subject to the requirements of the ratio of the length of the flap to its width, which is theoretically 5:1 for the face and scalp, 3:1 for the trunk and 1:1 for the lower limbs [18].

Presence of Scars

The presence of scars may interfere with the blood-supply of the flaps. After 3 weeks, a normally sutured

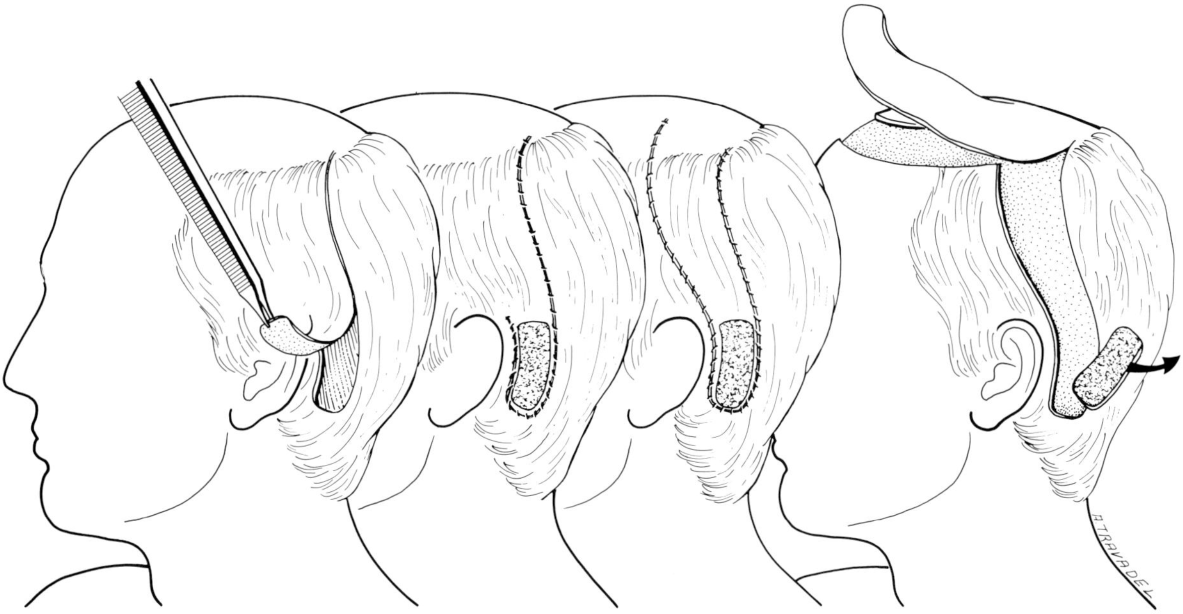

a b c d

Fig. 4a–d. Transposition after autonomisation of Nataf long retroauricular flap. **a** First stage: incision of posterior margin and apex of flap, stripping of apex between hypodermis and muscle plane, placement of silastic sheet, fashioning of apex of flap, replacement and suture. **b,c** Second stage: incision and suture of anterior margin of flap. **d** Third stage: transposition of flap; the silastic sheet is removed before suture of margins

linear incision is the site of revascularisation. On the other hand, the presence of multiple scarred areas, as after the taking of grafts, greatly compromises the blood-supply of the flaps.

Technical Factors

Besides the problem of delays, discussed above, and in the knowledge that placement of an expander is also a way of preparing a flap, several other factors may be involved in the vitality of a flap.

Traction–Torsion

Suture of a flap at the receptor site must always be made without tension. Similarly, plication of a flap or torsion of its pedicle may compromise its vitality, which explains why post-auricular flaps are more risky than pre-auricular flaps [18]. These two factors stress the importance of selecting the shape of the flap, the position of its pivotal point and the angle created by its mobilisation.

Compression

Compression of a flap or its pedicle by a pressure dressing, a haematoma (importance of drainage), oedema etc. may compromise its vascularisation and lead to partial necrosis.

Design

The design of the flap must be correct. It is especially important that it should not be too small.

Drugs

Numerous drugs have been proposed to improve flap survival, but there is little formal proof of their efficacy.

The application of dimethyl sulphoxide (DMSO) or minoxidil increases vascularisation of flaps. Anti-adrenergic agents (reserpine, guanethidine, phenoxy-benzamine) as well as beta blockers (propranolol) also increase the vascularisation of flaps.

Corticoids (prednisone, methylprednisone) given preoperatively and continued for 48 h afterwards, though reported as improving the vascularisation in the studies of Nakatsuka et al. [44], have not been objectively confirmed by the fluorescein test, the size of different flaps, radioactivity measurements etc.

Effects of Adrenaline Injection

Experimental study (essentially conducted in the rat and pig) shows that injections of saline, with or without lidocaine, do not affect flap survival, and that injections of adrenaline (1/100000, 1/200000 and 1/400000) do not have significant effects on survival (incidence of necrosis) of unprepared flaps, whereas they are significant in prepared flaps. However, recent studies seem to stress the value of adrenaline dosage, in that there is a great difference between doses of 1/100000, 1/200000, 1/400000 and that of 1/800000, particularly as regards the speed of reappearance of survival parameters (pO_2 and pCO_2, measurement of blood-flow) and their increase two- or threefold, whereas the haemostatic effects of adrenaline 1/800000 are the same. Thus, it is this last dilution that should be used in clinical practice. In man, it is therefore better not to use adrenaline with autonomised flaps and to use diluted doses for the same haemostatic effects.

Effects of Smoking

Clinical experience has shown that cigarette-smoking diminishes the survival of flaps, mainly through the effects of nicotine (increased degradation of prostacyclins and therefore increased vasoconstriction, especially in the micro-circulation). In our study, patients who smoked had an incidence of flap necrosis double that in the non-smokers (Table 1) [18].

Correlation with time (rat study) seems to indicate that the effects of nicotine are prolonged for up to 2 weeks and that this is the minimum period for cessation of smoking before the operation. Apart from this short-term effect, there is a chronic tobacco toxicity which provokes an irreversible degradation of the subdermal capillary network. Therefore, the simple measure of stopping smoking a few days before the operation seems inadequate.

Table 1. Effects of smoking on flap survival and outcome

	Necrosis + alopecia at 6 months		Good results		Total
	(*n*)	(%)	(*n*)	(%)	(*n*)
Smokers	9	25	27	75	36
Non-smokers	17	14	103	86	120
Total	26	16.5	130	83.5	156

Direction of Hair Growth

In the scalp, the direction of hair growth supplied by autoplastic coverage is a cardinal consideration (Fig. 2, chapter on "Anatomy", p. 3). At the forehead, it conditions the natural appearance and the visibility of the scar. Only forward growth will camouflage the scar, let alone obtain hair growth in front of it [7]. Furthermore, dressing the hair backward will give a more bouffant aspect.

At the back, the direction of the hair provided by transposition of a flap changes in relation to the remaining adjacent hair, producing a very visible parting. This is why the indications for flap procedures here are so difficult to state.

Description of Technique (Photos 1–10)

Preparation of Patient

The preparation of the patient is similar to the preparation used for major reductions. We use so-called heavy premedication: a suppository of secobarbital (120 mg) 45 min after the injection of 0.5 mg atropine and 0.5 mg alimemazine 90 min before the operation.

The design of the flap is made before the operation with an indelible felt pen, which allows shaving of the hair at the lines of incision. The patient is placed in the dorsal decubitus position, the head resting on a narrow support, which allows excellent access to the lateral and even posterior regions.

Sterilisation of the operative field is made by lavage with a quaternary ammonium compound (dilute Cetavlon) or an iodine derivative (Betadine), and then sterile towels are arranged under the patient's head and on the chest, while the entire face, which has also been prepared, is left exposed.

Anaesthesia

Local anaesthesia is usually used. The technique is very precise, as it has to contribute to the operative

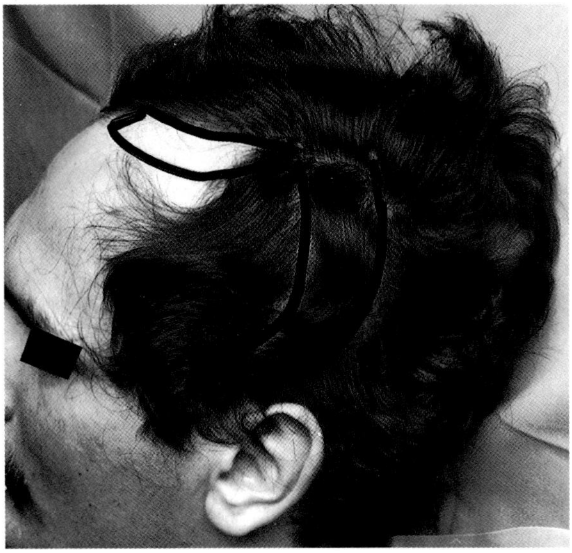

Photo 1. Design of vertical pre-auricular flap (Dardour)

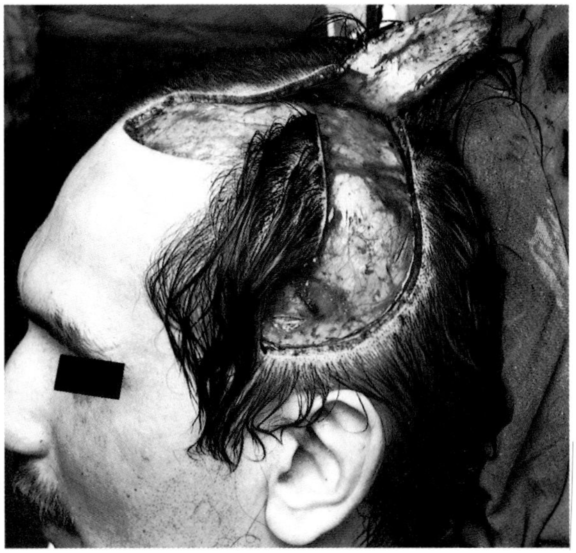

Photo 2. Excision of receptor zone and raising of flap

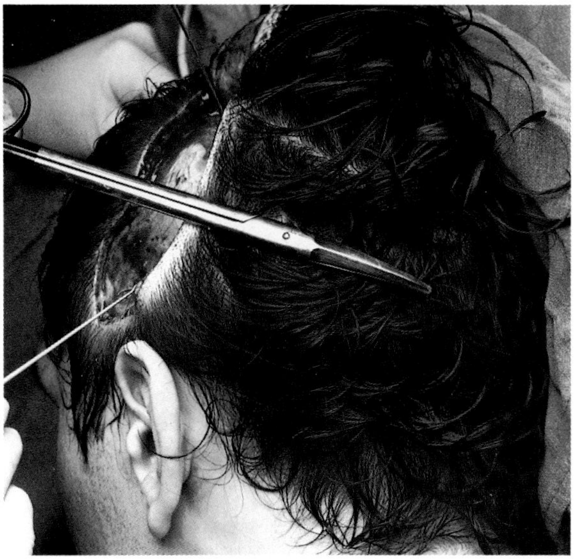

Photo 3. Posterior stripping must go to the point of the scissors

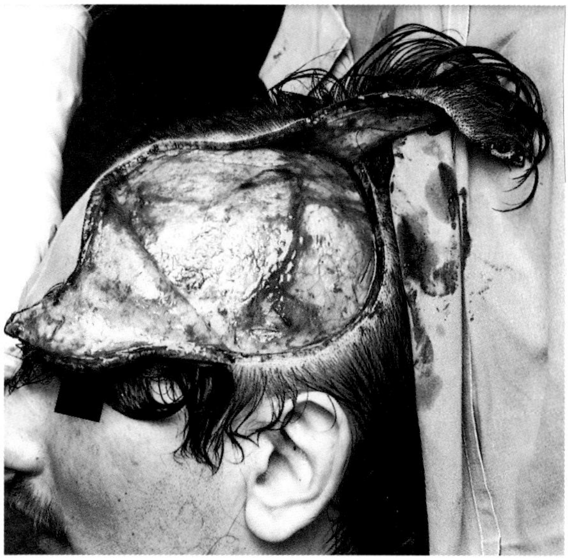

Photo 4. Anterior view of stripping

comfort of both patient and surgeon. We use 1% lidocaine with 1/100000 adrenaline, diluted to a half or third in normal saline; 40 ml 1% solution is adequate.

In the first stage, we perform a nerve trunk block of the supra-orbital, auriculo-temporal and occipital nerves and of C2 and C3 with an undiluted solution of lidocaine. We then perform coronal anaesthesia of the temporo-parietal region, circumscribing the flap and the zone of stripping. This infiltration is made with lidocaine diluted to a half or third in the plane of deep stripping under the galea.

The receptor site which must be resected is also infiltrated in the same plane. Finally, in a last stage, we perform a superficial infiltration in the supragaleal plane along all the incisional lines, which provides a virtually bloodless operative field. We do not hesitate to perform infiltration under the flap itself, since we do not believe that such infiltration endangers the flap; this is confirmed by the studies

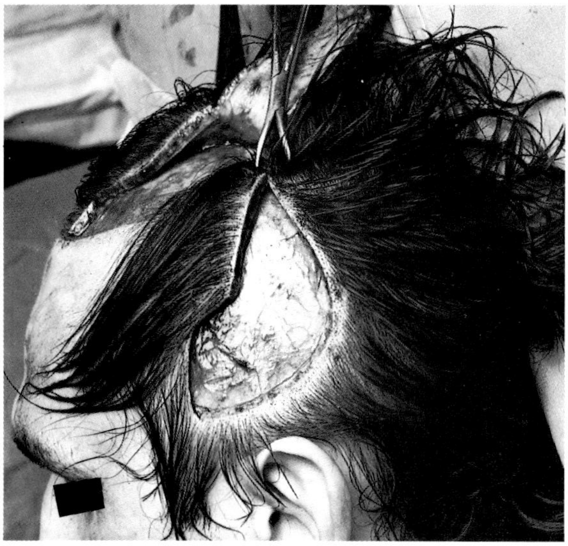

Photo 5. A towel clip is used to close the upper part of the donor zone

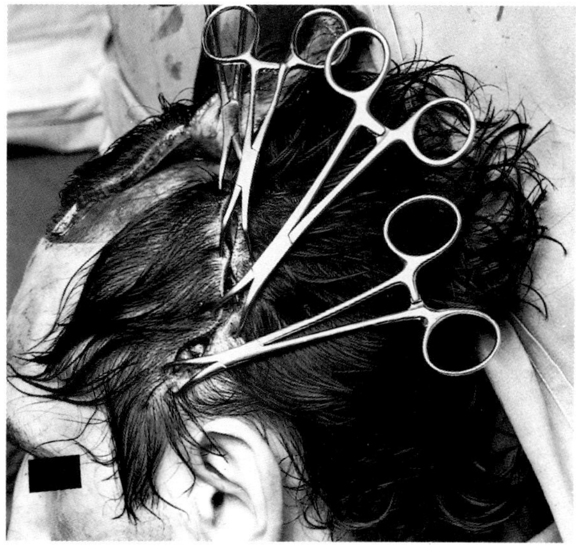

Photo 6. Three other towel clips complete the tacking

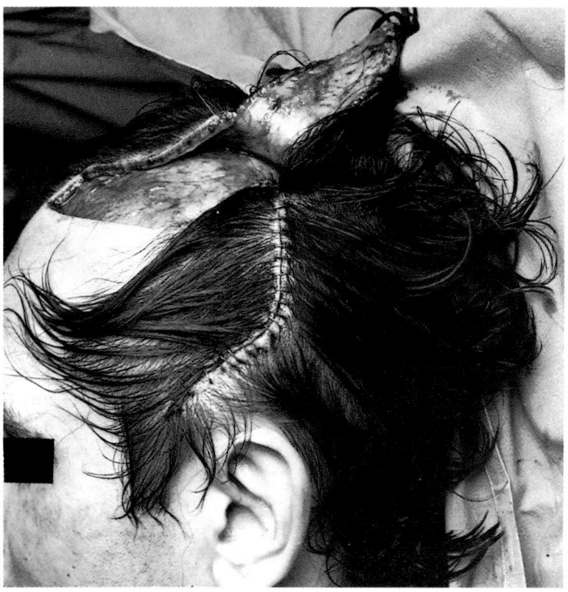

Photo 7. Closure of donor zone by staples

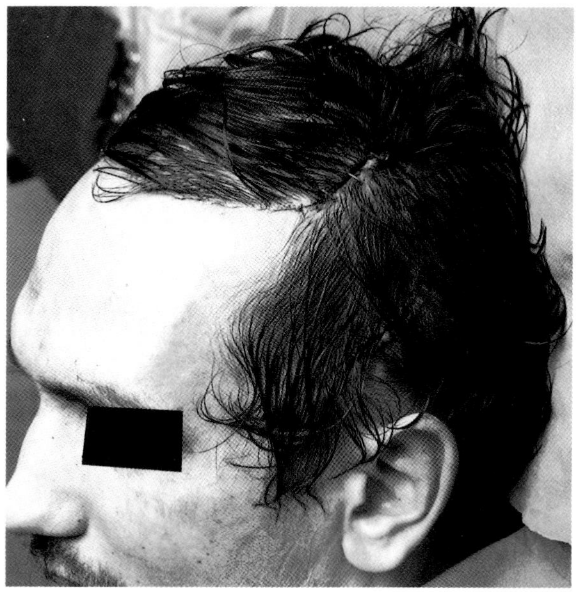

Photo 8. Positioning of the pre-auricular flap on the receptor site

cited above. On the contrary, we believe that such infiltration allows near-perfect haemostasis, which reduces the risks of haematoma and thus of necrosis.

Incision

The incision is made with the scalpel parallel to the follicles, i.e. in a direction varying with the region. Haemostasis is effected as the operation proceeds. The flap is then completely raised with scissors or scalpel. Bleeding at its extremity may be observed, but this test is of little value when negative because of the adrenaline infiltration. We then proceed to strip the margins, which must always be very wide, at least 8 cm on either side. This stripping is always made in the deep subgaleal plane, which is entirely bloodless. In the supra- and retro-auricular regions, the plane

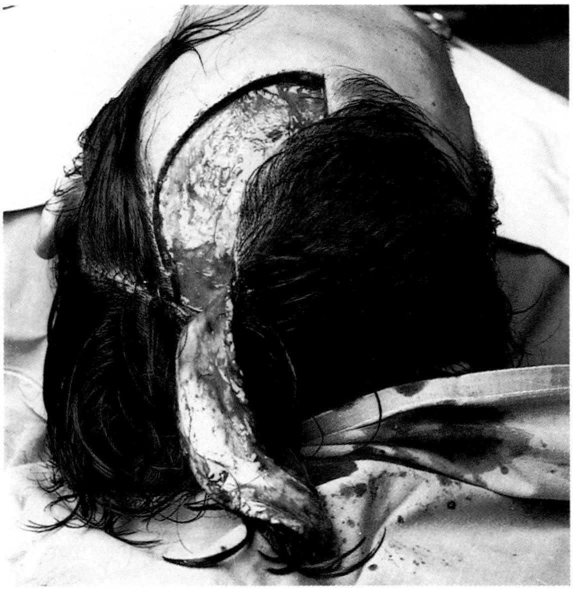

Photo 9. Superior view: the flap is raised and the receptor zone excised

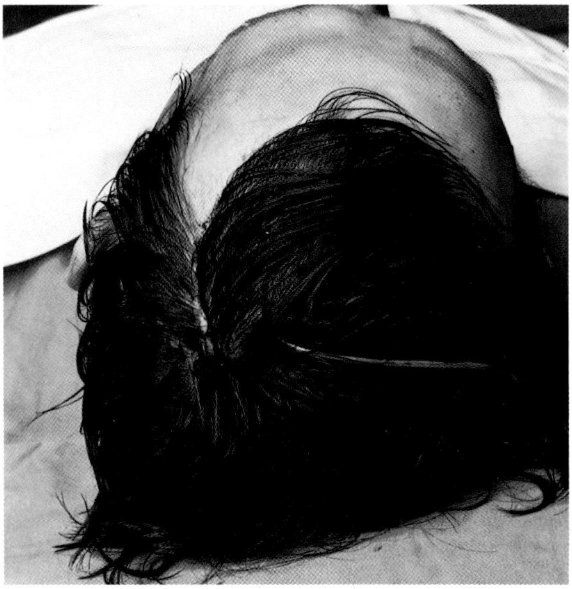

Photo 10. Superior view of flap in place: the hairs grow forward and the fronto-temporal recession is harmonious and deep

of stripping should always remain very deep, beneath the retro-auricular muscles, so as to avoid the perforating branches of the posterior auricular artery.

In the occipital region (solely for retro-auricular flaps), a change of plan is required in that part of the region situated at the external occipital protuberance, the stripping being made in a more superficial plane. The occipital vessels must be ligated here under observation.

When the wide stripping is completed, an attempt is made to close the donor zone. For this we use towel clips, which are not actually very traumatic, and tack the margins together very quickly. If the closure tension seems excessive, and in this case only, we perform galeotomies parallel to the lines of incision. To be effective these must be sufficiently deep and always require secondary haemostasis. Thus four towel clips temporarily close the donor zone and are immediately replaced by staples. We believe that closure in one layer is adequate and have shown in our statistics that the quality of this scar in the donor region depends only on tension. This quality can be greatly improved by the routine use of staples, but not by a second suture layer seizing the galea. Finally, we do not drain beneath the stripped donor zone, since the tension of closure on a spherical region prevents haematoma formation.

When the donor zone has been closed, the flap is positioned. It must be placed perfectly at the receptor site, avoiding all tension. This point is cardinal, since any distortion of the flap considerably increases the risk of necrosis. At the receptor site we advise excision of the smooth area rather than simple incision, as this allows better spreading of the flap, which in our view decreases secondary retraction of the flap and the risks of haematoma. The posterior margin is closed with staples in a single layer. The anterior margin, i.e. the frontal line, is closed with a continuous intradermal suture of 3/0 prolene. A suction drain is routinely inserted under the flap.

Dressing

Dressing consists of non-adhesive compresses and then absorbent pads held by a Velpeau bandage. The dressing should be firm but not compressive. It is retained for 24 h and removed the following day at the same time as the suction drain. The first shampooing is allowed on the second day and the patient is then asked to wash his head every day until removal of the staples on the ninth or tenth day. Any other local treatment is forbidden.

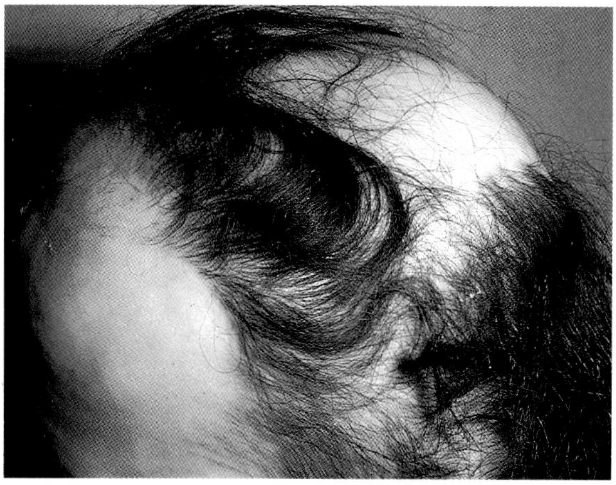

Photo 11. Alopecia of the anterior frontal line 7 years after transposition of a Juri flap due to continued alopecia

a

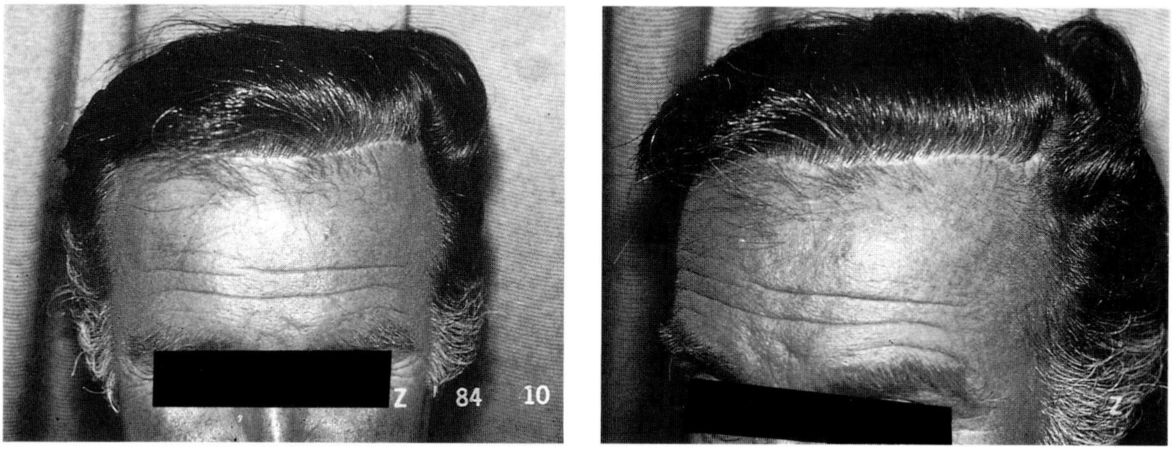

b

Photo 12a,b. Correction of baldness by Juri flap: the anterior scar is always visible because of backward hair growth

a

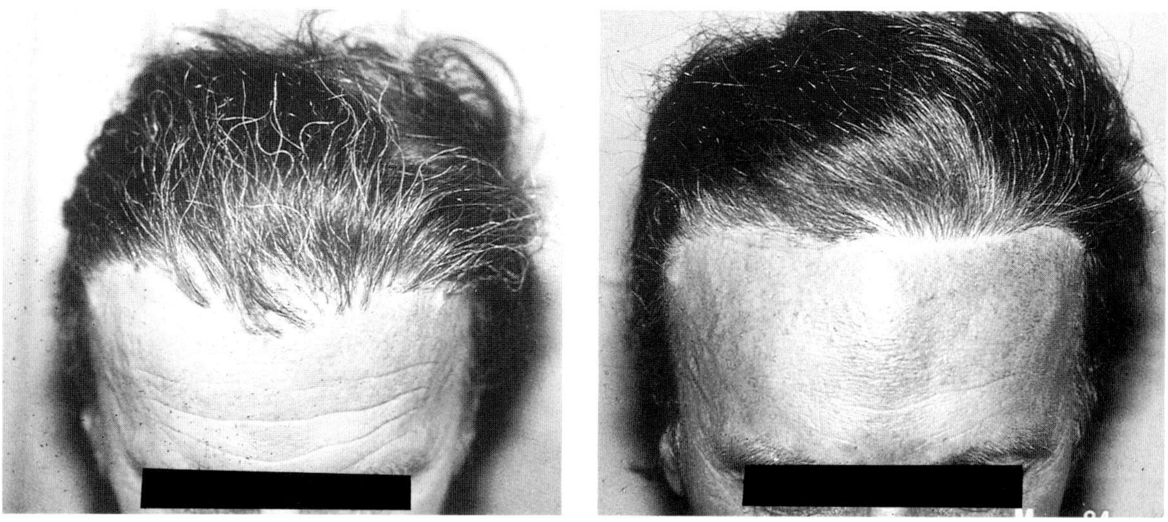

b

Photo 13a,b. Juri flap. **a** Placement behind autografts, unsatisfactory aspect. **b** Correction by excision of autografts, frontal lifting and harmonious reposition. The anterior scar remains visible since the hairs grow backward

Different Types of Flaps

Long, narrow transposition flaps are practically the only ones used in the surgery of baldness.

Inferior Pedicle Flaps

Flaps with an inferior pedicle are usually transverse flaps.

Advantages

They are centered on the superficial temporal artery, at least in their initial portion, which gives them the advantages of axial flaps, i.e. better reliability for equal length. The elasticity of the scalp being greater in the sagittal direction, they can be made wider (4 cm) than vertical flaps (3.5 cm).

Disadvantages

The upper border of the flap which will constitute the anterior frontal line is a zone where progressive hair loss of androgenic alopecia may continue. In this case, the reconstructed frontal line will be thinned to expose the anterior scar (Photo 11).

The 4-cm breadth of these flaps determines an amputation of the corona of more than one third (40% if HC=10 cm) and increases the breadth of the bald zone of the vertex.

Rotation of the flap by more than 90° creates a considerable "dog-ear", which often has to be tidied up subsequently.

The anterior frontal line thus created is usually straight. A second surgical stage is often needed to create deeper areas of fronto-temporal recession. However, the chief disadvantage of these flaps is the transposition into the frontal region of hairs which grow backward, leading to a visible frontal scar which, even when of good quality, attracts immediate attention (Photos 12, 13).

Superior Pre- and Post-auricular Flaps

Superior pre- and post-auricular flaps are flaps whose superior pedicle is situated in the temporo-parietal or parieto-occipital region, i.e. at the upper part of the crown. They do not therefore have an axial pedicle and survive only on the subdermal network, whose distribution is a matter of chance ("random flap"). These flaps are less richly vascularised than those with an inferior pedicle, whose origin is centered on a vascular pedicle, but they are no less reliable provided a different ratio between the length of the flap and the breadth of its pedicle is observed. In practice, only a randomised study of major series has allowed us to fix this ratio with maximum security. This has been determined in statistical terms and modified by certain risk factors which we shall discuss later.

Advantages

The main advantages of flaps with a superior pedicle compared with inferior pedicled flaps are:

- They allow easy provision of an anterior line and in particular of well-designed and natural fronto-temporal recession.
- They result in physiological implantation of the frontal hair, i.e. directed forward, whereas transverse flaps lead to a backwardly directed implantation whose appearance is always less pleasing. Often, this obliquity allows the hairs to traverse the frontal scar spontaneously (Photo 14).

The fact that they are raised over the entire level of the crown guarantees the absence of later balding of these flaps should the alopecic process continue. Only the pedicle of these flaps may possibly suffer such exposure, but this is a lesser evil, since this zone is set back from the apparent frontal line. The vertical raising of these flaps does not lead to amputation of the height of the crown and so does not accentuate the width of the bald zone at the vertex.

Disadvantages

Closure of the donor zone of a vertical flap is more difficult because, as we have seen, there is less elasticity in this direction, which calls for the raising of narrower flaps (between 3 and 3.5 cm) and often necessitates the performance of galeotomies to decrease the closure tension in the donor zone. The vertical orientation of the scar of the donor zone, parallel to the follicles at the crown, implies less satisfactory camouflage of this scar (Photo 6, chapter on "Surgical Techniques", p. 65).

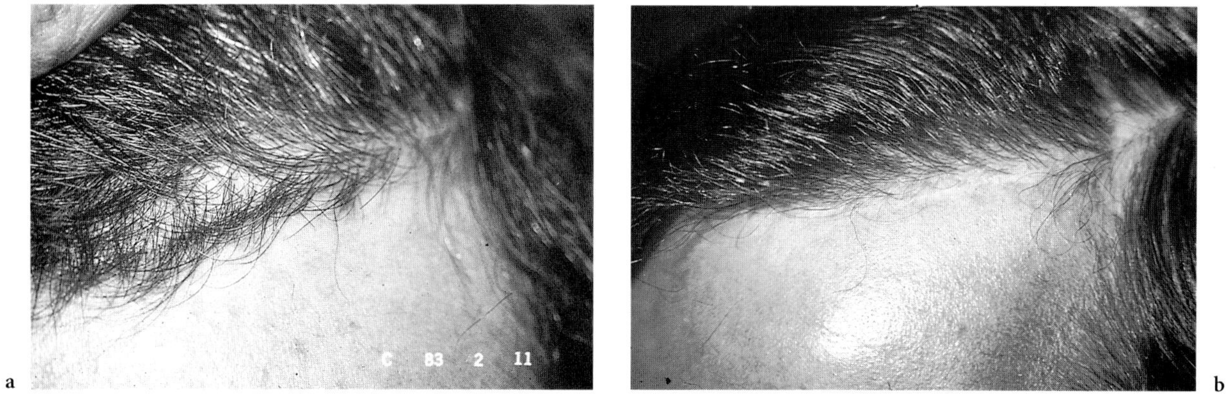

Photo 14. **a** Anterior scar after pre-auricular flap. Note that the hairs grow through the scar. **b** Pre-auricular flap: the anterior scar may be more obvious with stiff hair

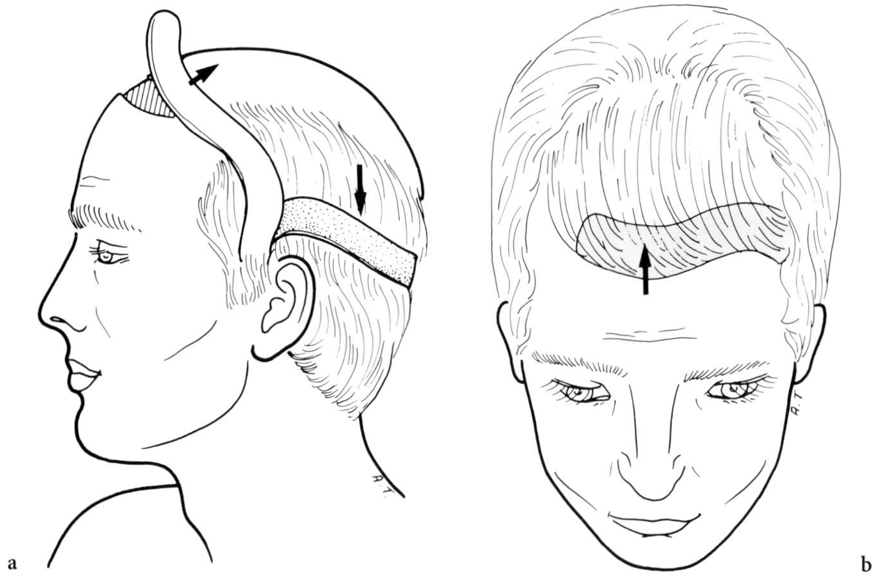

Fig. 5a,b. Passot flap. The *arrows* indicate the direction of the hair

Other Types of Flaps

Other types of flaps are not now used in the routine treatment of baldness, though they remain important in the treatment of alopecia due to other causes. We will now discuss flaps with an inferior pedicle and pre- and post-auricular flaps with a superior pedicle.

Inferior Pedicle Flaps

Transverse Flaps with an Inferior Pedicle

Surgical treatment by transposition of flaps with an inferior pedicle was recommended by Passot in 1920 [59] (Fig. 5). He described a transverse temporo-parieto-occipital flap with an anterior temporal

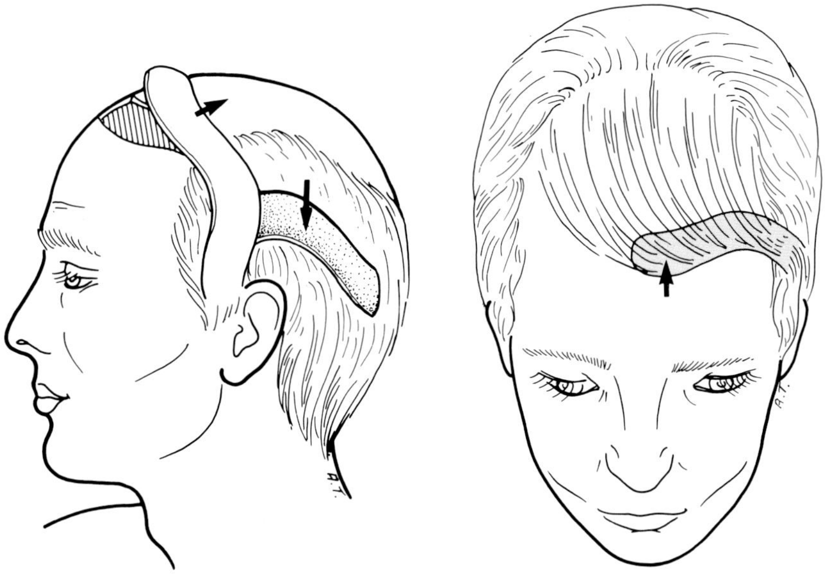

a b

Fig. 6a,b. Lamont flap. The *arrows* indicate the direction of the hair

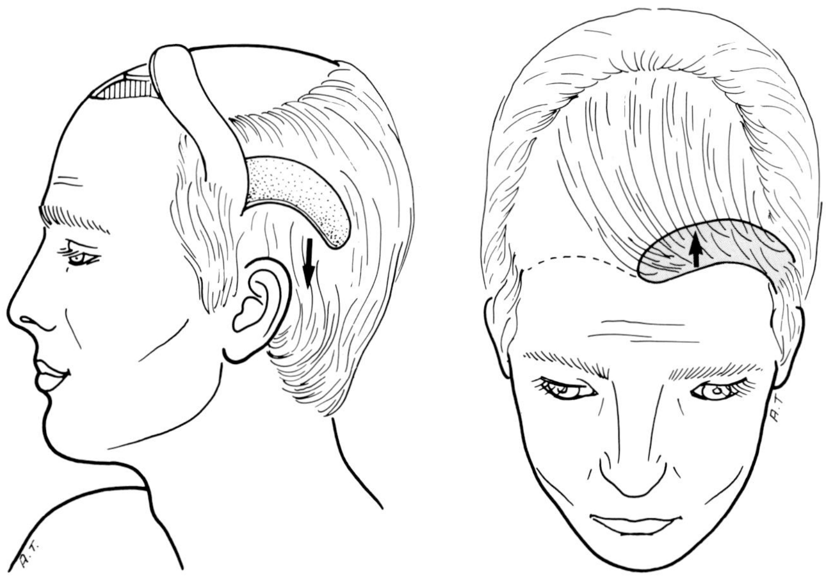

a b

Fig. 7a,b. Elliot flap. The *arrows* indicate the direction of the hair

pedicle, transposed to the frontal region, from which the flaps of Juri and Elliot were derived. This flap was transposed in one stage. In 1957, Lamont [38] advised transposition of two transverse temporo-occipital flaps with an anterio-inferior pedicle for the correction of frontal baldness. Autonomisation is performed 8 days before the transposition (Fig. 6). In 1977, Elliot [20–22] described a small transverse temporo-parietal flap with an inferior and anterior temporal pedicle, transposed without preliminary autonomisation towards the frontal region (Fig. 7). This type of flap is much smaller than that of Juri. Two small flaps are necessary to reconstruct the frontal line. Their management is easier since they are narrower and more flexible, and they do not need autonomisation.

Design of the Flap

The flap, 2.2–3 cm wide and 12–20 cm long, is designed to start from the same base as that described for Juri's flap. Its upper border runs parallel to and at some distance from the temporo-parietal limit of the crown.

Transposition of the Flap

Although transposition of this flap is simpler, the technique is similar to that described below for Juri's flap. The second flap, identical but contralateral, is transposed 3–4 months later. Some authors [35, 36] advise transfer of both flaps at the same time, but using very strict selective criteria.

Temporo-parieto-occipital Flap (Juri)

Published in 1975 [29], the temporo-parieto-occipital flap (Fig. 8) was the first technique to bring real progress in the surgery of baldness. Juri's flap is a transposition remarkable for its length (22–25 cm) and the narrowness of its pedicle (4–5 cm). This ratio can be explained by three factors:

1. A large part is centered at its origin on the superficial temporal artery.
2. The scalp is a particularly well-vascularised region.
3. The flap is performed after two preparatory stages of autonomisation.

The pedicle of the flap, 4–5 cm wide, is situated in the pre- and supra-auricular regions, centered on the superficial temporal artery. The flap then describes a curve with an inferior concavity situated in the middle part of the crown. It ends in the nuchal region, quite near the mid-line.

Design of the Flap

The anterior frontal line is designed following the usual rules set out above. The bounds of the flap are conditioned by the course of the superficial temporal artery, which is located by palpation or by some with the help of a Doppler type of detector. Such location is necessary only for the design of the proximal 3–4 cm of the flap. The lower border of the flap must begin at about 3 cm above the root of the helix. The upper border begins at 4 cm from this point along a straight line making an angle of 30°–45° with the horizontal. The base of the flap must be absolutely centered on the posterior branch of the superficial temporal artery. Two parallel lines 4 cm apart are drawn well away from the upper border of the crown. A type of compass with two pen-points can be used.

The length of the curves of the flap can be better determined by using a sort of rubber pattern. Usually, the length of the flap is 22–30 cm and corresponds to the length of the frontal line increased by 50%. The apex of the hairy frontal line is situated approximately between the second and third thirds of the flap. Thus, the last two thirds of the flap will become the frontal line, while the first third recreates a modified temporal line. It should be noted that the apex is the only part of the flap devoid of galea and that it remains on the supra-muscular plane.

Autonomisation of the Flap

Two sessions of autonomisation are made at 2 weeks and 1 week before transfer of the flap.

First Session of Autonomisation. The incision of the margins as designed, parallel to the hair roots, must be bold and deep down to the inferior part of the galea. Two parallel incisions are made and demarcate the proximal three quarters of the flap. Continuous suture or staple closure is done. This autonomisation procedure creates a bi-pedicled flap centered on the posterior branch of the superficial temporal artery and the occipital artery.

Second Session of Autonomisation. One week after the first session, the terminal 6–8 cm of the flap is incised. This portion is elevated above the supra-muscular plane. It is therefore essential to perform ligation of the occipital artery and haemostasis of the perforating vessels. The margins are sutured.

Comments on Autonomisation

These large flaps, whose length to breadth ratio is 7:1, require autonomisation. Some authors report the possibility of transfer of the flap after a single session of autonomisation or even without preliminary autonomisation at all [50, 51]. We believe that these operative procedures are nevertheless hazardous for such large flaps because of the great variability of the arterial network and especially of its quality. The

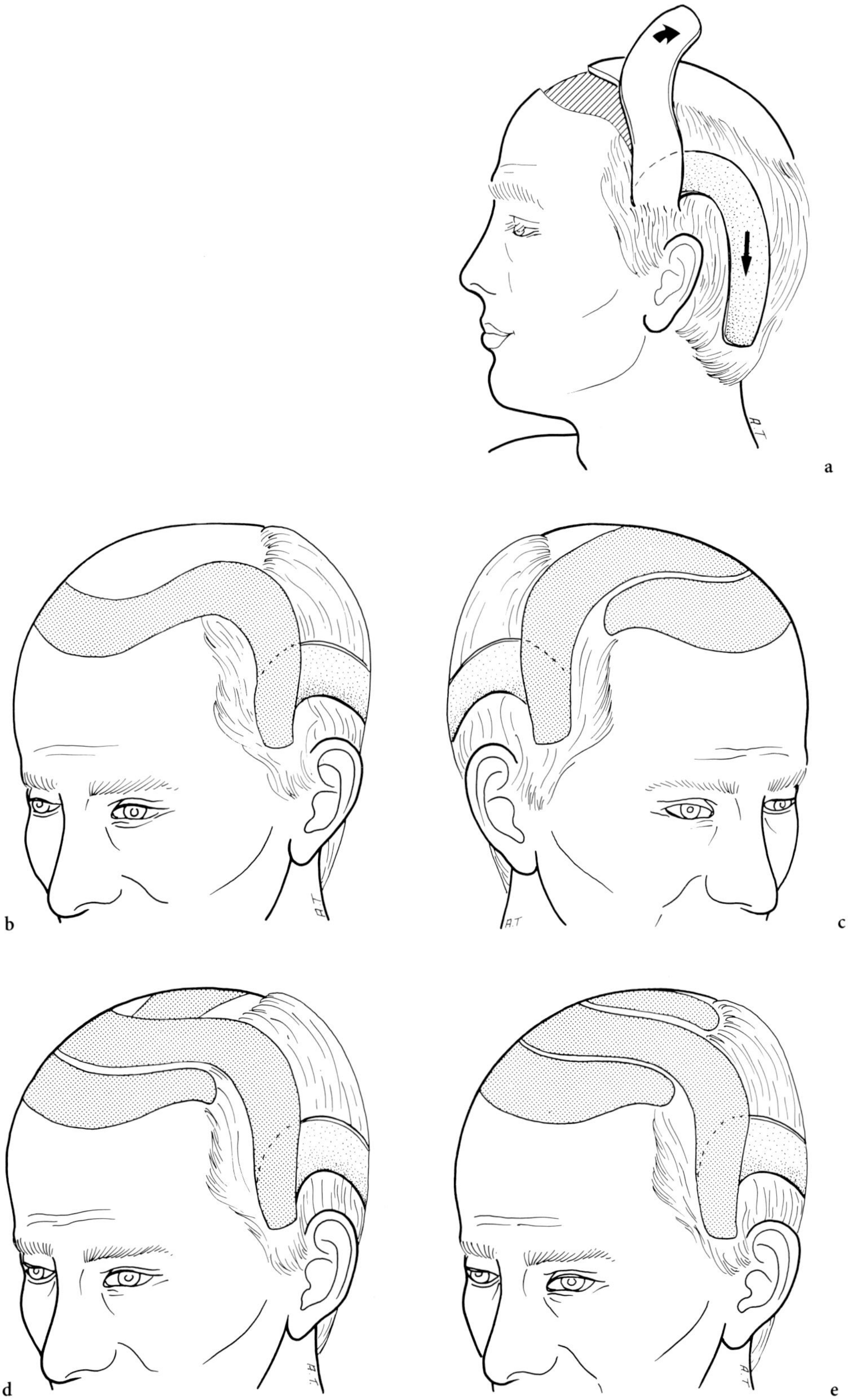

Fig. 8. **a** Juri flaps. **b** First flap of Juri. **c** Second flap of Juri. **d** Third flap of Juri. **e** Fourth flap of Juri (variant)

torsion of this flap during its transfer will further compromise the adequacy of the blood-flow. In fact, the sole aim of autonomisation is to allow proper vascularisation of the last third of this flap, considered as a random flap.

Transfer of the Flap

Transfer of the flap is performed under general anaesthesia with supplementary use of local vasoconstrictor anaesthesia. After elevation of the flap, the parietal scalp is completely stripped at the subgaleal space. Posteriorly, the stripping passes above the supra-muscular plane and then continues into the neck in a subcutaneous plane. The retro-auricular skin of the ear lobe is also stripped. The donor zone is then closed with suture in two layers. Some authors advise epidermal denudation of the anterior edge of the flap over a breadth of 1 mm. This procedure would allow the hairs to traverse the scar, giving a more natural appearance to the anterior line. (It is difficult to conceive that the hairs growing from the flap with a backward orientation can traverse an anterior scar.) The flap is sutured to the receptor site by monofilament material or staples, after excision of the excess of smooth skin, whose breadth is usually less than that of the flap. The frontal line is sutured by interrupted sutures with monofilament 5/0. A suction drain is inserted at the stripped zone of the neck. Two or three small drains are placed beneath the flap and between the sutures. A non-compressive dressing should be applied, avoiding compression of the ear, which forms the origin of the flap.

Incidents and Complications

The incidents and complications are common to all flaps:

- Oedema and ecchymosis of the forehead and eyelids disappear in 3–8 days.
- The "dog-ear" at the origin of the flap shrinks in 6 weeks, but often minor surgical correction is needed.
- Wide dehiscence of the donor zone is due to taking an excessively wide flap which requires closure under tension.
- Necrosis of the distal portion of the flap in the 6–10 days following operation has not been quantified in any statistics.

Two Other Flaps of Juri (Fig. 8b,c)

The second flap of Juri is made on the other side 3–4 months after the first. Its design is identical with the former but is raised higher up, at the crown. The autonomisation is similar, but its transfer is easier. It is placed 4 cm behind the first. Excision of the smooth zone is made in a second stage. The third flap of Juri allows coverage of the vertex, but its author

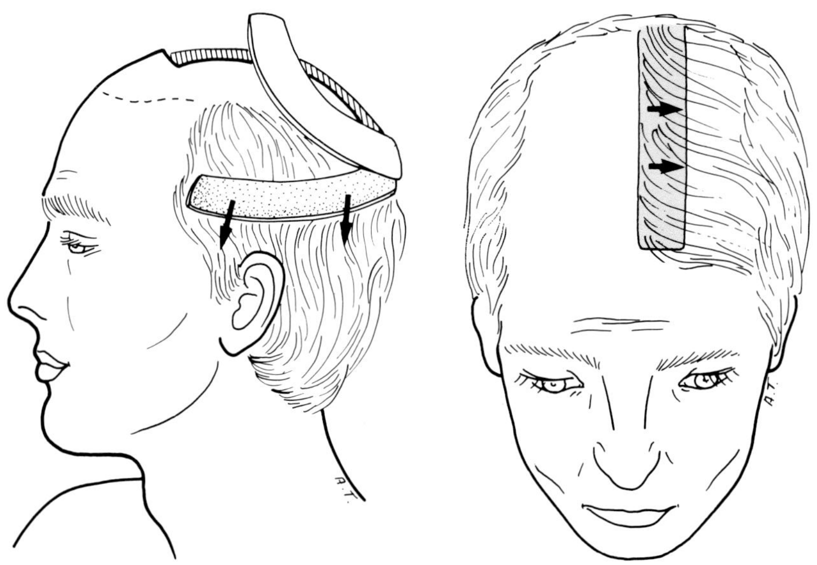

a b

Fig. 9. **a** Passot flap with superior pedicle. **b** Passot flap prefers the practice of vertical reduction and grafting to correct this region.

Superior Pedicle Flaps for Frontal Cover

Passot Flap (Fig. 9)

The first flap with a superior pedicle was also described by Passot in 1920 in the same article [59]. The pedicle of this flap is situated in the upper part of the crown, well posterior and near the external occipital protuberance, in such a manner that this flap, unlike other superiorly pedicled flaps, is almost entirely transverse. This flap is transposed sagittally to the mid-line.

Pre-auricular Flap of Nataf

The pre-auricular flap of Nataf was described in 1976 (Fig. 10) and revived by Bouhanna in his thesis [4, 5]; it is actually the first flap with a superior pedicle intended for reconstruction of the anterior frontal line. It is a vertical temporo-parietal flap with a superior pedicle. Its pedicle is situated at the upper part of the corona, 3–4 cm behind the line of the temporal muscle attachment. The width of the flap at its pedicle is 2.5–3 cm. The flap is slightly concave backward and ends vertically at the sideburn in front of the ear. Its average length is 12 cm. The author describes this flap in three stages, with two stages of autonomisation preceding its final placement; these are performed at 3-month intervals. However, the

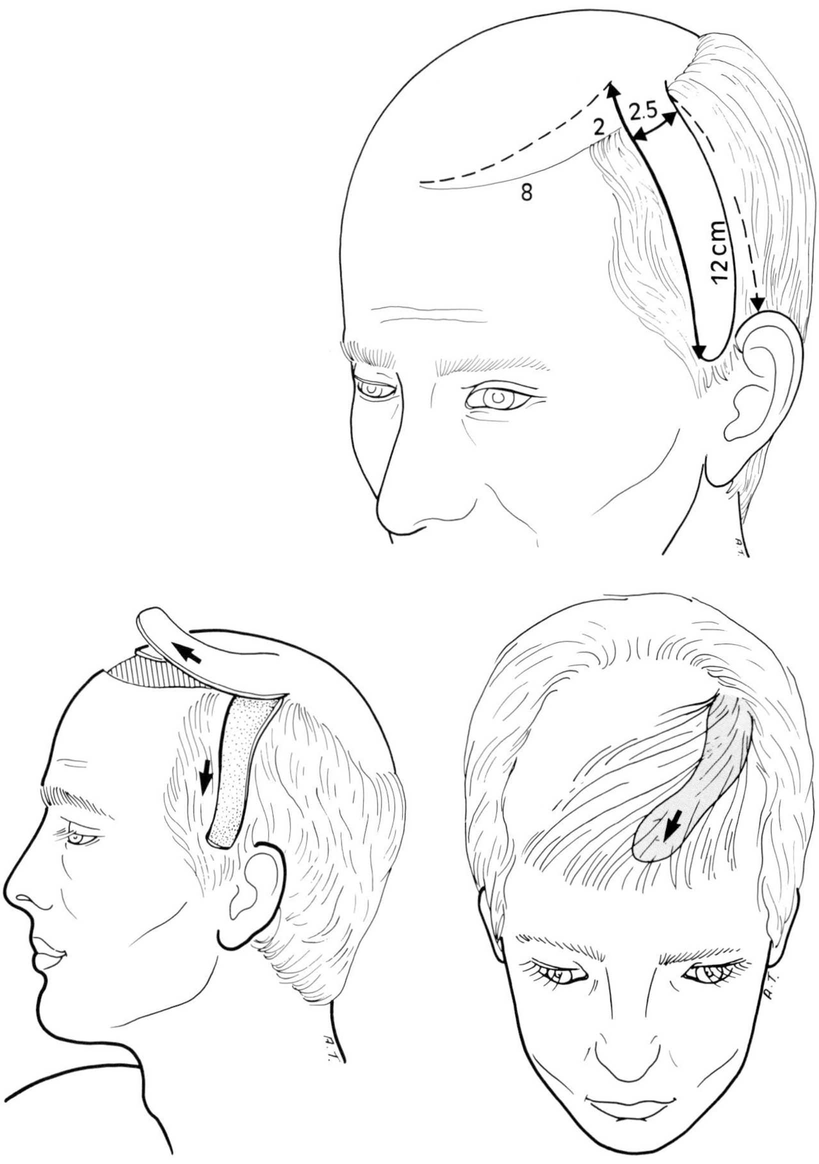

a

Fig. 10a–c. Nataf flap b c

article mentions that in certain cases autonomisation is unnecessary.

However, this flap, original in conception, presents certain disadvantages:

- The area of the scalp transposed is small, between 30 and 33 cm^2.
- The extremity of the flap being tapered, it supplies very few hairs at the mid-frontal line.
- The quality of these terminal hairs is sometimes mediocre, as they may derive from the sideburn itself in which the flap terminates, and this is a transitional zone where the beard has often already replaced the scalp hair.
- The direction of the flap remains parallel to the axis of the hairs when the flap is positioned, so that the hairs grow toward the opposite side and not forward; this may be a nuisance when a second and similar opposite flap is performed.
- Lastly, the shape of the flap with a backward concavity and its direction of rotation implies that, when it is positioned at the receptor site, the longer side becomes the shorter and vice versa, which always leads to a considerable "dog-ear".

Bouhanna [1] has suggested a flap with a straight upper pedicle (Fig. 11), oblique downwards and forwards. The dimensions are identical to those of the above-mentioned flap (12 × 3 cm). The extremity, 2.5 cm wide, is square on its inner side and rounded on its outer side in order to allow better adaptation with the contralateral flap; in practice, this flap has been proposed as a possible supplement to the flap described by Dardour, with which it intermeshes.

Retro-auricular Flap

The retro-auricular flap is described in the same article (Fig. 12):

- Its pedicle is slightly posterior in relation to the preceding one.
- The length of the flap is therefore greater, about 17–18 cm.
- Its breadth is 2.5 cm.
- Its shape resembles an italic "*S*" with its first segment convex forward and its second segment concave forward, and it ends vertically in the retromastoid region.

As for the previous flap, the author advises two preliminary autonomisation stages but records the possibility of a single-stage procedure. These two flaps reach the mid-frontal line when they are positioned.

Long Retro-auricular Flap of Nataf and Bouhanna

First described in 1984 [8, 47], the long retro-auricular flap of Nataf and Bouhanna has the same shape as the previous one (Fig. 13). Its pedicle is situated above and behind the ear, sometimes therefore above the crown. The flap is initially directed down-

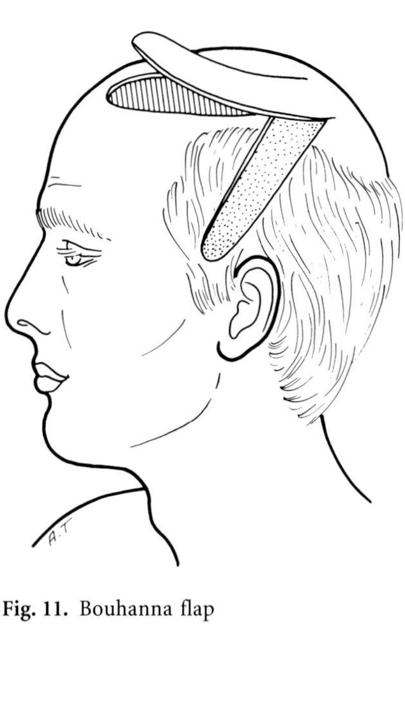

Fig. 11. Bouhanna flap

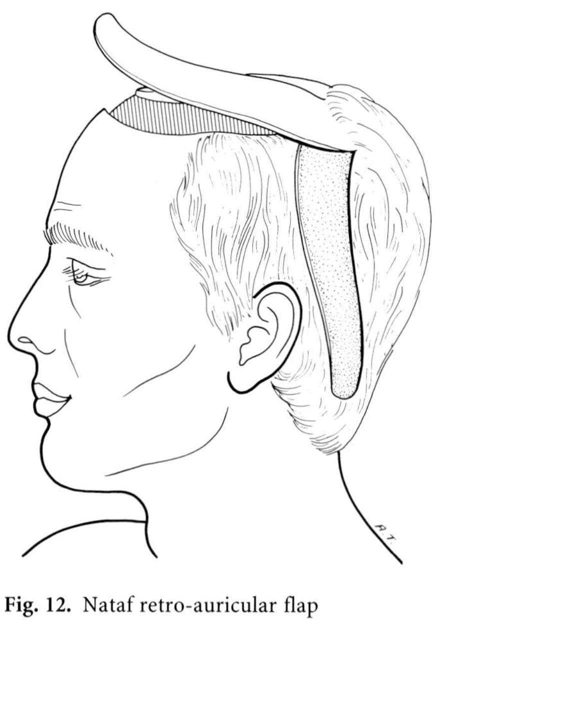

Fig. 12. Nataf retro-auricular flap

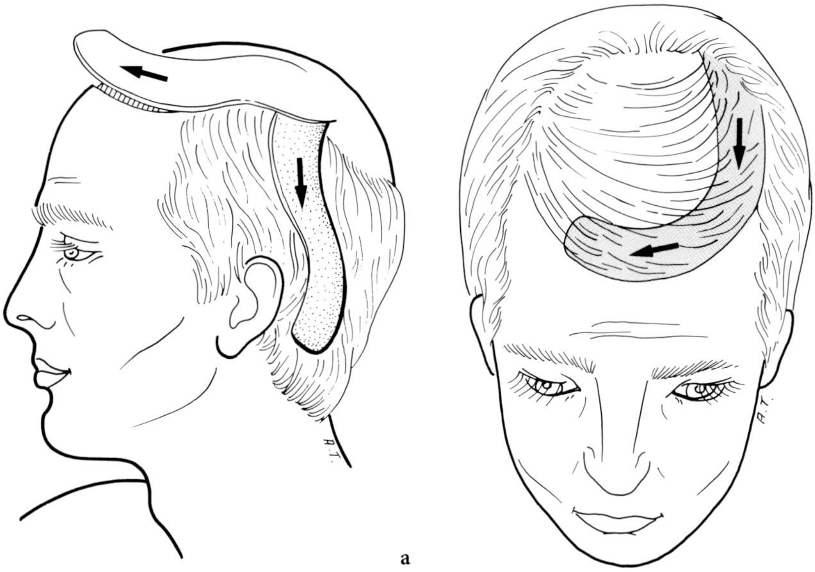

a b

Fig. 13a,b. Long retro-auricular flap (Nataf and Bouhanna)

wards and forwards and then curves backwards to descend behind the ear. In all, this flap is 22–24 cm long and 3 cm wide. Given the length of the flap, two autonomisation stages are always needed during its preparation.

Of course, the value of this flap lies in the fact that, once put in place, it transgresses the mid-line by 3–4 cm, which obviates any need for a contralateral flap. However, the author has never published any statistics on the results of this very long flap of at least 22 cm. Therefore there remains a doubt, especially as regards the incidence of necroses to which this technique may lead. It is true that this flap provides a more extensive hairy area in front, of the order of 60–70 cm^2, but it is always quite narrow, which facilitates closure of the donor site. Actually, this is not really a criticism, if one considers that it is often necessary to perform grafting behind the flap. The shape of the flap seems much more open to criticism, since it is globally concave towards the back, whereas, once in position, this curvature must be reversed. We have already seen that this produces a very large "dog-ear" at the origin of the flap which always has to be surgically dealt with subsequently.

Pre- and Retro-auricular Flaps of Dardour

The pre- and retro-auricular flaps of Dardour were described in 1983 [15, 18] and have a concave shape which avoids the disadvantages.

Pre-auricular Flap

The pre-auricular flap is the most commonly used since it is safer and easier to perform (Fig. 14, Photo 15). Its pedicle is situated more or less vertical to the ear in the upper parietal region. The most anterior line of incision is situated about 4 cm behind the line of the temporal attachment. The breadth of the flap at the pedicle is 3.5 cm on average. It may reach 4 cm when the elasticity is excellent or be as little as 3 cm when elasticity is mediocre. Such a flap, if it is to reach the mid-frontal line, must measure between 14 and 16 cm on average. It will be shown that this size provides maximal security. Based on this pedicle, the flap comprises two more or less equal segments. The first is vertical and the second transverse, of such a nature that it terminates above the ear 1–2 cm behind the lower part of the temporal line. The extremity of the flap is almost square, with a breadth of 2.5 cm.

Advantages of the flap include the following:

- As the hairs are parallel to the flap in its first part and perpendicular in its second part, when the flap is positioned on the forehead they all remain directed forward throughout its extent, which allows natural reconstruction of the frontal line.
- The extremity being square and sufficiently large, the amount of hair transposed to the mid-frontal line is considerable.
- The anterior flap of the donor zone is rectangular and not tapered, which makes it less fragile. The

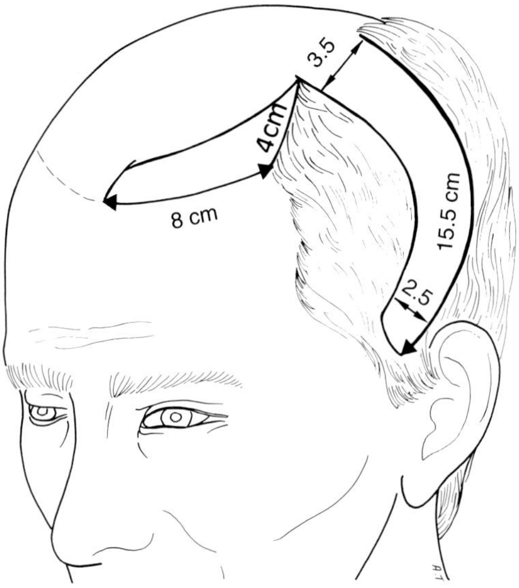

a

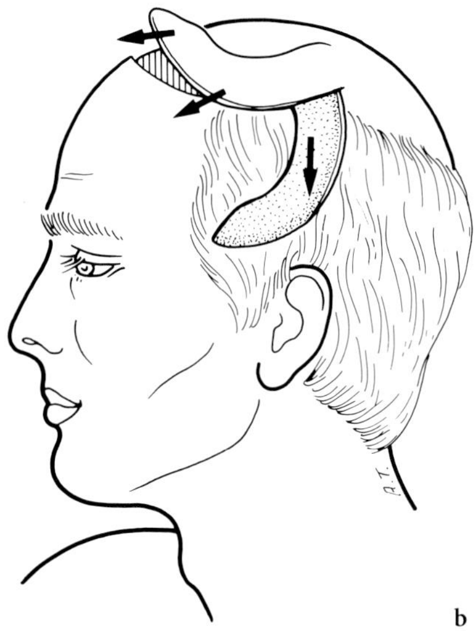

b

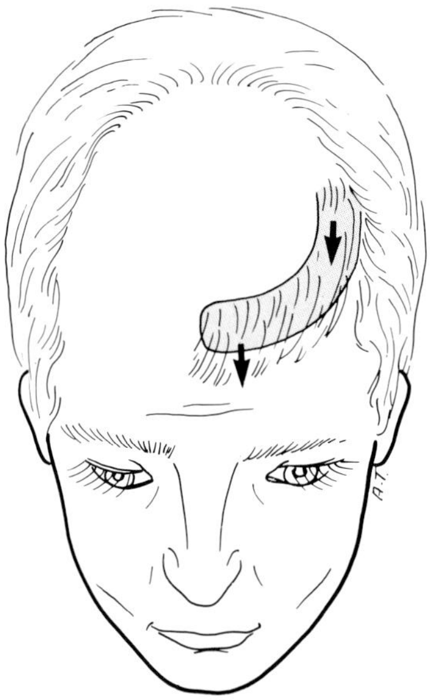

c

Fig. 14. **a** Pre-auricular flap of Dardour. **b,c** Pre-auricular flap. *Arrows* show direction of hair

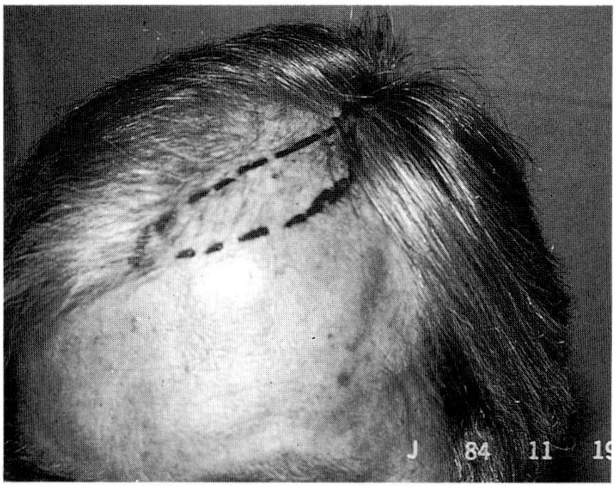

a

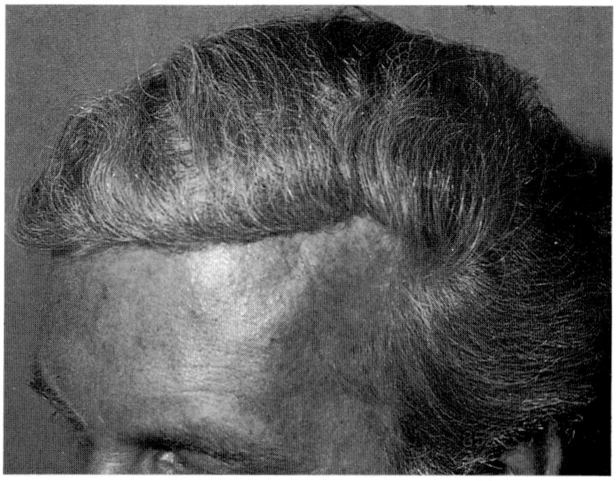

b

Photo 15. **a** Frontal baldness. **b** Correction by Dardour pre-auricular flap in one stage

design of the flap has exactly the shape of the receptor site and there is therefore no distortion and no "dog-ear" at its origin and certainly less risk of necrosis.
- Lastly, this flap transfers on average between 45 and 55 cm² of hairy area.

Closure of the donor site does not lower the crown, but it displaces the upper extremity of the anterior temporal line of insertion backward by 0.5–1 cm, which is usually negligible. However, when the line of temporal insertion is very posterior (t=3), and in these cases only, we advise the use of the retro-auricular flap.

Retro-auricular Flap (Fig. 15, Photo 16)

The pedicle of the retro-auricular flap is slightly posterior compared to the pre-auricular flap. The length of the flap is therefore greater on average (18 cm). Its breadth is the same, 3.5 cm on average, and its shape is still concave towards the front. However, the initial vertical segment is considerably longer than the second segment, which ends obliquely downward and forward in the retro-mastoid region. The angle of rotation of this flap for its positioning is greater than in the previous flap. Thus it forms a larger dog-ear at the origin of the flap, which sometimes – but not always – requires secondary resection. Because of its major length and torsion, this flap is less reliable than the pre-auricular flap, as confirmed by our statistics; it should therefore always be made after two autonomisation stages.

Vertical Mini-flaps of Dardour (Fig. 16)

Based on the same principle as the previous flap, these flaps differ in their shape and size. Their use is reserved for patients with simple fronto-temporal recession; the precise indication is discussed in the

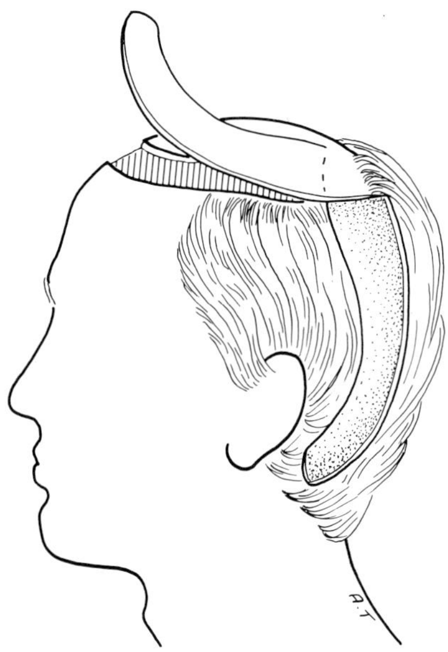

Fig. 15. Dardour retro-auricular flap

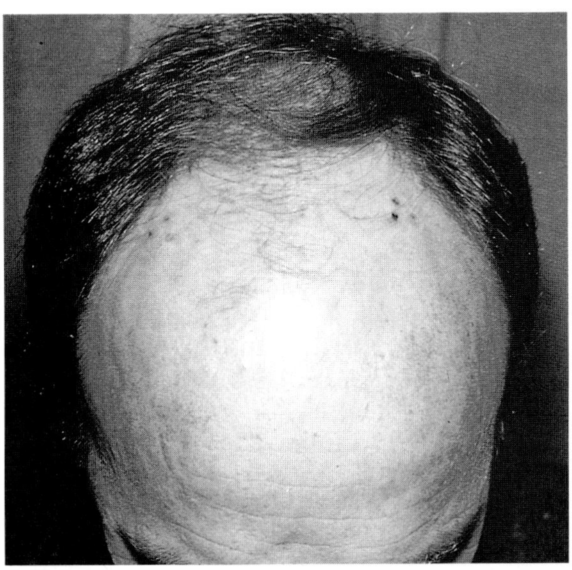

a

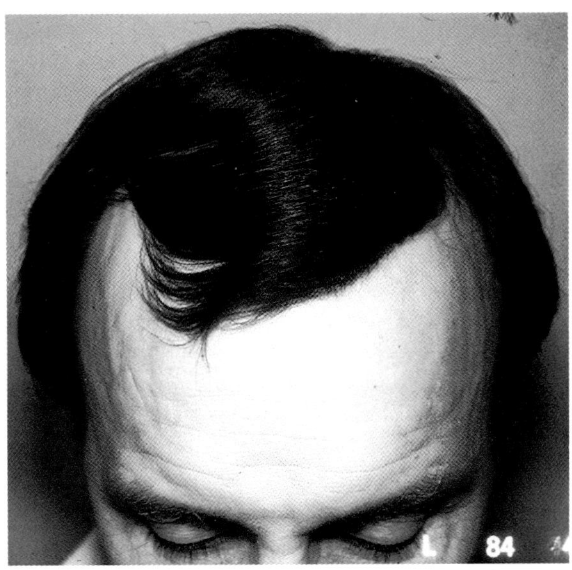

b

Photo 16. **a** Baldness grade F4 T4, H=13 cm. **b** Result after retro-auricular flap

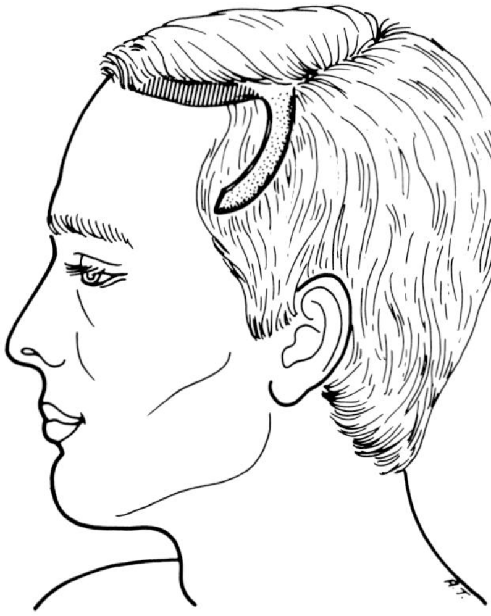

Fig. 16. Dardour mini-flap

chapter on "Operative Indications" (p. 189ff.). The baldness does not reach the mid-frontal line in these patients, and the flap can terminate 2 cm before it. As the implanted hairs always remain in the axis of the flap, this is therefore fashioned strictly vertically. Its breadth is 2 cm and its extremity tapered. Such a flap remains very reliable if its length does not exceed 10 cm. This implies that its pedicle is situated very far forward, the residual scar of the donor zone being situated 2 cm behind the temporal line of insertion.

Closure of such a flap is naturally very easy, provided very extensive posterior stripping has been done, in order to avoid recession of the temporal line as far as possible. This mini-flap allows perfect and very rapid filling of a slightly recessed fronto-temporal area (stage 1). Both sides can be done at a single stage, but our tendency is to advise the patient to have two procedures.

Vertical Flaps of Bouhanna

The vertical flap of Bouhanna, a mixed occipital flap with a superior pedicle [10] described in 1990, is derived from the flap of Passot (Fig. 17a,b). The author has introduced modifications of size and site at the receptor zone for reasons of reliability and cosmetic appeal and for a more rational planning of the indications. Its pedicle is situated more or less at right angles to the mid-occipital line. It is 16 cm long and 3.5 cm wide on average. This flap is concave towards the front and comprises two segments, the first vertical and the second almost transverse, ending above the ear. Its extremity is almost square and 2.5 cm broad. The shape and dimensions of this flap are similar to those of Dardour's flap, and it possesses the same advantages but at the vertical level.

Straight Occipital Flap with Superior Pedicle

The straight occipital flap with a superior pedicle was described as possibly complementary to the previous flap, with which it can be intermeshed. Its design and dimensions are similar to those of the straight frontal flap. Its pedicle is situated at the sagittal line, 7–8 cm above the inferior occipital line of hair insertion. It is on average 12 cm long and 3 cm broad. This flap, almost straight, necessarily terminates behind the auricular line. Its extremity is square on its inner side and rounded on its outer side (Fig. 6b, chapter on "Operative Indications", p. 199). The flap, concave towards the front, with a superior occipital pedicle, is transposed backwards at the vertex. Its pedicle is situated at the upper part of the crown, vertically above the external auditory meatus (Fig. 18).

Statistical Study of Two Types of Superior Pedicle Flaps (Dardour)

Between 1976 and 1986 we always performed flaps in a single operative stage. This gave us uniform statistics dealing with 156 flaps reviewed with a minimum follow-up of 6 months. These were one-stage pre- and post-auricular flaps. The two main complications were necrosis and alopecia.

Alopecia

Alopecia may exist without necrosis of the flap (Photo 17). It is evidenced by a secondary loss of hair around the third week. This alopecia is the sequel to partial ischaemia of a more or less extensive part of the flap, sufficient to produce damage or sometimes death of the hair follicles, but not enough to produce skin necrosis. Such an alopecia was observed in 15% of cases ($n=24$) at the first month; it lasted to the sixth month in 5% of the cases ($n=8$), i.e. in a third of all cases. Actually, regrowth was heralded from the end of the first month by the early appearance of a fine down visible under the lens. It should be noted that this alopecia without necrosis was always totally regressive at 6 months in the 14- and 15-cm flaps, unlike the 16- to 18-cm flaps, whether they were pre-

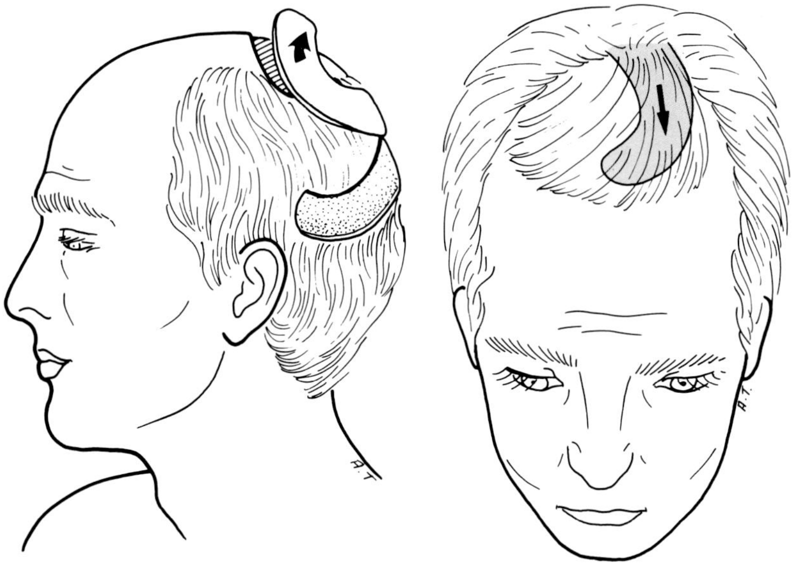

a b

Fig. 17. **a** Mixed occipital flap (Bouhanna). **b** Mixed occipital flap (Bouhanna)

or retro-auricular (Table 2). It is possible and even probable that the application of minoxidil may accelerate this regrowth, though one cannot yet be certain.

Necrosis

Necrosis of the distal extremity of the flap does not affect the final outcome when it is less than 2 cm (Photo 18). The following results therefore include as complications only those necroses of 2 cm or more. In this same series of 156 flaps made at one stage, there were 8% of distal necroses for 14- to 15-cm flaps and 12% for 16- to 18-cm flaps (Table 2).

If, as usual, the alopecias without necrosis are included, the incidence of overall complications was 8% for flaps of less than 16 cm and 18% for those over 16 cm.

To refine these results we have separated the pre- and retro-auricular flaps, in the knowledge that the latter never measure less than 17 cm (Table 3). The

Table 2. Results at 6 months related to length of flap

Length of flap	Necrosis >2 cm		Alopecia without necrosis >2 cm		Good results		Total
(cm)	(*n*)	(%)	(*n*)	(%)	(*n*)	(%)	(*n*)
14–15	2	8	0	–	23	92	25
16–18	16	12	8	6	107	82	131
Total	18	11.5	8	5	130	83.5	156

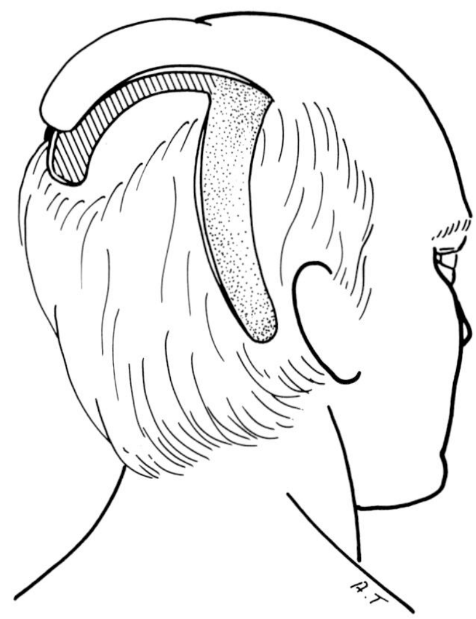

Fig. 18. Vertical flap (Bouhanna)

Table 3. Necrosis and alopecia in pre-auricular and retro-auricular flaps

Length	Necrosis	Alopecia at 6 months	Total number of flaps	
(cm)	(*n*)	(*n*)	(*n*)	(%)
Pre-auricular flaps				
14–15	2	0	25	8
16–18	11	4	111	13.5
Retro-auricular flaps				
16–18	5	4	20	45

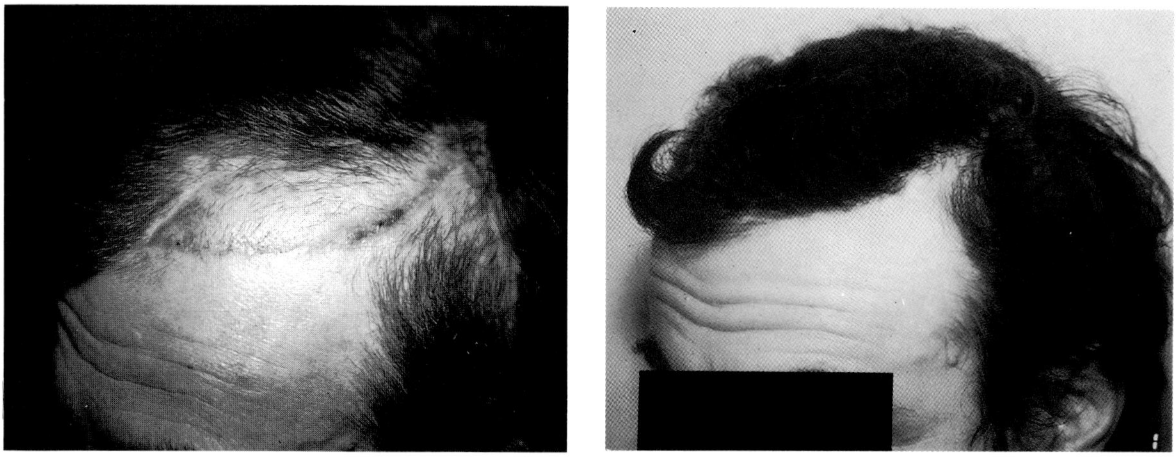

a b

Photo 17. **a** Early transient total alopecia on pre-auricular flap done in one stage. **b** Complete regrowth of hair after several months

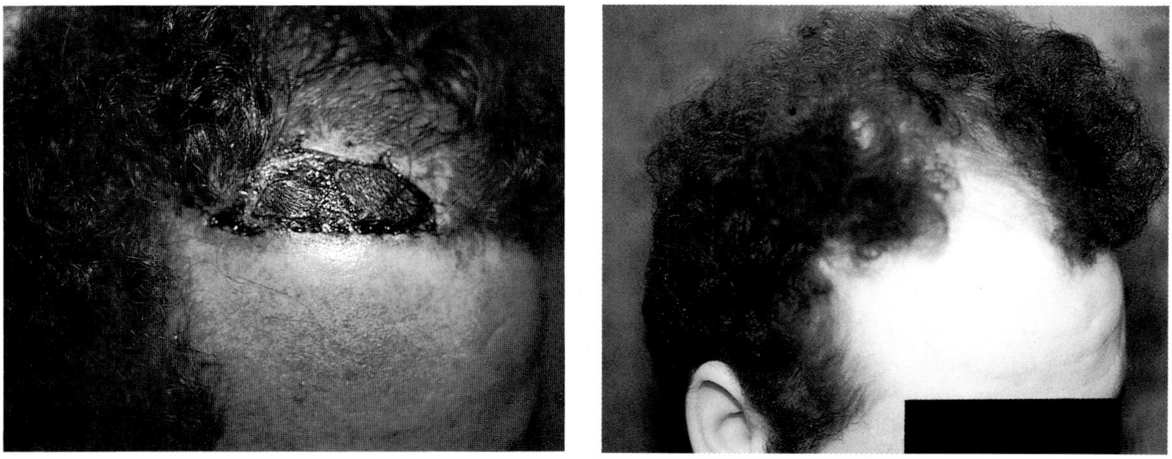

a b

Photo 18. **a** Necrosis of pre-auricular flap exceeding 2 cm at tenth day. **b** Result without revision after spontaneous healing

results for the short flaps are unchanged, but the incidence of necrosis of the long flaps is 10% for pre-auricular flaps and 25% for retro-auricular flaps. If we add definitive alopecias without necrosis to these figures, the overall incidence of complications rises to 13.5% for the pre-auricular flap and 45% for the retro-auricular flap, a considerable difference. Our first conclusion must be that the pre-auricular flap can be made in one stage, whereas the retro-auricular flap must be made in two or three stages.

We then attempted to assess the influence of certain risk factors: smoking, emotional state and degree of anxiety. Table 1 (p. 120) shows that, overall, smokers have twice as many complications (25%) as non-smokers (14%). Further, the two sole complications for the short pre-auricular flaps of 14–15 cm occurred in smokers. In other words, no case of necrosis of 2 cm or more was found for short pre-auricular flaps in non-smokers.

The emotional state and anxiety of the patient seems to increase the risks in the same proportions (Tables 4, 5). Of course, it is probable that the majority of the patients may have been smokers, but it is also possible that these patients were sensitive to stress and had a greater adrenaline output. This provokes repeated vasoconstriction, which is responsible for necrosis of flaps whose vascularisation was initially limited.

Finally, when all the risk factors are excluded, the incidence of complications in pre-auricular flaps, whatever their length (14–18 cm), is 7% as against 25% in subjects with one or more risk factors (Table

Table 4. Influence of emotional state on complication rates and results

	Necrosis + alopecia at 6 months		Good results		Total
	(*n*)	(%)	(*n*)	(%)	(*n*)
Emotional	7	23.3	23	76.6	30
Non-emotional	19	15.0	107	85.0	126
Total	26	16.5	130	83.5	156

Table 5. Influence of anxiety on complication rates and results

	Necrosis + alopecia at 6 months		Good results		Total
	(*n*)	(%)	(*n*)	(%)	(*n*)
Anxious	11	26.8	30	73.2	41
Non-anxious	15	13.0	100	87.0	115
Total	26	16.5	130	83.5	156

Table 6. All risk factors related to complications

	Necrosis + alopecia at 6 months		Total
	(*n*)	(%)	(*n*)
Risk factors excluded	7	7	97
Risk factors included	19	32	59
Risk factors included except retro-auricular flap	10	25	39

Table 7. Specific risk factors related to complications

	Necrosis of flap >2 cm		Total
	(*n*)	(%)	(*n*)
Age			
<25 years	3	10	33
25–45 years	13	11	112
>45 years	2	18	11
Thickness			
Considerable	0	0	6
Moderate	12	10	115
Minor	6	18	35
Bleeding from extremity			
Considerable	1	1.5	70
Moderate	10	20	52
None	7	21	34
Haematoma			
Considerable	4	23.5	17
Moderate	6	17	35
None	8	11	70

6). Other risk factors have been studied but without leading to definite conclusions:

- Although Table 7 suggests a relationship between age and incidence of complications, the small number of patients aged over 45 years makes the percentage differences non-significant.
- The same applies to the relationship between scalp thickness and the incidence of complications. The figure of 0% of necroses in thick scalps is not significant, since the number of patients was too small. On the other hand, the difference in incidence between scalps of medium thickness and very thin scalps seemed very significant: the risks of necrosis were greater when the scalp was thin.

  If there is marked perioperative bleeding from the end of the flap (nearly half the cases), the risk of necrosis may be considered nil. However, the absence of bleeding has no absolute negative significance (Table 7), since this may be expected after adrenaline infiltration. Further, we have seen that such infiltration does not affect the end-result.
- The presence of a haematoma under the flap, even if evacuated the following day, considerably adds to the risk of complications. In the absence of a haematoma the incidence of necrosis was 11.5%, whereas the incidence rose to 17% with a moderate haematoma and to 23.5% with a major haematoma. These findings compelled us to use a suction drain, drainage by strip proving ineffective.

The conclusions from this study are as follows:

1. The vertical retro-auricular flap, with an average length of 18 cm, has the highest percentage of complications (45%). It should therefore never be performed in a single stage, but after one or two preparatory stages.
2. A preauricular flap 16 cm long or less in a non-smoking, non-anxious and unemotional patient, if correctly performed and well drained, carries virtually no risk of necrosis. Our experience has shown that such a flap of 15–16 cm can always reach the mid-frontal line.
3. Smoking, anxiety or emotionality undeniably constitute risk factors which must be allowed for, since they double the incidence of complications. We do not believe that they necessitate the routine use of a multi-stage procedure, but we ask the patient to stop smoking in the week following the operation.
4. A risk factor that was not included in this study is the presence of scars near the flap pedicle. Though they may not be an absolute contraindication to transposition of a flap, they are an

argument for operating in two or three stages. We are particularly wary of patients who have previously had numerous grafts. The presence of grafts in the vertical region seems to be a contraindication to the construction of a vertical flap with a superior pedicle.

5. Lastly, we do not believe that the vertical pre-auricular flap need be routinely constructed in two or three stages, for several reasons:
   - The baldness treated is often major and requires several procedures for complete coverage. A flap in several stages further increases the number of visits to the operating room, which may be very upsetting for the patient.
   - Technically, the preparation of a flap provokes some degree of deterioration at the margins, which may lead to final scars of poorer quality, while the flap itself is much less elastic and supple and its performance is more difficult. Our experience has shown that this is the quickest and most cosmetically successful technique for the treatment of anterior baldness. Patients who have had no complications are presentable in public at the eighth day, a claim that can be made for no other treatment. It is always possible to reduce the remaining baldness by other procedures, the hair of the anterior flap helping to overcome their disadvantages.

A distal necrosis is best repaired by fusiform grafts (Photo 19), which will lead to a perfect final result by 6 months. Thus, even a flap with distal necrosis gives a better and faster result than two grafting sessions. An equivalent result can be obtained only after a minimum of four sessions, which, since the operative site is very exposed, implies an unpleasing appearance for at least a year.

At the donor site (Photos 20, 21) there is an undeniable relationship between the closure tension and the quality of the final scar (Tables 8, 9). The greater the tension of closure, the greater will be the bald area around the scar and the less tendency for it to regress. At most, it may form bald patches 4–5 cm wide, which always regress in 3–4 months but which constitute a very serious physical handicap for the patient throughout this period. We have already seen (in the chapter on "Surgical Techniques") that 1 month after operation 41% of patients in whom the donor site was closed under great tension exhibited marked alopecia around the scar, whereas this was found in only 4% of patients in whom closure was made under minor tension. At the sixth month the scar was perfect in only 59% of patients of the former group, whereas this was the case in 96% of patients of the latter group, the residual 4% having a scar of medium quality and none a scar of poor quality.

Table 8. Elasticity of the scalp

Tension at donor zone	Elasticity					
	Excellent		Moderate		Nil	
	(*n*)	(%)	(*n*)	(%)	(*n*)	(%)
Great	0	0	24	24	10	40
Moderate	11	30	52	50	14	60
Minor	20	70	25	25	0	0
Total	31	–	101	–	24	–

Table 9. Relation of tension at donor zone to subsequent alopecia at 1 and 6 months

Alopecia of donor zone	Tension at donor zone					
	Great		Moderate		Minor	
	(*n*)	(%)	(*n*)	(%)	(*n*)	(%)
At 1 month						
Major	14	41	21	27	2	4
Moderate	9	26	27	35	12	27
Negligible	11	33	29	38	31	69
Total	34	–	77	–	45	–
At 6 months						
Major	5	15	10	13	0	0
Moderate	9	26	27	35	2	4
Negligible	20	59	40	52	43	96
Total	34	–	77	–	45	–

Statistical Study of Four Types of Superior Pedicle Flaps (Bouhanna)

Between 1976 and 1988 Bouhanna studied 207 flaps with a superior pedicle transposed in 132 male patients aged between 21 and 62 years with androgenic alopecia. This study was aimed at assessing the cosmetic value and complications of each type of flap.

Different Types of Flaps (Table 10)

Four types of flaps were followed up for between 6 months and 10 years:

1. Fifty-eight long, vertical retro-auricular flaps (Figs. 12, 13). These parieto-occipital flaps with a superior pedicle (Nataf) measured 18–22 cm in length and 3.5–4 cm in breadth. They were transposed 3 months after two autonomisation procedures. These were the only flaps in which a silastic sheet was placed under the apex.

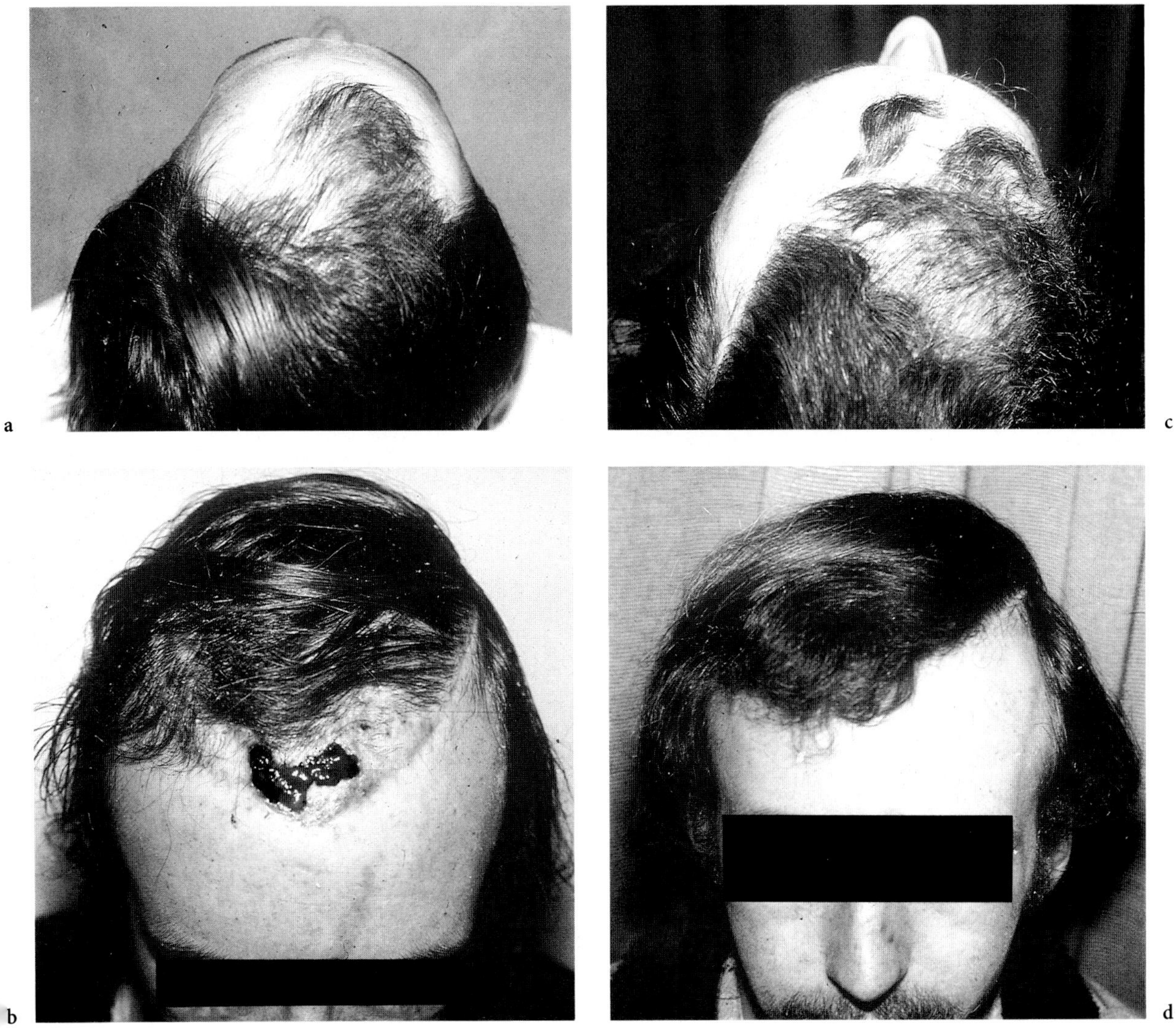

Photo 19. **a** Anterior baldness, grade C1 T1 F3. **b** Terminal necrosis of pre-auricular flap transgressing mid-line. **c** Correction by three fusiform grafts after spontaneous hair regrowth on proximal part of flap. **d** Satisfactory final result

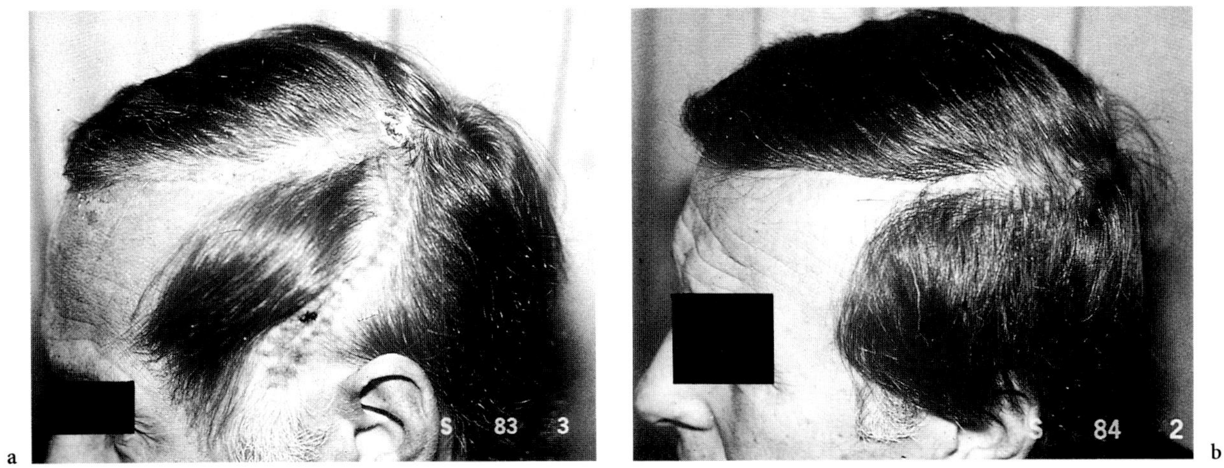

Photo 20. **a** Alopecic scar secondary to closure of donor zone of pre-auricular flap without great tension. **b** Result after 3 months with spontaneous regrowth

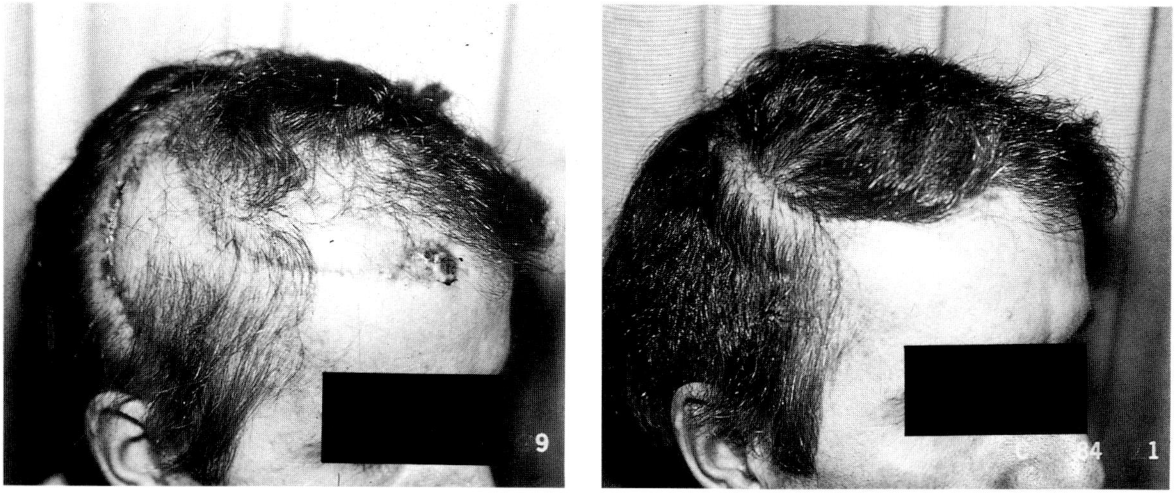

a b

Photo 21. **a** Secondary alopecia due to moderate ischaemia of flap and donor area. **b** Spontaneous complete regrowth of hair after 3 months

Table 10. Different characteristics of transposed superior pedicle flaps

Type	Author	Size (cm)	Autonomisation	Patients (*n*)
Long vertical retro-auricular (Figs. 12, 13)	Nataf	18–22×3.5–4	Autonomised	58
Mixed, short occipital, superior pedicle (Fig. 17a,b)	Bouhanna	16–18×3.5	Autonomised (*n*=18) Not autonomised (*n*=10)	28
Short, vertical pre-auricular (Fig. 10a–c)	Nataf	10–12×3	Autonomised (*n*=44) Not autonomised (*n*=38)	82
Mixed, short pre-auricular (Fig. 14a–c)	Dardour	10–12×3	Not autonomised	39

2. Twenty-eight short, mixed flaps with a superior occipital pedicle (Bouhanna) (Fig. 17a,b). These occipito-parieto-temporal flaps had a superior pedicle situated near the mid-occipital line as described by Passot. However, for reasons of safety and other indications, we reduced their length to 16–18 cm. The breadth was 3.5 cm. Transposition was done without previous autonomisation for flaps less than 16 cm long and after two autonomisation procedures for those over 18 cm. The results, as will be seen later, have confirmed that autonomisation is unnecessary if the 5:1 ratio is observed and if there are none of the contraindications mentioned above. In our study, these flaps were the only ones advised for vertical cover.
3. Eighty-two short, pre-auricular vertical flaps (Nataf) (Fig. 10a–c). The superior pedicle was situated vertical to the ear. These parieto-temporal flaps, 10–12 cm long and 3 cm wide, were transposed with previous autonomisation in 44 cases and without in 38 cases. The results once again confirmed the lack of need for autonomisation.
4. Thirty-nine mixed, short pre-auricular flaps (Dardour) (Fig. 14a–c). The superior pedicle was situated vertical to the ear. These parieto-temporal flaps, 10–15 cm long and 3 cm wide, were transposed without previous autonomisation. The results confirmed the reliability of these flaps. However, the slight additional incidence of necrosis compared with the results in the short vertical flap of Nataf led us not to exceed a length of 13 cm if the transfer was made without previous autonomisation [6, 7].

Results

Cosmetic Results. Each of these four types of flaps have important cosmetic advantages. Thus it was confirmed that each flap, depending on its size and the density of the donor zone (between 100 and 200 hairs cm^2) allows the transposition of 3000–17000 hairs. By comparison, a session of 60 cylindrical 4-mm grafts allows an average transplantation of 600 hairs, which do not become long until 6–9 months after the operation [9, 10].

Complications. At the donor site (Table 11), possible complications include temporary hair loss 2–6 weeks after operation. This alopecia is due to a dystrophic type of damage to the hairs in the anagenic stage, as confirmed by trichography. The operative trauma, the circulatory impoverishment due to marginal tension after closure, but also a degree of individual susceptibility seem to be the factors underlying this hair loss (according to Bouhanna, the psychological profile of these patients is similar to that of patients affected by patchy alopecia). The histological picture shows a similar dystrophy. There are no significant differences between the types of flap. Spontaneous regrowth occurs after 2–3 months, and regrowth is hastened by twice-daily application of a 2% minoxidil lotion.

The scars are often not very marked. Sometimes they are obvious and require correction, either by excision and suture if adequate elasticity has redeveloped or by transplantation of some minigrafts. These scars are statistically commoner and more obvious in zones where flaps have been taken vertically.

The "dog-ear" aspect is usual after transposition of a flap (Table 12) but usually settles down in 4–6 weeks; correction is simple but rarely necessary. Alopecia without necrosis of the apex of the flap is infrequent and often transient (Table 13). Tidying up by transplantation of minigrafts was rarely needed. The phenomenon of complete necrosis was never seen. Necrosis of the apex of less than 2 cm occurred in 3%–10% of flaps, but left only minor scar sequelae (Table 14). Necrosis of more than 2 cm leaves scarred areas which can easily be corrected by transplantation of ten to 30 minigrafts or by simple excision. The incidence of apical necrosis is statistically greater for flaps whose length exceeds 18 cm. However, we confirm that improved autonomisation techniques, particularly by placing a silastic sheet under their apex, improve the reliability of these flaps.

Table 11. Complications such as temporary hair loss and quality of scar at donor zone in superior pedicle flaps

Flap type	Temporary hair loss	Scars	
		Satisfactory	Unsatisfactory
	(%)	(%)	(%)
Long, vertical retro-auricular	8.6	82.7	17.2
Mixed, short, occipital, superior pedicle	7.1	92.8	7.1
Short, vertical, pre-auricular	4.8	90.2	9.8
Mixed, short, pre-auricular	5.1	89.7	7.6

Table 12. "Dog-ear" complications in different types of superior pedicle flaps

Flap type	Temporary "dog-ear" (%)	Permanent "dog-ear" (%)
Long, vertical retro-auricular	86.2	13.8
Mixed, short, occipital, superior pedicle	42.8	0
Short, vertical, pre-auricular	85.1	1.3
Mixed, short, pre-auricular	53.8	0

Table 13. Incidence of temporary or definitive alopecia at the apex of superior pedicle flaps

Flap type	Temporary alopecia (%)	Permanent alopecia (%)
Long, vertical retro-auricular	15.3	3.8
Mixed, short, occipital, superior pedicle	7.6	3.8
Short, vertical, pre-auricular	2.5	1.2
Mixed, short, pre-auricular	5.4	2.7

The conclusions of this second study have allowed a better idea of the possible indications for each flap and a more precise assessment of the factors capable of producing the different complications, the better to prevent them. The importance of each of these flaps will be studied in detail in the chapter on "Operative Indications" (Figs. 19–21).

Table 14. Incidence of necrosis in different types of superior pedicle flaps

Flap type	Necrosis <2 cm (%)	Necrosis >2 cm (%)
Long, vertical retro-auricular	10.3	3.4
Mixed, short, occipital, superior pedicle	7.1	0
Short, vertical, pre-auricular	3.6	0
Mixed, short, pre-auricular	5.12	2.5

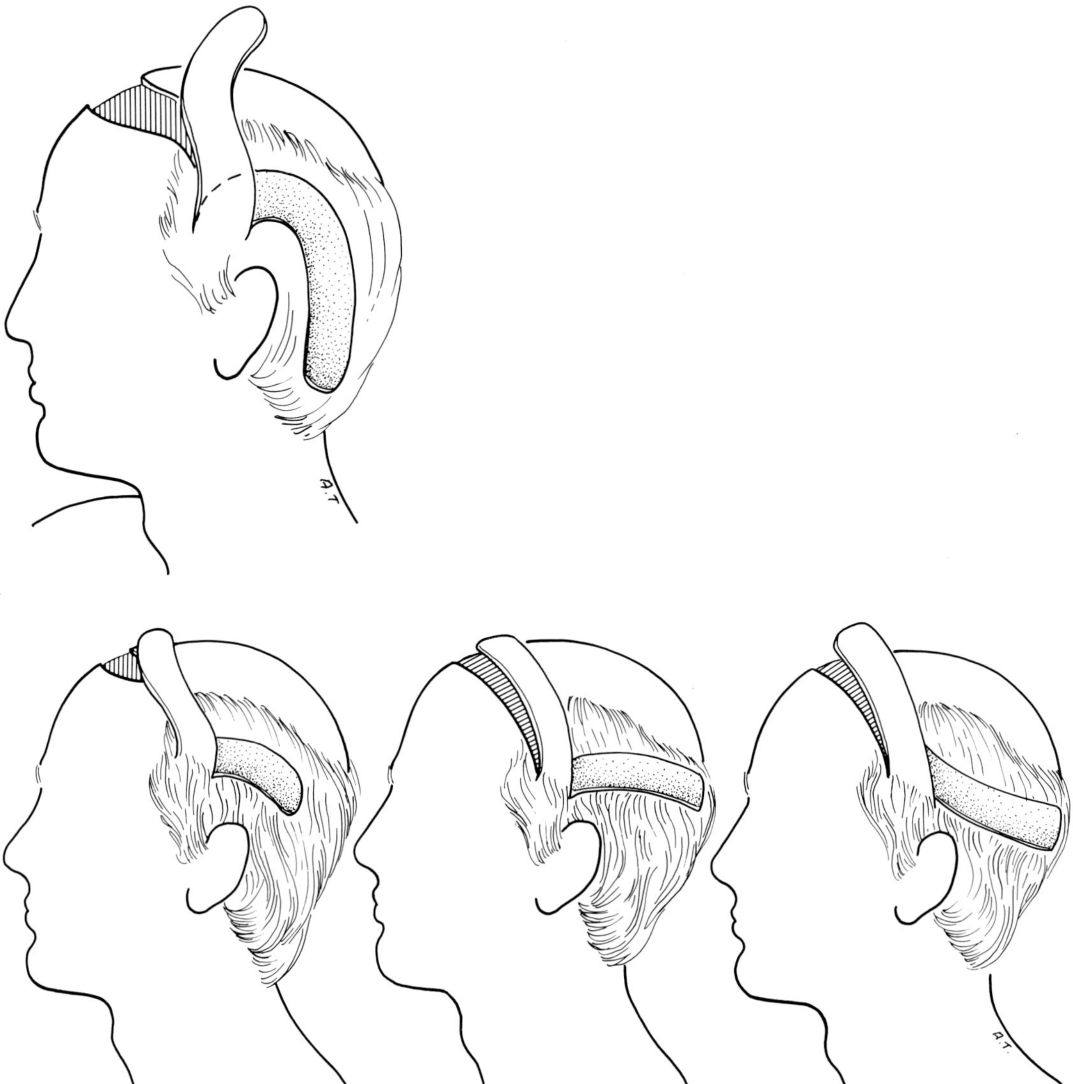

a b c d

Fig. 19a–d. Flaps with inferior pedicle. **a** Juri (1975). **b** Elliot (1977). **c** Passot (1920). **d** Lamont (1957)

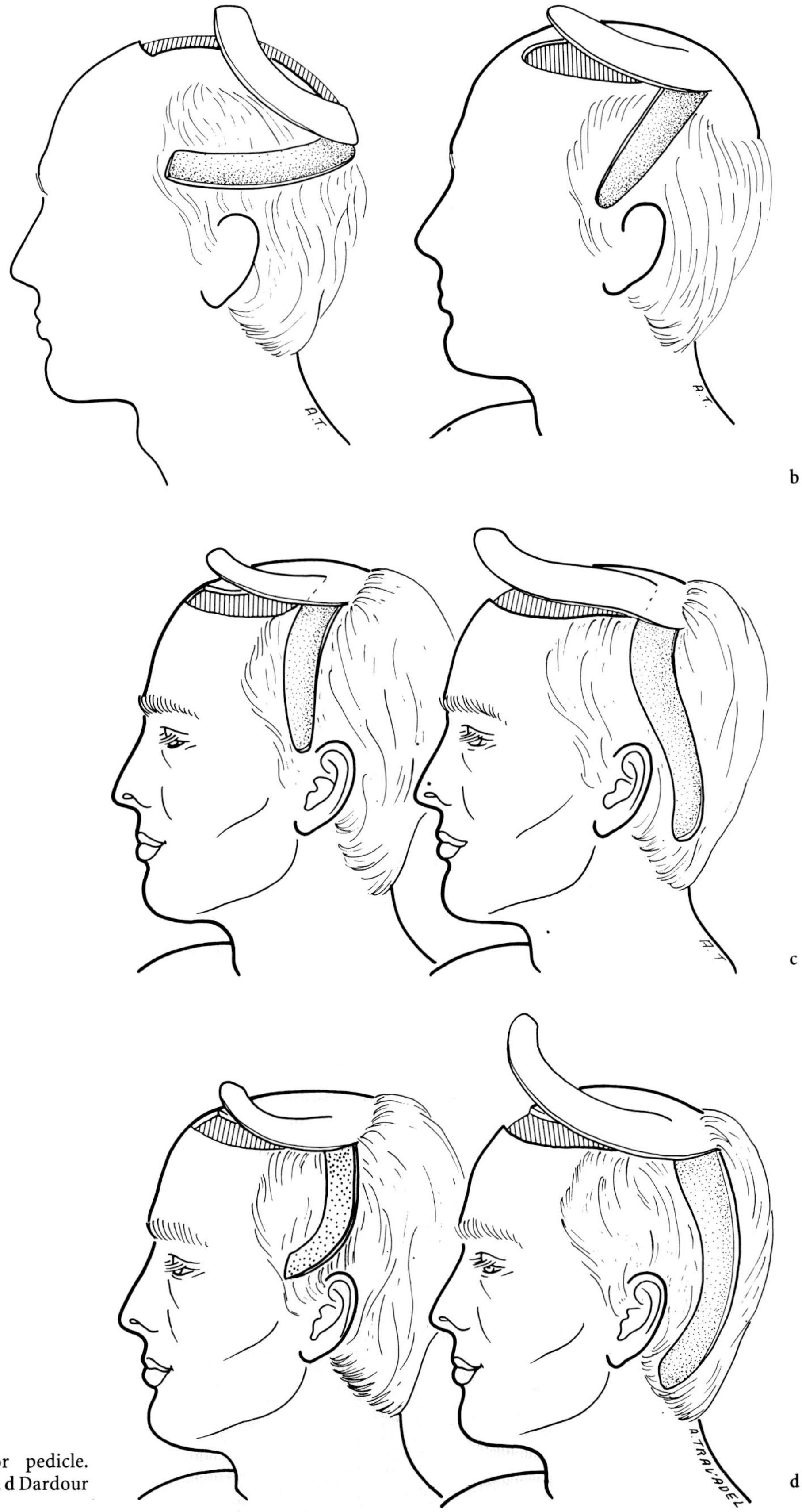

Fig. 20. Flaps with superior pedicle. **a** Passot. **b** Bouhanna. **c** Nataf. **d** Dardour

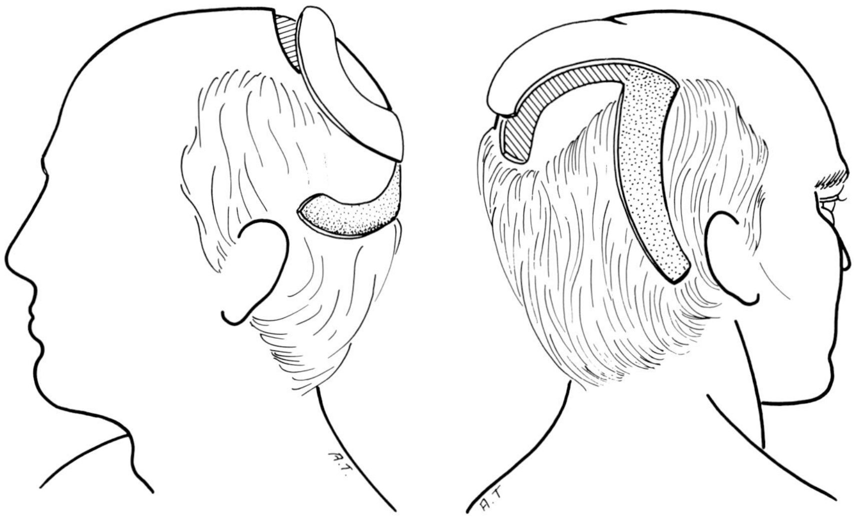

Fig. 21. Vertical flap (Bouhanna)

References

1. Baudet J, Lemaire JM, Legroux PH et al. (1974) Transfert par micro-anastomoses d'un lambeau de cuir chevelu dans un cas d'alopécie cicatricielle. Ann Chir Plast 19(3): 213
2. Blanchard G, Blanchard B (1977)Obliteration of alopcia by lifting: a new concept and technique. J Natl Med Assoc (Canada) 69: 639
3. Bonnefon A (1981) Le lambeau de Juri nos problèmes. Ann Chir Plast 26(3): 286–288
4. Bouhanna P (1976) Le cuir chevelu: les alopécies définitives et leurs traitements. Thesis, Paris
5. Bouhanna P, Nataf J (1976) À propos des transplantations de cuir chevelu. Critiques et propositions. Rev Chir Esthet 7(2): 17–23
6. Bouhanna P (1981) Considérations su le traitement chirurgical des alopécies masculines. J Med Esthet Dermatol 2(9): 182–184
7. Bouhanna P (1982) New flaps and fusiform grafts for male pattern baldness. In: Transactions of the international advanced hair replacement symposium. Birmingham, Alabama, February 3–4
8. Bouhanna P (1984) The post-auricular vertical hair-bearing transposition flap. J Dermatol Surg Oncol 10(7): 551–554
9. Bouhanna P (1988) The phototrichogram: an objective technique used for hair replacement surgery evaluation. In: Unger WP, Nordström REA (eds) Hair transplantation, 2nd edn. Dekker, New York, pp 68–76
10. Bouhanna P (1990) Les lambeaux de cuir chevelu à charnière haute. Ann Chir Plast Esthet 35(5): 397–404
11. Chavoin JP, Rouge D, Costagliola M (1987) Lambeau axial temporo-occipital en un temps. pour alopécies avec repérages Doppler. À propos d'une série homogène de 21 cas. Ann Chir Plast Esthét XXXII, 3: 247–253
12. Chajchir A, Benzaquen I (1982) Surgical treatment for baldness. Aesthetic Plast Surg 6(1): 33
13. Correa-Iturraspe M, Arute HN (1957) Plastic surgery of partial alopecia. Semana Med 19: 937
14. Dardour JC (1978) Des alopécies – des lambeaux. Ann Chir Plast Esthet 23(4): 231–33
15. Dardour JC (1983) Treatment of male baldness with a one stage flap rotation. In: Transactions of the VIII Congress of Plastic Surgery, Montreal, June 26–July 1, pp 680–681
16. Dardour JC (1985) Treatment of male pattern baldness with a one stage flap. Aesthetic Plast Surg 9: 109
17. Dardour JC (1986) Treatment of male baldness. Ann Plast Surg 17: 267
18. Dardour JC, Pugashe, Aziza R (1988) The one stage preauricular flap for male pattern: long term results and risk factors. Plast Reconstr Surg 81(6): 907–912
19. Elbaz JS, Zummer A (1978) À propos des lambeaux du cuir chevelu, le lambeau en filet, Ann Chir Plast 23(2): 112–114
20. Elliot RA (1977) Lateral flaps for instant results in male pattern baldness. Plast Reconstr Surg 60(5): 699–703
21. Elliot RA (1980) Lateral scalp flaps for baldness. In: Rees T (ed) Aesthetic plastic surgery. Saunders, Philadelphia
22. Elliot RA (1982) The lateral scalp for anterior hair line reconstruction. Clin Plast Surg 9(2): 241–253
23. Flemming RW, Mayer TG (1981) Short and long scalp flaps in the treatment of male pattern baldness. Arch Otolaryngol 107(7): 403–408
24. Flemming RW, Mayer TG (1985) Scalp flaps reconstruction of the unfavorable result in hair replacement surgery. Head Neck Surg 7(4): 315–331
25. Gilles H (1944) Note on scalp closure. Lancet 2: 310
26. Harii K, Ohmori K, Ohmori S (1974) Successful clinical transfer of 10 free flaps by microvascular anastomoses. Plast Reconstr Surg 53(3): 259–270
27. Harii K, Ohmori K, Ohmori S (1974) Hair transplantation with free scalp flap. Plast Reconstr Surg 53: 410
28. Himburger RA (1977) Single stage rotation of arterialized scalp flaps for male pattern baldness: case report. Plast Reconstr Surg 60(5): 789–791
29. Juri J (1975) Use of parieto-occipital flaps in the surgical treatment of baldness. Plast Reconstr Surg 55(4): 456–460
30. Juri J, Juri C, Arufe HN (1978) Use of rotation scalp flaps for treatment of occipital baldness. Plast Reconstr Surg 61(1): 23–26

31. Juri J, Juri C (1981) Two new methods for treating baldness: temporo-parieto occipito-parietal pedicled flap and temporo parieto occipital free flap. Ann Plast Surg 6(1): 38–47
32. Juri J, Juri C (1981) Aesthetic aspects of reconstructive scalp surgery. Clin Plast Surg 8(2): 243–254
33. Juri C, Juri J, Colnago A (1980) Monopedicled transposition flap for the treatment of traumatic scalp alopecia. Ann Plast Surg 4(5): 439–454
34. Kazanjian UH, Webster RC (1946) The treatment of extensive losses of the scalp. Plast Reconstr Surg 2: 360
35. Kabaker SS (1978) Experience with parieto-occipital flaps in hair transplantation. Laryngoscope 88(1): 73–84
36. Kabaker SS (1979) Juri flap procedure for the treatment of baldness arch. Head Neck Surg Otolaryngol 105(9): 509–514
37. Lafaurie P (1988) Progrès recents dans la chirurgie du cuir chevelu. Thesis, Paris
38. Lamont ES (1979) A plastic surgical transformation – report of a case. West J Surg 65: 164
39. Langè, Boyd (1942)
40. Lauzon G. Transfer of a large single temporo-occipital flap for treatment of baldness. Plast Reconstr Surg 63(3): 369–371
41. Limburger S (1959) Die operative Behandlung des Haarverlustes. Med 35: 155–159
42. Marchac D (1978) Complication des lambeaux du cuir chevelu dans le traitement de la calvitie. Ann Chir Plast 23(3): 183–185
43. McGregor, Morgan (1963)
44. Nakatsuka et al. (1985)
45. Nataf J (1981) Particular techniques of hair transplantation. In: Orfanos CE, Montagna W, Stutten G (eds) Hair research status and future aspects. Springer, Berlin Heidelberg New York, pp 655–659
46. Nataf J (1978) Lambeaux du cuir chevelu et étude comparative avec les autres techniques de transplantation. Ann Chir Plast 23(3): 176–182
47. Nataf J (1984) Surgical treatment for frontal baldness: the long temporal vertical flap. Plast Reconstr Surg 74: 628
48. Nataf J (1984) Reflexions sur 7 années d'utilisation du lambeau "enfoui". Ann Chir Plast 29(1): 53–57
49. Nataf J, Elbaz JS, Pollet J (1976) Étude critique des transplantations du cuir chevelu et proposition d'une optique. Ann chir Plast 21(3): 199–206
50. Ohmori K (1980) Free scalp flap. Plast Reconstr Surg 65(1): 42–49
51. Ohmori K (1980) Free scalp flap surgery. Ann Plast Surg 5(1): 17–23
52. Ohmori K (1982) Application of micro-vascular free flaps to scalp defects. Clin Plast Surg 9(2): 263–268
53. Ohmori K (1984) Hair transplantation with micro-surgical free flap. J Dermatol Oncol Surg 10(12): 974–978
54. Onizuka T, Ohmori S (1965) Treating of alopecia cicatricosa using an artery flap. Plast Reconstr Surg 35(3): 338–341
55. Ohtsuka H, Nara Y, Niki Y (1982) Successful transposition of a large scalp island flap based on the superficial temporal artery with no obvious venous drainage: case report. Br J Plast Surg 35(5): 300–301
56. Orticochea M (1969) Application de la technique des quatre lambeaux dans la reconstruction du front et des régions pariétales. Ann Chir Plast 14(2): 153–158
57. Orticochea M (1971) New three flap scalp reconstruction technique. Br J Plast Surg 24(2): 184–188
58. Passot R (1920) Les autoplasties esthétiques dans la calvitie. Presse Med 23: 222–223
59. Passot R (1920) Un cas d'autoplastie esthétique du cuir chevelu pour calvitie. Presse Med 48: 408
60. Passot R (1931) Chirurgie esthétique pure. Technique et résultats. G Doin et Cie, Paris
61. Rabineau P (1980) Surgical treatment of baldness using Juri's technique. cutis 25: 511
62. Rizzetto-Stubel A, Ellen Bogen R (1986) Male baldness: immediate single-stage rotation of very long arterialized temporo-parieto-occipital flaps. Plast Reconstr Surg 77(2): 215–220
63. Sawhney CP (1980) Transposition flaps of inextensible skin such as the scalp. Br J Plast Surg 33(1): 119–121
64. Silverman et al. (1985)
65. Stough DB, Cates JA, Dean AJ (1982) Updating reduction and flap procedures for baldness. Ann Plast Surg 8(4): 287–295
66. Stough DB, Cates JA (1980) Transposition flap for the correction of baldness: a practical office procedure. J Dermatol Oncol Surg 6(4): 286–289
67. Stur et al. (1982)
68. Svensson et al. (1985)
69. Walker WD (1982) An alternative flap in the treatment of baldness. Aesthetic Plast Surg 6: 75–79

Reduction Procedures

Repeated reduction is theoretically the best technique for the treatment of baldness. It is the most simple procedure, consisting essentially of excision and suture; it is the quickest, the result being immediate, and the safest, complications being rare. It is also the most cosmetically successful, since the zone of coverage is perfectly uniform at the cost of a single scar. However, the main deficiencies of this technique are inability to routinely cover the frontal region and the displacement of hair-bearing zones, which may become partly bald in the future.

General Considerations

Before embarking on the problems of the different techniques employed, it may be useful to recall certain factors:

1. Usually, some months after a first procedure, the scalp fully or almost fully regains its initial laxity, allowing a second procedure to be carried out. Assessment of the initial laxity of the scalp is essential in this technique, as this determines the prognosis and the value of the operation. In fact, the speed of recovery of scalp laxity is a function of the initial laxity, allowing rapid re-operation; the number of possible procedures is greater when initial laxity is great. Four or even five sessions may be performed in cases with extreme laxity, whereas in marginal cases sometimes only one procedure is possible. In practice, the best interval between two reductions is 3–4 months. A longer delay does not allow the performance of wider excisions.

   The amount of smooth skin resected at each stage is also a function of scalp laxity and the extent of the stripping; it varies from 2 to 5 cm. The difference in results obtained in two patients with the same degree of baldness may be very variable, from 2 to 10 cm of total gain in some cases.
2. The laxity of the scalp is greater in the sagittal than in the antero-posterior direction. Sagittal reductions with lifting of the temporal crown therefore allow more extensive excisions than transverse reductions.
3. In the superior occipital region, the extensibility of the scalp is very limited, both vertically and transversely. Lifting of this region by a transverse fusiform reduction is therefore not a profitable exercise. Moreover, taking account of the clinical course, it must be remembered that this superior occipital region is the first to suffer hair loss with the passage of time.
4. The occipital region, situated below the external occipital protuberance, in contrast, allows very considerable expansion after stripping, since the dissection at this site is subcutaneous [11, 12, 14]. However, this stripping necessarily involves dissection, and sometimes the sacrifice, of the greater occipital nerve of Arnold and the occipital vessels, which results in anaesthesia of the entire scalp. The long-term recovery of this sensation has not been studied.
5. Usually, reductions do not create problems of necrosis due to inadequate vascularisation. However, in certain types of very major reductions (so-called giant reductions or lifting of the scalp) with sacrifice of the occipital vessels, it becomes necessary to preserve the superficial temporal arteries, since these are known to be capable by themselves of ensuring the vascularisation of the entire scalp [13, 17, 20, 29]. However, when grafts have been taken in the stripped zones, the risks of necrosis are certain. They increase with the extent of the stripping and when a considerable number of grafts has been taken. For this reason, we believe – unlike some authors [1] – that it is preferable to perform reductions before grafting, whenever possible, and that to proceed in the opposite way calls for great caution.
6. The equation according to which the residual smooth area is equal to the total smooth area minus the resected smooth surface is false. Actually, it may be considered that the entire area

gained by the stripping and therefore the expansion of a smooth zone is nil. Thus, a vertex 10 cm wide, treated by a median sagittal reduction and stripping of the margins of each side over 5 cm would give a result of nil, even if the resected zone were 4 or 5 cm wide. It is therefore more useful to perform a reduction at the boundary between smooth and hairy zones, rather than in the middle of a smooth zone.

7. Calculation of the resected area is made in different ways by different authors (Fig. 1). Some assimilate the resected zone to the shape of a rectangle, which allows them to calculate the area by simply multiplying the length by the breadth. Thus they consider that, in removing a fragment of 20×4 cm, they have resected 80 cm^2 of smooth skin. Others assert that they remove a spindle whose shape they assimilate to that of a lozenge. The geometric calculation then shows us that the area is reduced by 50% (40 cm^2 for the same example). Some authors [2] consider that the area of the spindle is inferior by 40% to that of the rectangle (48 cm^2 for the same example). We ourselves believe that the resected area must be assimilated to a rectangle, of which only the extremities taper over the last 2 or 3 cm, which modifies the area of the latter by 16–20 cm^2 only (i.e. 60–64 cm^2 for the same example). However, since in practice, as the preceding paragraph has shown, the residual smooth area is not equal to the original area minus the resected area, only a very approximate mathematical approach to the problem can be claimed.
8. Secondary enlargement in the months following reduction of a residual smooth zone is a particular phenomenon, difficult to predict and very variable. The loss may be estimated at between 0% and 70% of the gain originally obtained. This has been particularly studied by Nordstrom [21, 22], who concludes that a third or half of the effect of the reduction is lost postoperatively, that most of this loss occurs in the 2 months after operation and the rest during the third month and that the greater part of the recurrence occurs at the zone adjacent to the scar. However, Nordstrom studied this phenomenon only in median sagittal reductions. Furthermore, he did not study the factors influencing it. One of these factors, the elasticity of the scalp, seems particularly important. Study of our cases showed variations of this phenomenon of between 0% and 70% of the gain obtained at reduction. In general, this is proportional to the laxity of the scalp.

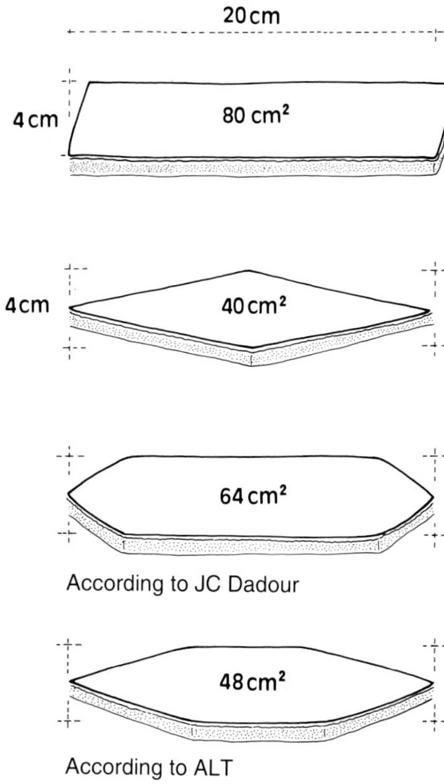

Fig. 1. Different ways of calculating area of resection

On the other hand, it is clear that a marginal reduction at the boundary of the smooth and hairy zones reduces the effect of this phenomenon by half, since one of the two margins which suffers the effects of secondary stretching is hairy. Insofar as this phenomenon is due to secondary stretching of the smooth zone adjacent to the reduction, its extent can be minimised by reducing the capacity of this alopecic zone for secondary stretching as much as possible. This may be done by a maximum excision, with stripping of this region too, even if this stripping leads to no immediate gain in the effect of the reduction.

Lastly, the extent of the secondary enlargement of the residual smooth zone as related to the degree of tension at the time of closure has not been studied to our knowledge. However, it is very probable that the greater this tension, the greater the enlargement.

9. The appearance and course of the scars depend on the tension at the suture region and the position of the scars on the scalp. Closure tension must be minimal. Any excess leads to marginal ischaemia, which results in the loss of hair follicles over an area proportional to the degree of

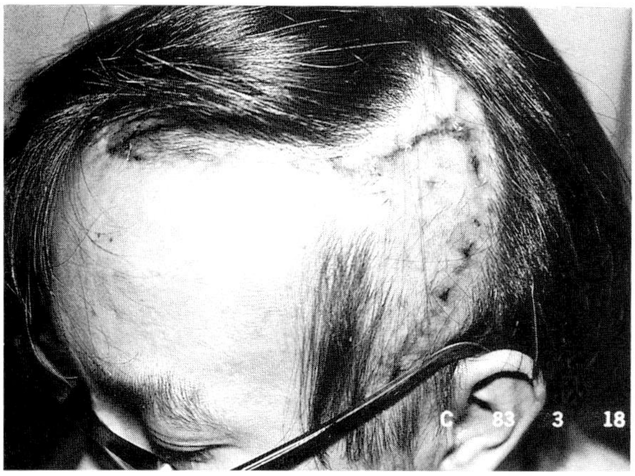

Photo 1. Premature alopecia due to closure under excessive tension

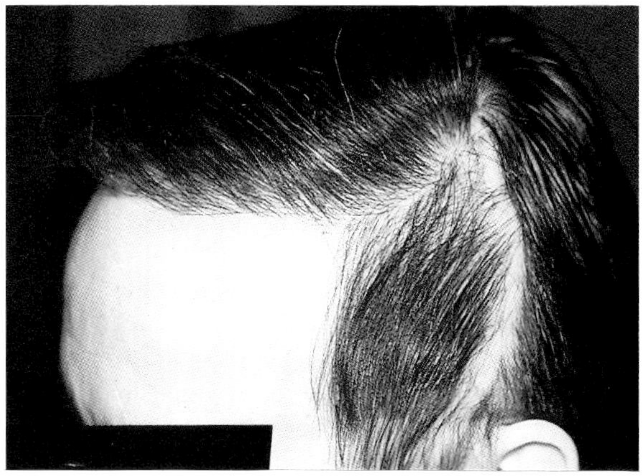

Photo 2. Complete regrowth of hair between third and sixth month

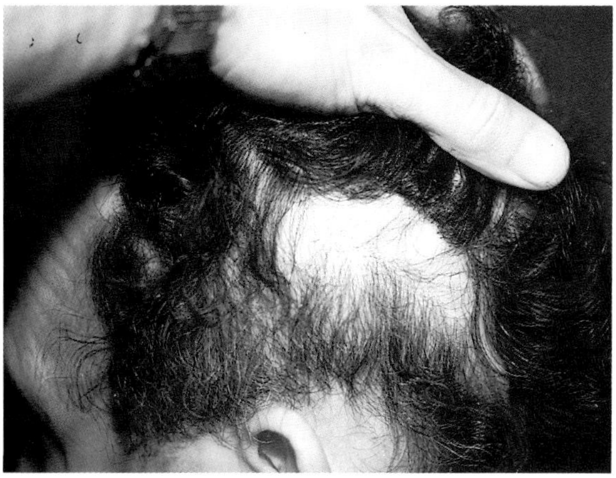

Photo 3. Delayed scar alopecia without necrosis due to prolonged ischaemia

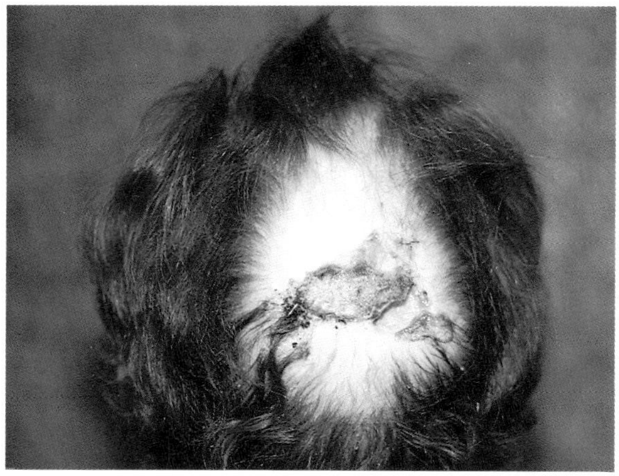

Photo 4. Skin necrosis evident at eighth day

tension (Photos 1, 2). If the ischaemia is not great, the follicles are damaged but do not die, as evidenced clinically by secondary hair loss around the third week (anagenic defluvium). With higher tension, the ischaemia of the follicles is greater and prolonged and leads to their necrosis (Photo 3). The hair loss is irreversible, whereas the skin remains normal. Lastly, if the tension is even greater, the necrosis of the follicles is accompanied by skin necrosis, as indicated by the early appearance of blackish crusts or plaques visible by the eighth day (Photo 4).The performance of galeotomies has been advocated to increase the effect of reductions [2], but we do not advise them for several reasons:

- They impair the marginal vascularisation by eliminating the galea, which protects the vessels and prevents their overstretching.
- They notably add to the length of the procedure, as careful haemostasis is essential after galeotomy.
- Lastly, the gain so obtained is minimal, around 0.5 cm. This gain, which might be very important for closure of the donor site of a flap, seems negligible in terms of a reduction. In practice, we always advise excision as required and never laid down in advance, since it is impossible to predict the extent of a reduction to within 0.5 cm. When closure tension is excessive, it also produces stretching of the scar itself, which be-

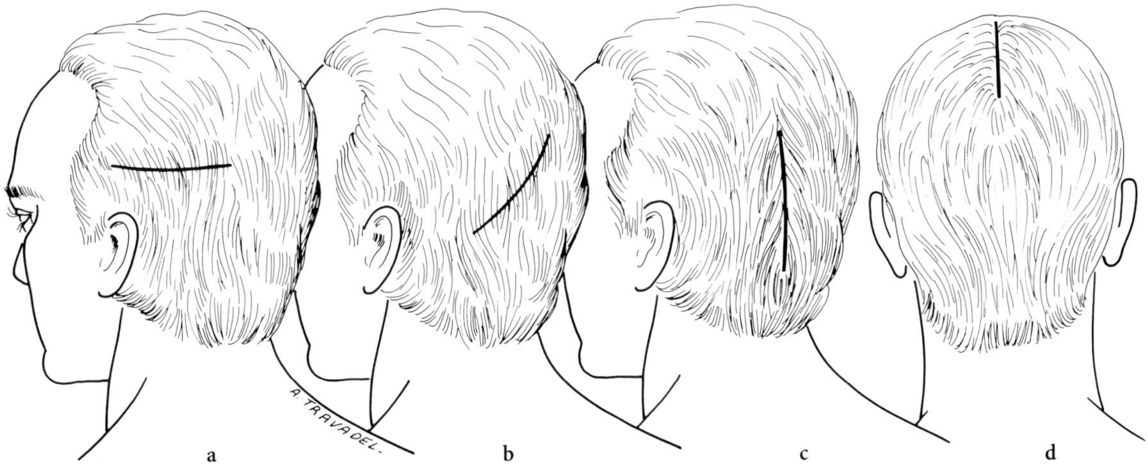

Fig. 2a–d. Position of scars related to direction of follicle implantation. **a** Excellent. **b** Correct. **c** Moderate. **d** Poor

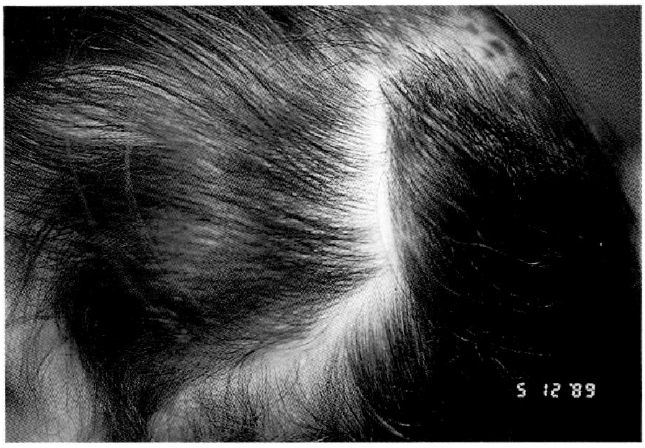

Photo 5. The vertical portion of the scar is more obvious than the transverse portion

comes dehiscent. The area gain obtained by increase of closure tension is therefore fully lost again by this double phenomenon.

The position of the scars affects the possibilities of camouflage. Transverse scars at right angles to the direction of implantation of the hairs are always less obvious than vertical ones (Fig. 2, Photo 5). A scar should not be created in a zone where the hairs grow in a divergent fashion, which would lead to a permanent parting. This may occur during transverse reduction of a vertex with excision of the central point and is found at the posterior end of the scar secondary to several sagittal reductions (Photo 6). Lastly, it is important to avoid an elementary technical error, which consists of incising the scalp at right angles to the skin. The scalpel should always be parallel to the implantation of the follicles in order to prevent loss of the hairs situated at the margin of the incision and all the more so when the follicles are more obliquely aligned.

Description of Technique

Preparation of Patient

Preparation of the patient is always the same and has been described in preceding chapters. The patient is premedicated 90 min beforehand with a suppository of secobarbital (Nembutal; 60 mg) or Sedol and 45 min later an intramuscular injection of 0.5 mg atropine and 0.5 mg alimemazine (Theralene). The design of the excision is made with an indelible felt pen before positioning the patient, which we consider allows better assessment of the resection zone in terms of scalp elasticity. Usually, the patient is placed in the dorsal decubitus position, a position which allows excellent approach to the lateral zones, though the approach to the posterior region is more difficult. However, we prefer this position to the ventral decubitus position, even if stripping is mainly occipital, as in transverse fusiform reductions and in large reductions which call for posterior

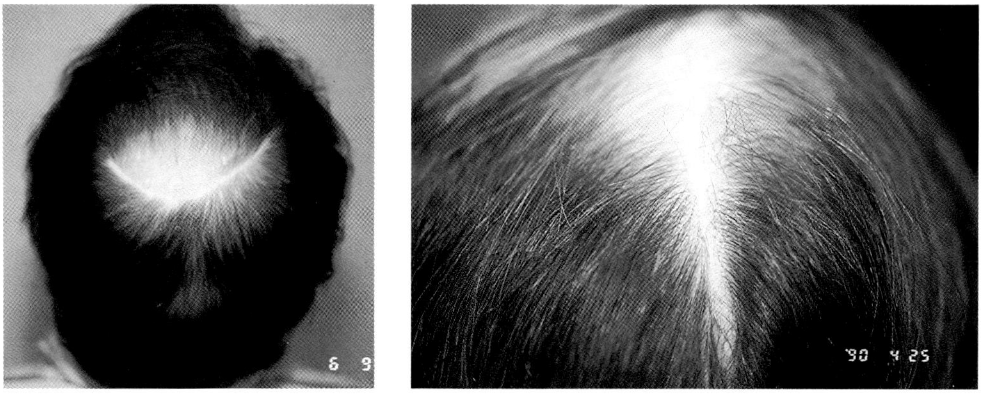

a b

Photo 6. **a** Vertical scar in a region where the follicles diverge. **b** Scar subsequent to several sagittal reductions

cervical stripping down to the lower limit of the hair.

Sterilisation of the operative field is done by shampooing with a quaternary ammonium compound (dilute Cetavlon), and sterile towels are arranged under the head of the patient and over the chest, while the face, also previously sterilised, is freely exposed.

Local Anaesthesia

Local anaesthesia is carried out by infiltration of 1% Xylocaine with adrenaline, diluted to a third with normal saline. In practice, 40 ml Xylocaine usually suffices with an added 80 ml saline. However, in major reductions an additional 20 ml Xylocaine may be needed. We first perform a block of the greater occipital nerve and sometimes of the supra-orbital nerve. We then make a peripheral circular block to anaesthetise the entire scalp. Finally, systematic infiltration of the whole zone to be stripped is made, which facilitates subgaleal stripping and decreases bleeding. In some cases we also perform superficial dermal infiltration at the lines of incision in order to diminish bleeding at the margins.

Incision

The incision is made with the scalpel, at right angles to the skin in the smooth zone and obliquely and parallel to the follicles for marginal incisions at the boundary of the scalp. Stripping is always made between the galea and periosteum with long, curved, blunt-ended scissors. We have found this instrument as effective as any of the strippers described, and they do not need to be changed whenever adhesions have to be divided, which represents an enormous saving of time. The stripping must always be pursued as far as possible. At the temporo-parietal and upper occipital regions it is very easy and quite bloodless. It is more difficult in the supra-auricular region, where it must be done in a deep supra-periosteal and inframuscular plane if there is to be no bleeding. It is then possible to almost reach the external auditory meatus. It will be seen that posterior stripping under the attachments of the occipital muscle is very difficult.

Resection

Resection is carried out as required. The stripped scalp is placed under tension using towel clips. Damage of the margins is not important since these will be resected in any case. We then use an instrument commonly employed in the surgery of lifting, the forceps of Assumpcao or Pitanguy. This makes it possible to mark out exactly the amount of skin to be resected with the desired tension. Progressively, as the marks are made, the skin is incised by transfixion with a scalpel blade and by making an incision perpendicular to the margin and joining it. The two margins are then immediately approximated with a towel clip acting as a temporary suture, a procedure no more traumatising for the hair follicles than a suture. The same action is repeated every 3 or 4 cm until the tacking is completed, and the skin is then resected between the temporary sutures. This technique, normally practised during lifting, is the only one that permits real excision “as required”, by an exact regulation of the desired tension.

Drainage

Drainage is usually unnecessary except in cases of low posterior stripping, since this region contains numerous perforating vessels. A suction drain is then essential. Closure is made in a single layer by staples. This technique seems much preferable to more classical closure in two layers, as it is not only quicker but also yields scars of better quality, even with closure under tension.

Dressing

Dressing is not always essential; however, we think it preferable for the first night. It is removed on the following day and the first shampooing is allowed on the second day. In the following days we ask the patient to rinse his head under a warm shower every day and to shampoo as often as necessary. The staples are removed between the eighth and 12th days.

Classical Reduction Procedures

Sagittal Fusiform Reductions

Median Sagittal Fusiform Reduction [5, 6, 7]

The median sagittal fusiform reduction is very easy. The design of the excision is spindle-shaped centered on the mid-line (Fig. 3). This technique is the simplest and allows good ascent of the crown in the middle part, but it has many disadvantages:

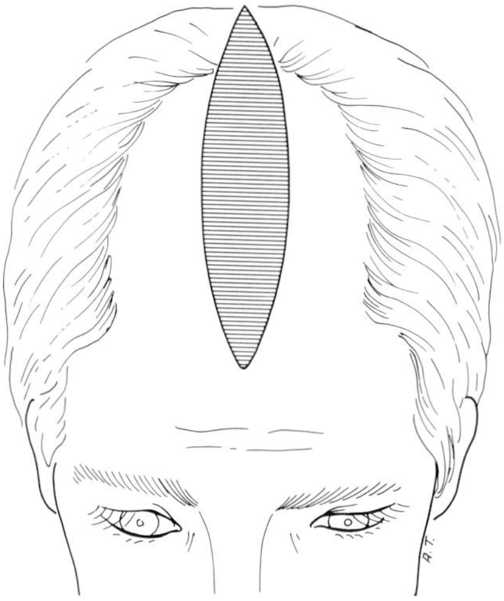

Fig. 3. Sagittal reduction

- If the posterior end of the spindle is situated at the upper limit of the occipital crown, the amount of smooth area resected in this region will be minimal; if the posterior end of the spindle is situated lower down, a hairy zone is sacrificed.
- Again, if the anterior end of the spindle does not transgress the anterior temporal line, the anterior part of the crown will not be subject to the ascent desired. Of course, it is possible to advance this extremity to the level of the future frontal line. But in these cases this produces deformation of the fronto-temporal recession if the frontal region is naturally hairy, either after grafting or after a flap (Photo 7), or a visible scar in front if this zone is smooth. Further, even if three or four procedures

a 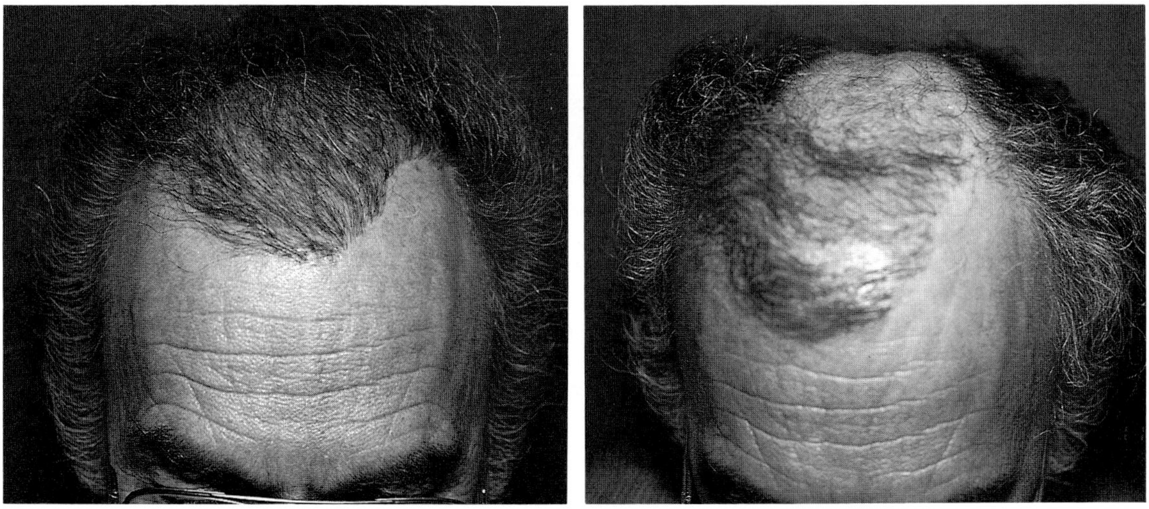 b

Photo 7a,b. Deformation of fronto-temporal recession after reduction in a previously grafted patient

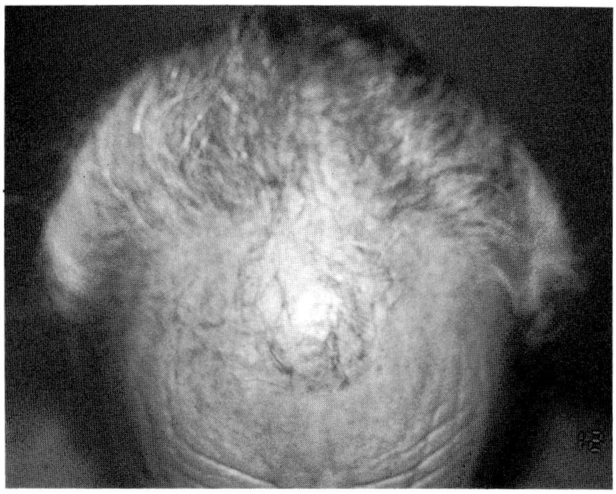

Photo 8. Residual smooth frontal zone after four sagittal reductions

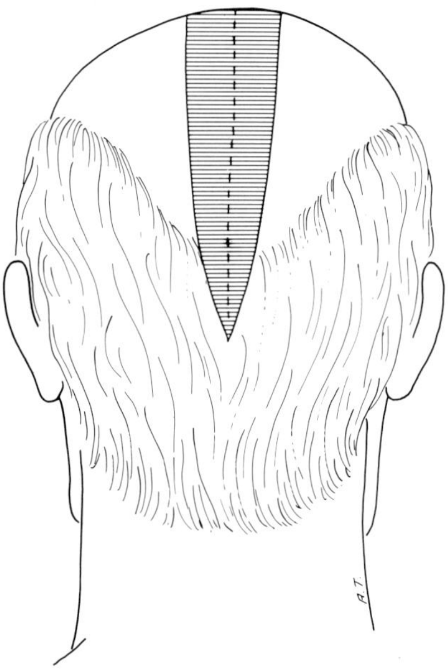

Fig. 4. Sagittal reduction, posterior view

allow total reduction, a smooth frontal zone will still remain which can only be covered by three or four autograft sessions, i.e. seven or eight procedures in all to cover the entire bald area (Photo 8).

- Though the smooth area resected is often considerable, closure is made partly by stretching of the residual smooth area, which notably limits the true efficacy of the procedure. In other words, the ascent of the crown on either side is not equal to half the width of the zone resected. On the other hand, the secondary skin stretching is made to a great extent at the expense of the smooth zone.

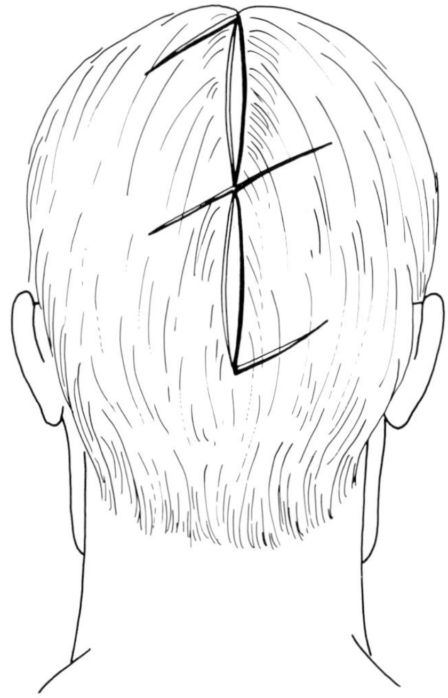

Fig. 5. Posterior Z-plasties to camouflage scar

- In the rare favourable cases, or after several procedures, it is possible to obliterate the vertical region completely. This produces at the posterior part of the scar a lowering of the occipital crown with an outward rotation of the hair follicles, leading to a permanent visible scar in this region, one that is impossible to conceal by hair-styling (Fig. 4, Photos 9, 10). To palliate this disadvantage, one must either make the posterior part of the incision 45° oblique or perform a Z-plasty at the posterior end to change the direction of the hairs (Fig. 5).

Lateral Sagittal or Paramedian Reduction [1, 2]

At the boundary of the bald and hairy zones, a lateral sagittal or paramedian reduction allows better ascent of the crown, the lateral stripping being pursued lower down than with a mid-line incision (Fig. 6). However, it is subject to the same disadvantages as the preceding technique, since it leads to an equivalent excision. Moreover, after two or three procedures a median flap with a narrow straight pedicle is left (Fig. 7, Photo 11). However, the secondary skin stretching is done on one side at the expense of the smooth area, but on the other at that of the hairy scalp. Some authors [1, 2] state that this technique allows closure under great tension without risk of

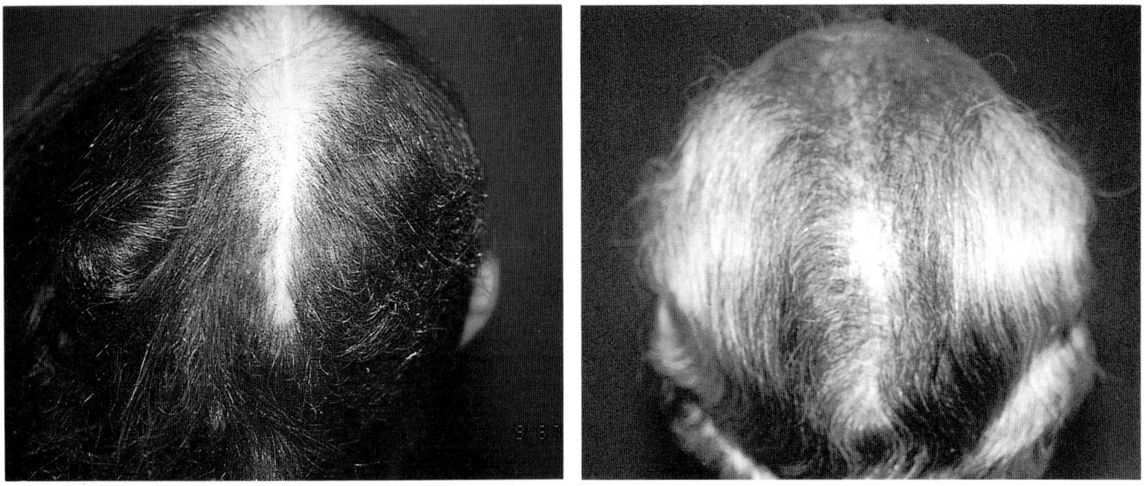

Photo 9a,b. Visible posterior scar forming a parting, secondary to divergent orientation of follicles

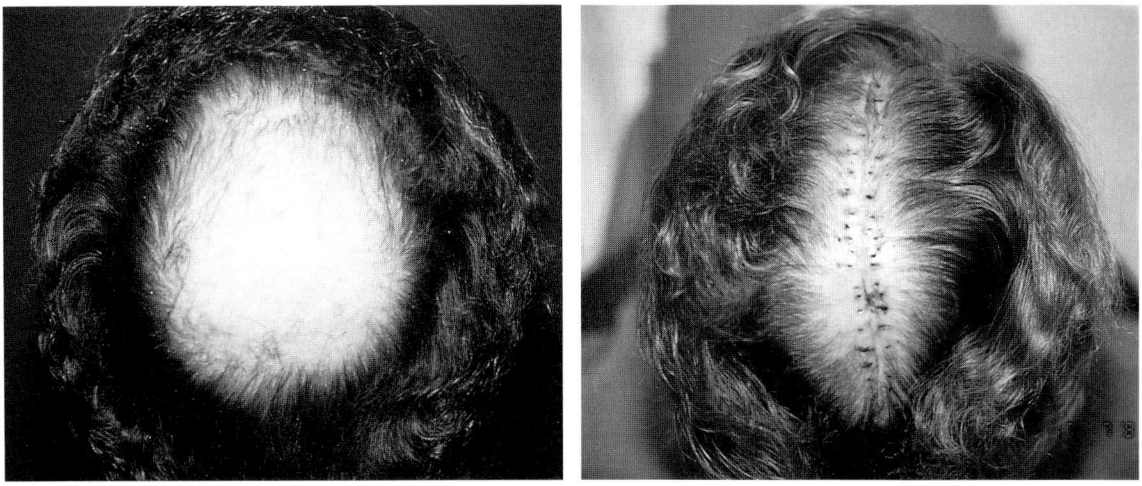

Photo 10. **a** Isolated vertex. **b** Vertex treated by three sagittal fusiform excisions

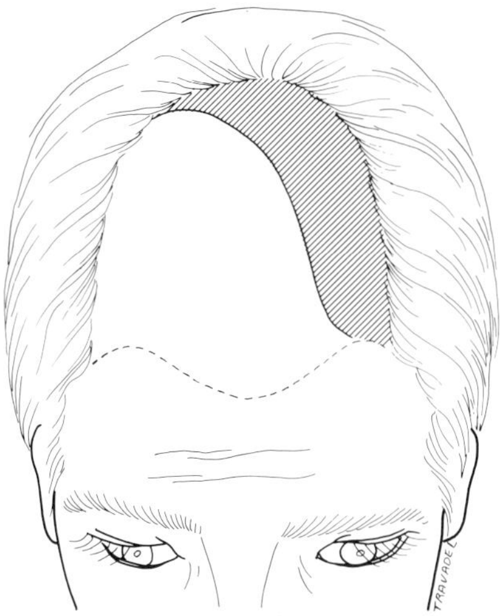

Fig. 6. Paramedian reduction

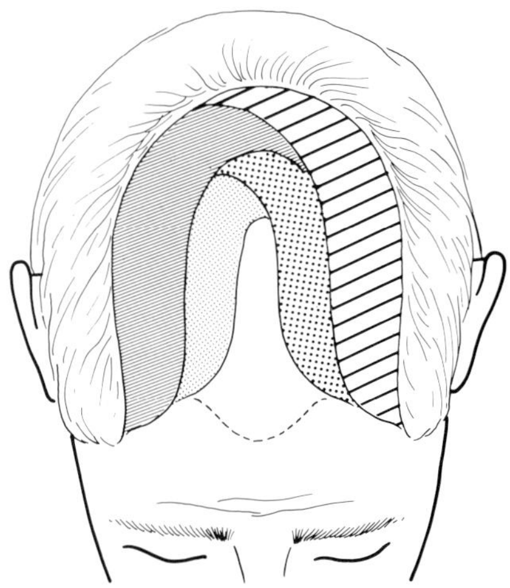

Fig. 7. Residual median flap after four reductions

a 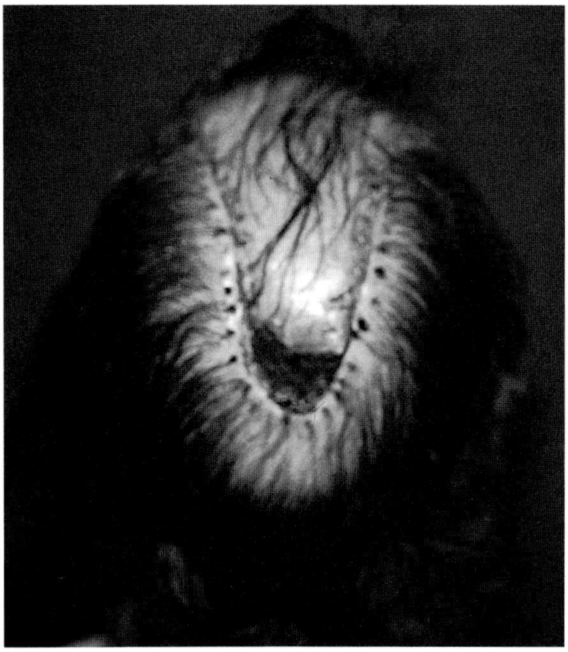 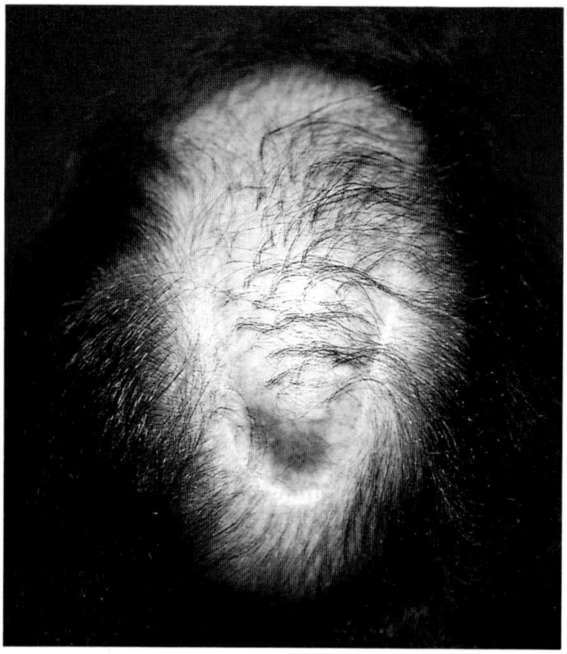 b

Photo 11. **a** Necrosis of residual median sagittal flap after paramedian reduction. **b** Final scar

necrosis, which also allows performance of galeotomies under the hairy flap. We do not favour either of these devices, for the reasons given above.

Transverse Fusiform Reductions (Fig. 8, Photo 12)

Transverse fusiform reductions are usually made at the summit of the crown, in the occipital region, given the poor elasticity of the scalp in this region, and thus the gain obtained is always small (at most 2–3 cm). Moreover, because of the convexity of the cranial vault, it is difficult to sufficiently extend the stripping downwards. It is possible to improve the yield of this technique by making two lateral vertical incisions, one on either side, which constitute a rectangular flap with an inferior pedicle, thus allowing more extensive downward stripping under observation. This more extensive stripping implies the sacrifice of the occipital arteries and thus some weakening of the flap, which is not incompatible with its survival but does incur additional risk. The two lateral incisions can be replaced by a mid-line vertical incision. Lastly, we have seen that the upper incision must not obliterate the transition zone, when it exists, i.e. when there is hair at the vertex.

Mixed Fusiform Reductions (Fig. 9, Photo 13)

Mixed fusiform reductions combine a sagittal and a transverse spindle. These procedures, more attractive in theory, are of only minor additional value in practice. Indeed, contrary to what might be expected, they do not allow the excision of greater areas of smooth skin than a purely sagittal excision. They may, in some cases, lead to a scar that is cruciform, anchor-shaped or Y-shaped. There is always then a risk of necrosis at the junctional angles whenever there is some degree of closure tension. The indications for these reductions are relatively rare, but they may in some cases meet the criteria for a vertex of a particular shape. In such cases the surgeon must know how to adapt the shape of the excision to that of the bald area. These excisions are dictated by the classical rules of plastic surgery.

The reduction described by Fleming [15] in 1965 (Fig. 10), which combines a median sagittal spindle with a transverse spindle anterior to the bounds of the frontal zone, can also be classed under this heading. The design allows ascent of the crown and advancement of the temporal lines at the same time. Actually, the gain obtained is usually quite small, as we have seen that what is gained in advancement is

Fig. 8. **a** Transverse reduction. **b** Transverse reduction combined with two lateral incisions producing a rectangular flap. **c** Transverse reduction combined with median vertical incision

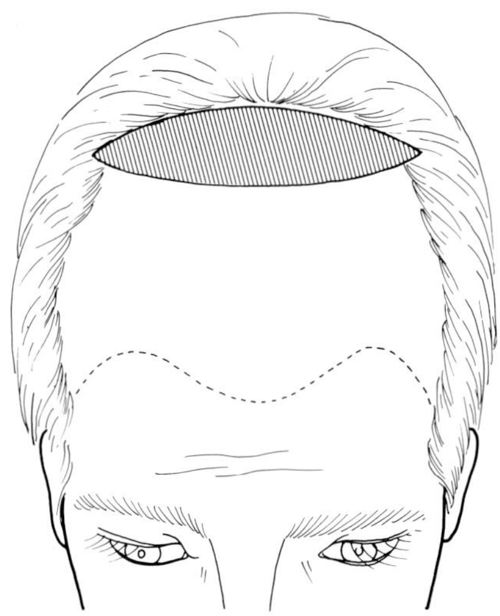

a

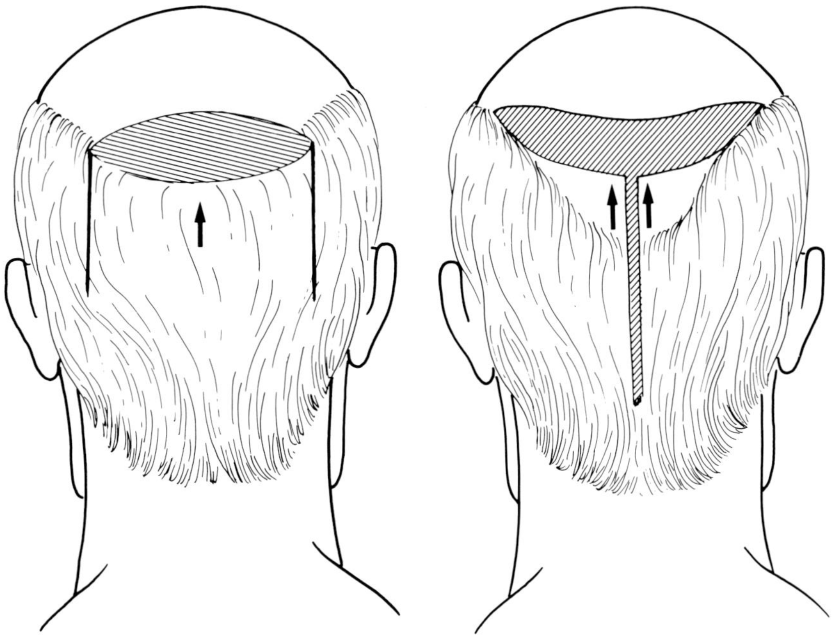

b c

mostly lost in ascent of the crown. Therein lies all value of giant reductions.

Giant Reduction Procedures

Techniques Originally Described by Marzola and Brandy

The techniques originally described by Marzola and Brandy have a twofold principle: total stripping of the entire scalp and occipital stripping extended below the hair-bearing zone in the posterior cervical region. These techniques involve sacrifice of the occipital vessels and preservation of the superficial temporal vessels, and it is not surprising that the authors of these reductions have described partial necroses of the distal part of the occipital flap. The shape of these reductions resembles that of the modified flap of Fleming, described by the brothers Blanchard [5].

Marzola's Technique

Marzola's technique [16] requires at least three stages (Fig. 11):

1. The incision begins at the anterior part of the sideburn and ascends along the temporal line of hair insertion. It then turns backward and skirts

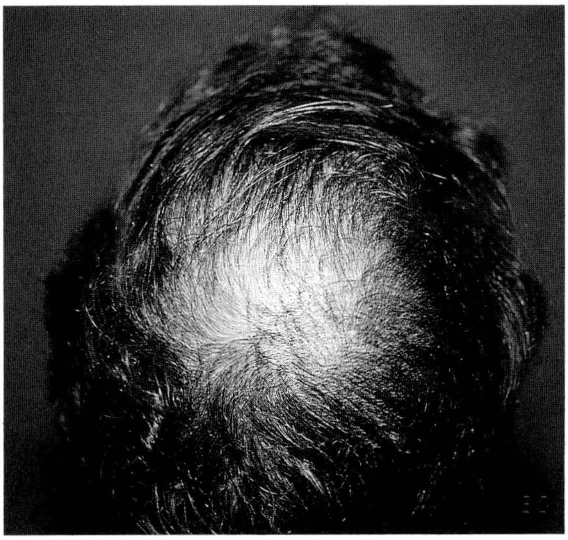
a

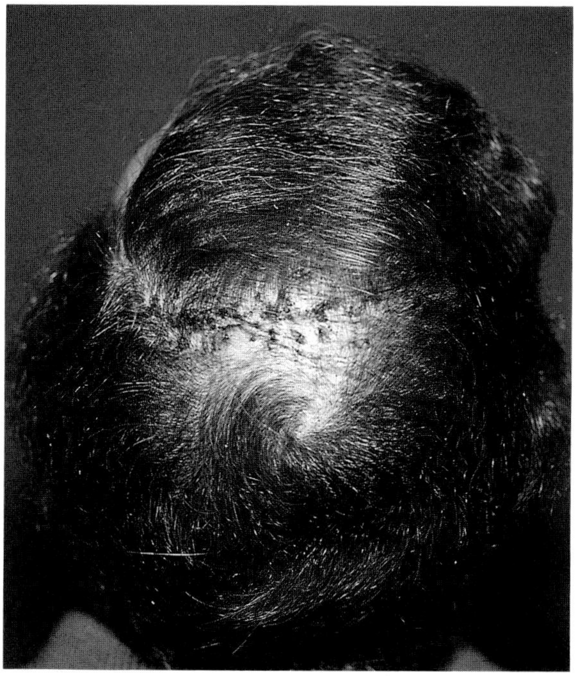
b

Photo 12. a Baldness C1 F1 T4. **b** Result after classical transverse reduction

the upper border of the crown and ends in the occipital region after having transgressed the mid-line by 5–6 cm. This incision must allow preservation of the superficial temporal vessels.

The subgaleal stripping extends over the entire temporal scalp and extends below as far as the attachment of the pinna. At the back, it is easily continued in the same plane as far as the external occipital protuberance. Below this limit the dissection plane must be changed to cross the galea and continue at the subcutaneous level. The vast parieto-occipital flap thus defined must then undergo superior and anterior translation. The ascension of the scalp may thus exceed 4 cm in the occipital region and 4 cm in the temporal region. Advancement of the anterior temporal line by 1–3 cm is possible, depending on cases and requirements.

2. The second stage consists of performing the same procedure on the other side, which allows a decrease in the width of the vertex by as much as 6 cm.
3. The third stage is virtually a sagittal reduction aimed at joining the margins of the crown at the mid-line. To avoid a visible vertical mid-line scar, the author advises extension of the excision backwards and quite far laterally in the occipital region.

Brandy's Technique

Brandy's technique [11, 12] is based on the same principle, but the author performs a bilateral reduction at the same operative stage (Fig. 12, Photos 14, 15). The procedure takes longer, but this technique saves an operative stage and especially allows better monitoring of the occipital pedicles. The final stage is identical in both techniques.

These two techniques, apart from the not inconsiderable difficulty of their performance, also have the disadvantage of leaving a vulnerable median flap with a long narrow pedicle at the summit of the cranium after the penultimate procedure. Furthermore, these reduction techniques, which allow excellent coverage of the vertical region, do not cover the frontal region. For this, Marzola advises the use of a small, vertical temporal flap 10 cm long and 2 cm wide, situated at the anterior limit of the temporal region. While attractive in theory, this small flap actually has several disadvantages; the temporal line of attachment has to be moved back, coverage is minimal and it is ill-suited to the region to be covered.

As for the coverage of the frontal region advised by Brandy during the final operative stages, this is possible only if scalp elasticity is excellent. Of course, it is always possible to perform cylindrical grafting to

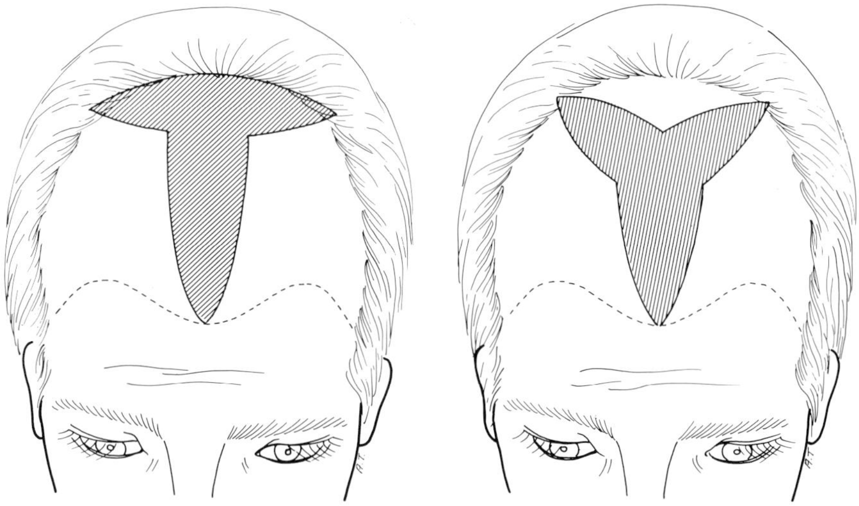

a b

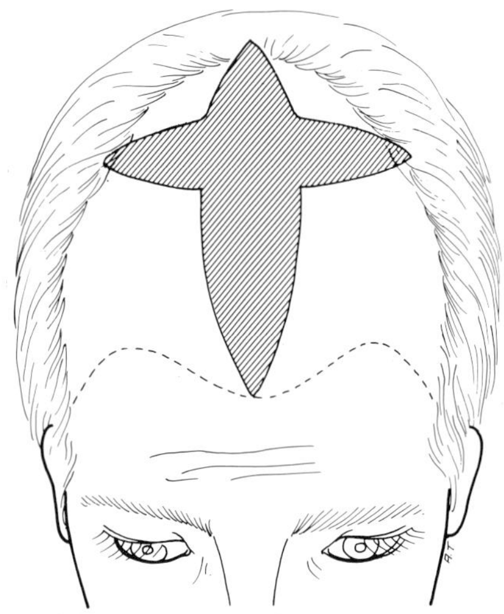

c

Fig. 9a–c. Mixed fusiform reduction. **a** T-shaped scar. **b** Y-shaped scar. **c** Cruciform scar

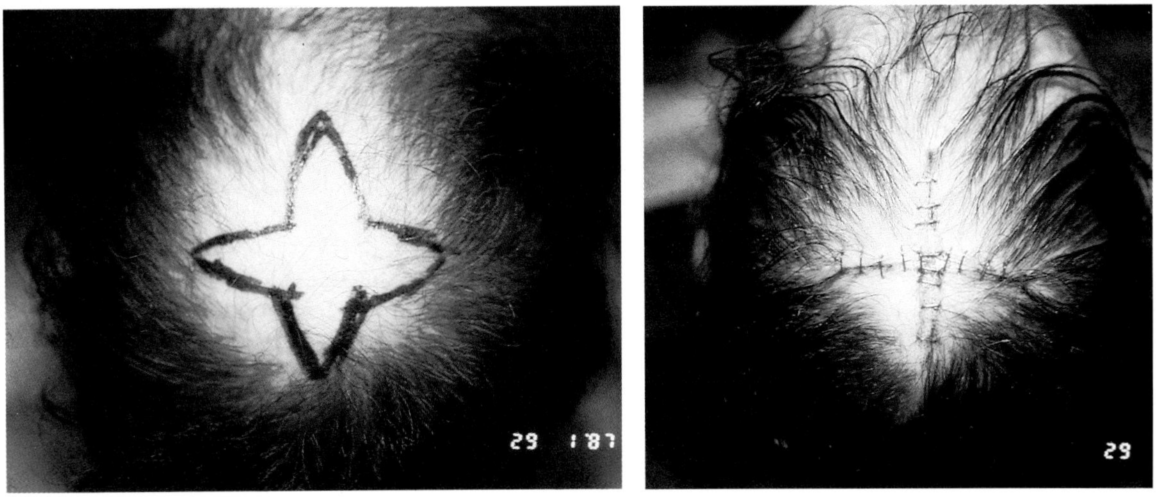

a b

Photo 13a,b. Mixed reduction

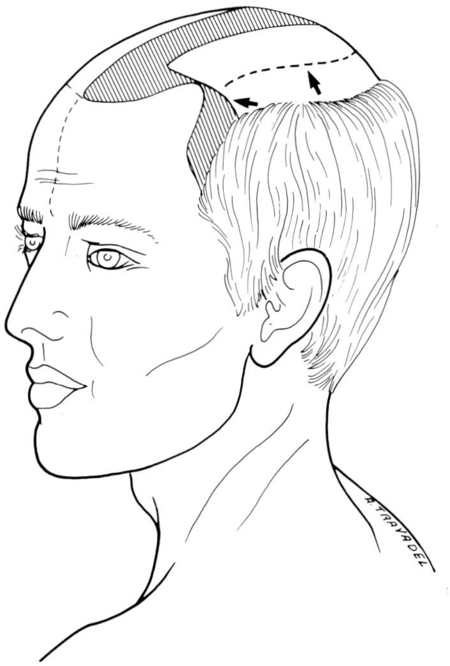

Fig. 10. Fleming type of reduction

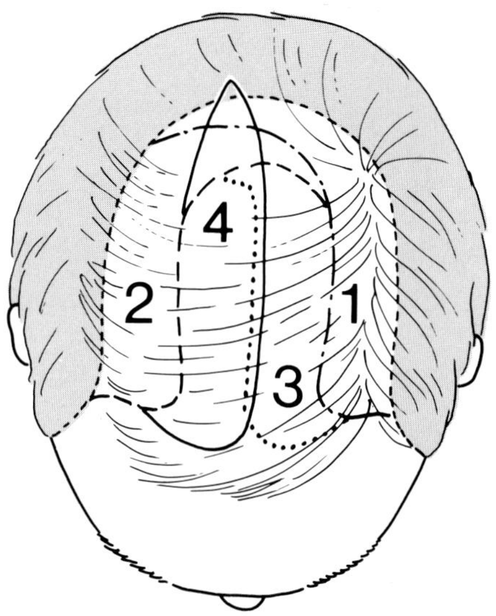

Fig. 11. Marzola's four-stage technique

cover this region, but we have seen its disadvantages: the need for three or four supplementary procedures and the difficulty of obtaining a final cosmetic aspect of good quality.

Dardour's Techniques for Lifting the Scalp [14]

Necroses have been reported with the preceding techniques and are due to failure to observe certain fundamental rules:

- Preservation of at least one superficial temporal artery
- Failure of too many grafts in the stripped zone to take
- Inferior occipital stripping that is too superficial

In theory, on reaching the external occipital protuberance, the change of plane should be made at the superior curved occipital line where the occipital muscle is attached. In practice, it is easier to work slightly above this. This change of plane occurs in a zone where the adhesions are very dense. It is easier to control the occipital artery slightly after its emergence in the muscle, which avoids the risk of retraction. The artery and the greater occipital nerve are intimately apposed at this level (Photo 16, Fig. 13). Unlike previous authors, who divided them, we believe that with careful dissection the occipital vessels and nerves can be preserved, so that after their freeing they permit adequate stretching.

Once past this zone, the subcutaneous attachments are looser and dissection is easier. It is continued in a deep subcutaneous plane, respecting the subjacent perimysium as far as the mid-cervical region, below the zone of hair implantation, and in the mastoid region behind the ear. Since observing these principles, we have encountered no necroses in several hundred cases. Once we were sure of the safety of this extensive stripping, we developed three new techniques with spectacular results.

Lifting of the Scalp by the Marginal or Peripheral Route Combined with One or Two Vertical Flaps in One Operative Stage [14] (Fig. 14)

Brandy's technique advances the temporal line and causes frontal skin loosening, which sometimes even leads to ptosis of the eyelids and accentuation of the frontal creases; this has obliged us in some cases to consider subsequent frontal lifting. This is why we thought of combining lifting of the scalp with a small, vertical anterior marginal flap, 2 cm wide and

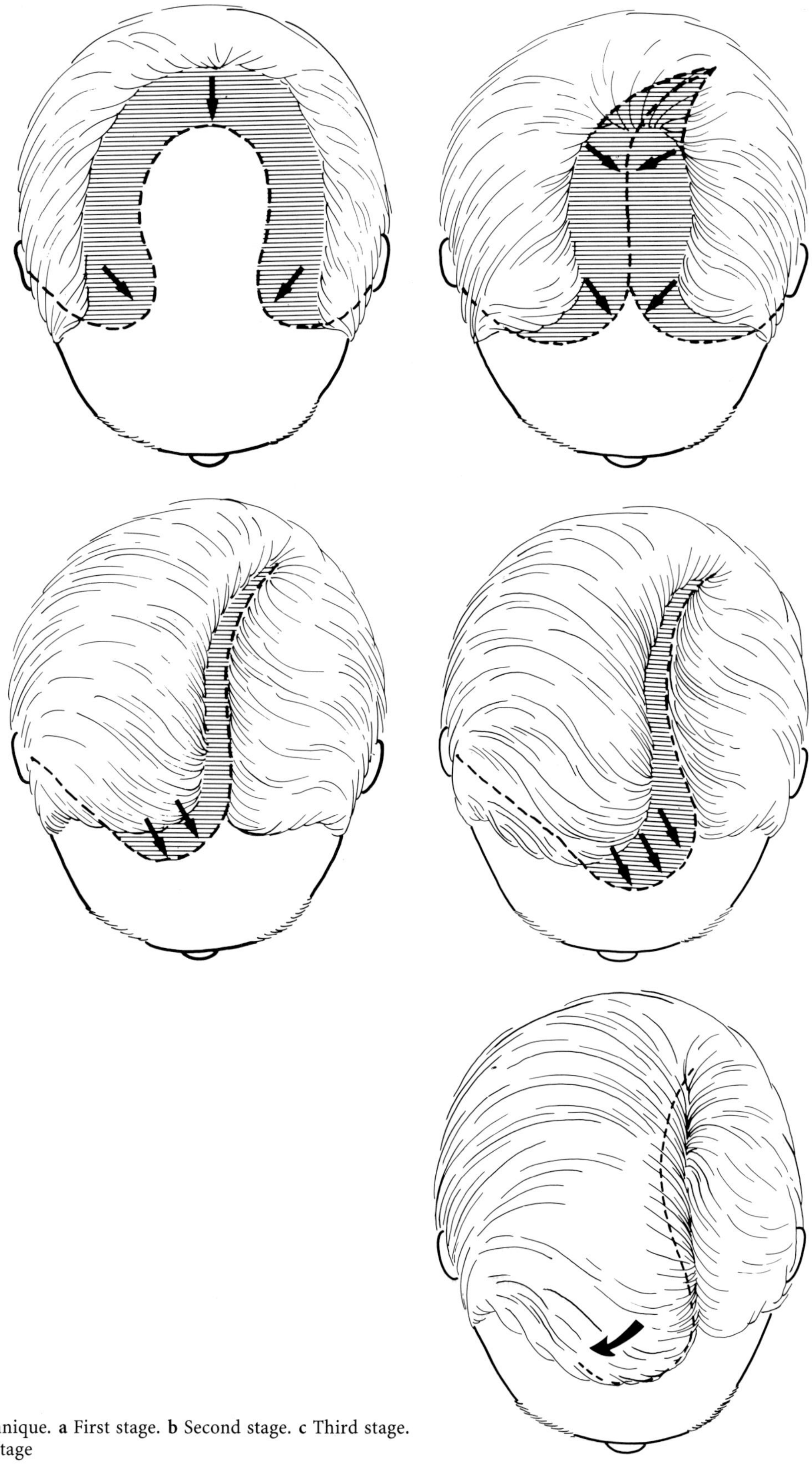

a b c d e

Fig. 12a–e. Brandy technique. **a** First stage. **b** Second stage. **c** Third stage. **d** Fourth stage. **e** Fifth stage

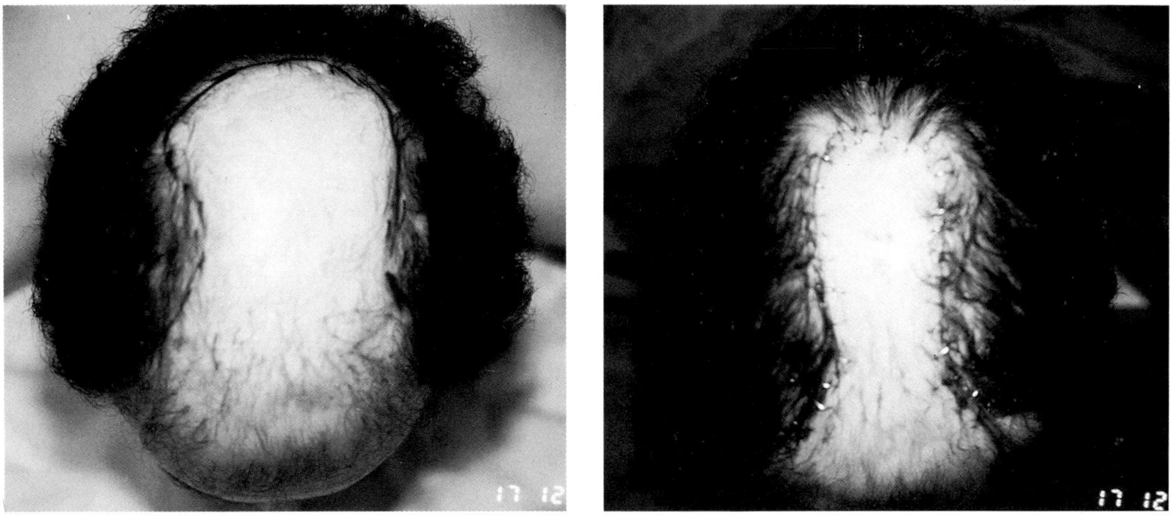

Photo 14. **a** Brandy-type reduction. **b** Result after one procedure

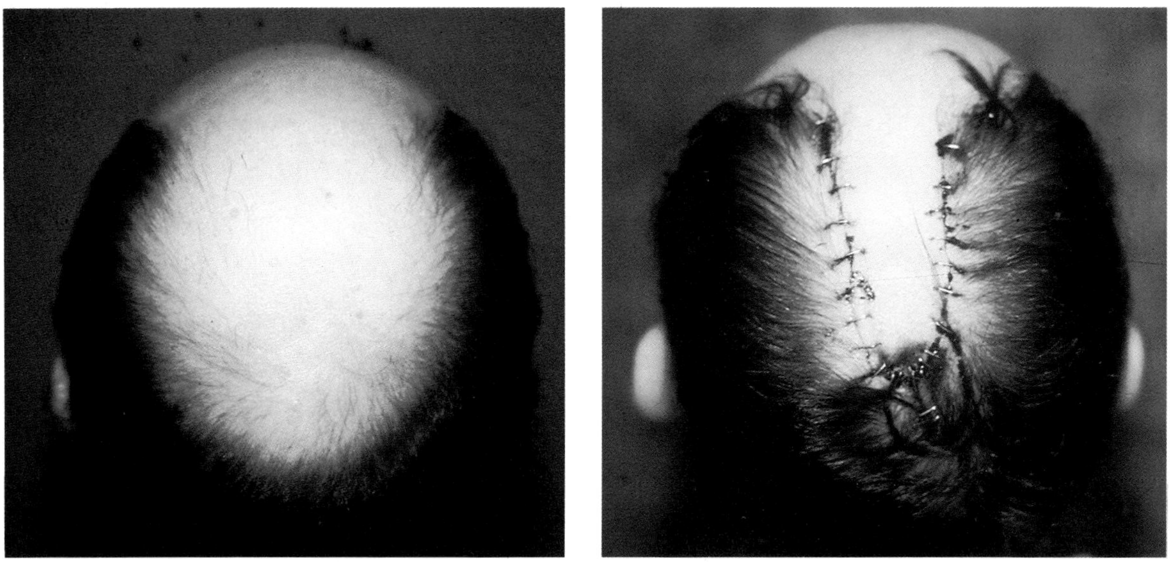

Photo 15. **a** Brandy technique. **b** Result after one procedure in a patient with a very lax scalp (S2). Note damage to residual median flap

10 cm long, ending at the mid-line and providing a small but not negligible frontal coverage (Photo 17). The incision begins on one side at the lower part of the anterior temporal line, which it follows from below upwards. It then skirts the upper border of the crown throughout its length and redescends along the opposite temporal line. Unfortunately, the construction of a flap reaching the mid-line is possible only on one side, since two flaps joining at this point would isolate a posterior skin island deprived of all vascularisation. If the surgeon wishes to make a flap on each side, each must be about 2 cm shorter, such that there will be a persisting mid-frontal bridge of skin 4 cm wide to ensure the blood supply of the residual median smooth zone (Photo 18).

This technique is very valuable since it allows coverage of the vertex and frontal region at the same time, but it is not possible except in patients in whom the temporal line is sufficiently anterior (*t*1 or *t*2). The design of the anterior marginal temporal incision is slightly concave towards the front, so as to construct a mini-flap as already described (see the chapter on "Flaps", p. 135).

At the closure stage, after having performed complete stripping of the entire scalp, it is essential to begin by positioning the flap(s) at the frontal region

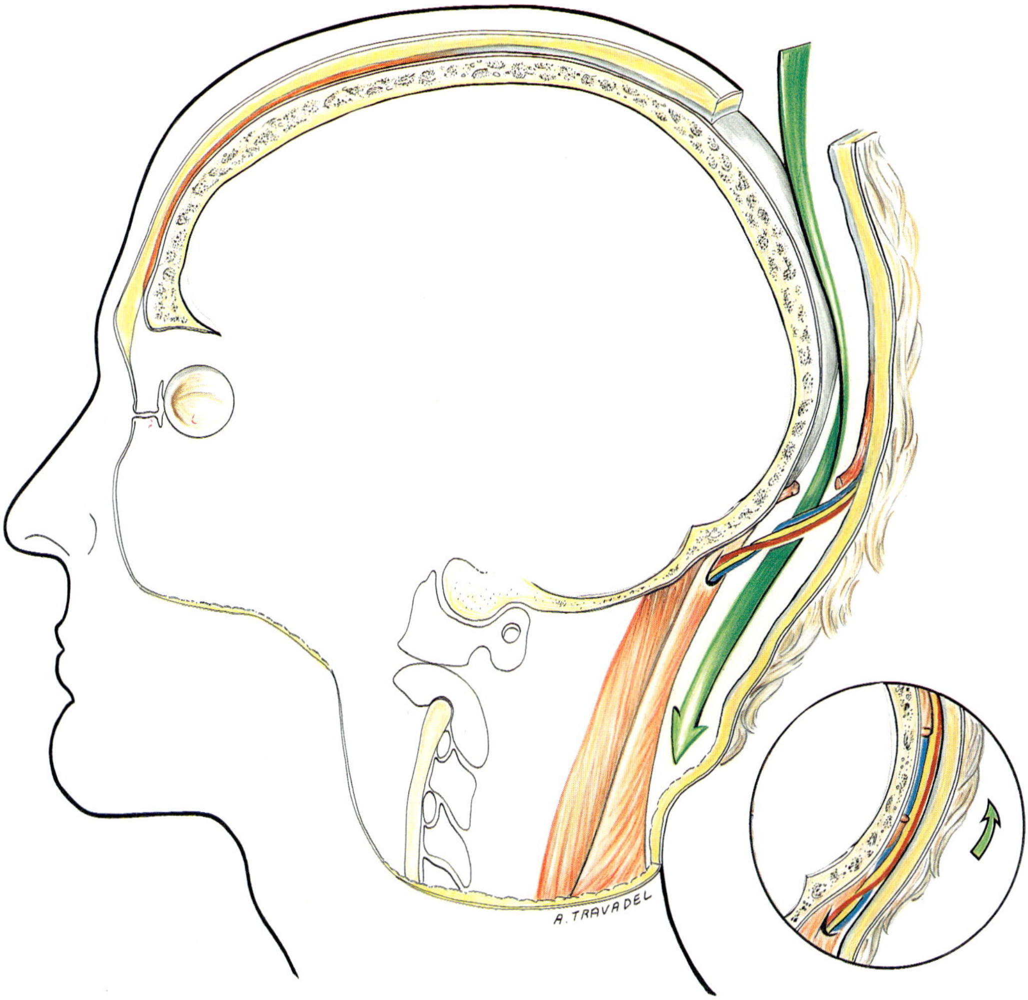

Fig. 13. Paramedian sagittal section passing through occipital pedicle and showing plane of cleavage of scalp, lifting and change of plane below pedicle

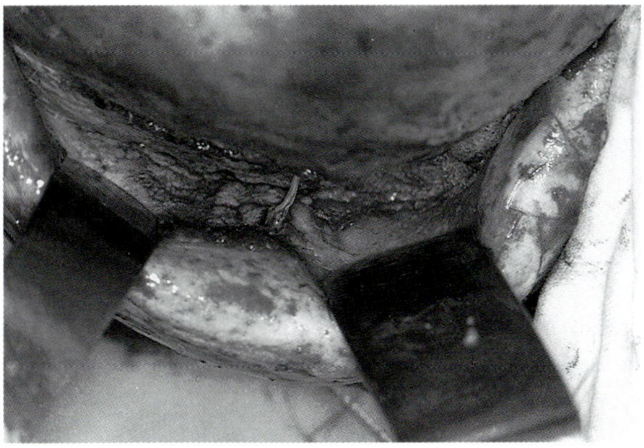

Photo 16. Dissection of occipital pedicle: the artery and nerve have been preserved

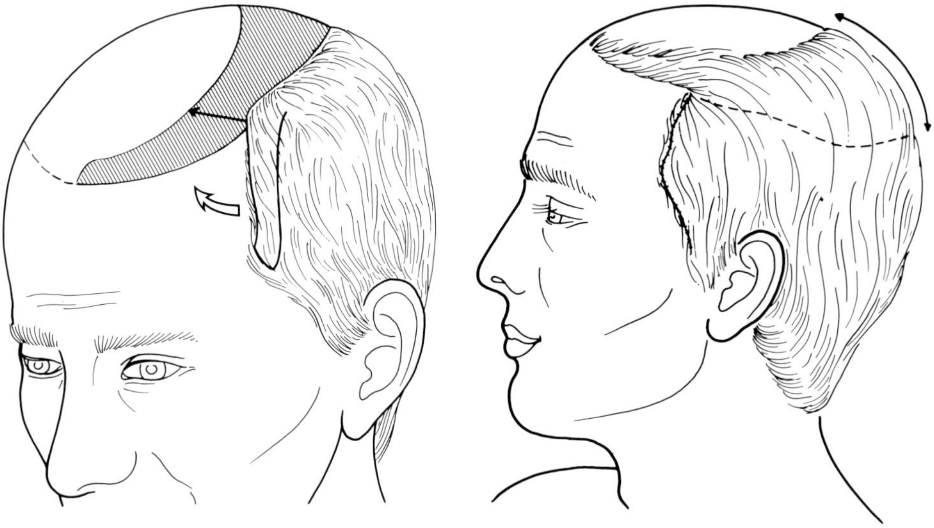

a b

Fig. 14. **a** Lifting of scalp combined with vertical pre-auricular flap. **b** Result after first operation

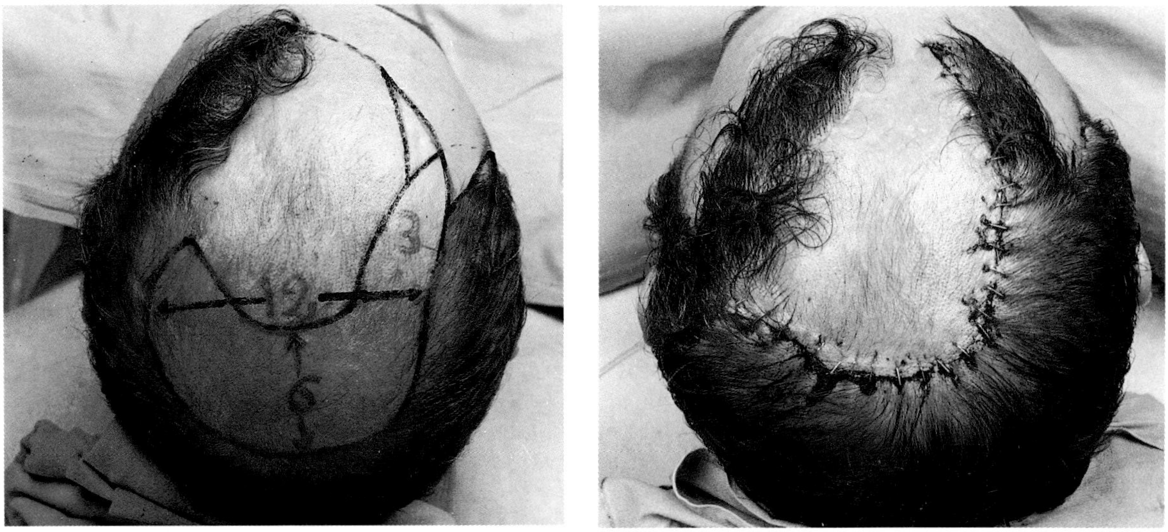

a b

Photo 17a–h. Lifting of scalp combined with pre-auricular flap: very severe baldness (height of crown, HC=9 cm) treated at first stage by left pre-auricular flap

and then to effect ascension of the occipital scalp and fix its mid-point. This usually allows a resection of 6 cm of the smooth posterior zone. Then the reduction must be made from the front backwards to avoid a "dog-ear" at the origin of the flap.

Four months after this first procedure, the scalp has practically regained its initial laxity and it is possible to re-do the same procedure. The incisions and stripping must then allow re-elevation of the anterior flaps and their inward shifting by 2 cm, leaving a loss of substance to be filled by two new vertical flaps identical to the previous ones (Photo 19). Thanks to this technique, after the second procedure the patient will have two frontal flaps 4 cm wide, a lateral ascension of the crown by at least 4 cm on each side, i.e. a reduction of the width of the vertex by 8 cm, and a posterior ascent of the crown by 8 or sometimes 10 cm.

Lifting of the Scalp by a Mid-line Incision Combined with Two Vertical Mini-flaps in One Stage

This technique (Fig. 15, Photo 20), much like the preceding one, may suffice in itself for the treatment of major baldness. It palliates the chief disadvantage

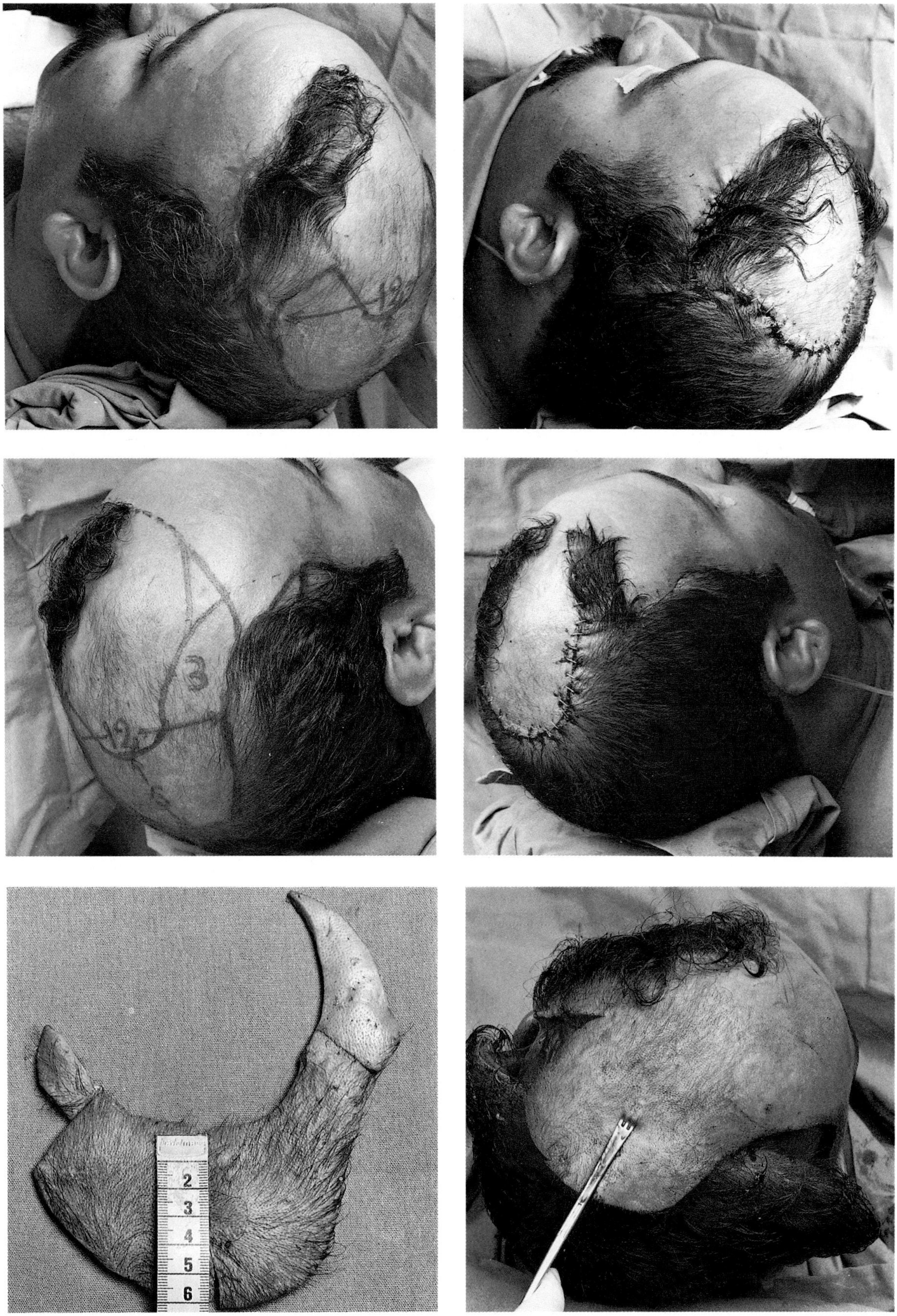

Photo 17c–h.

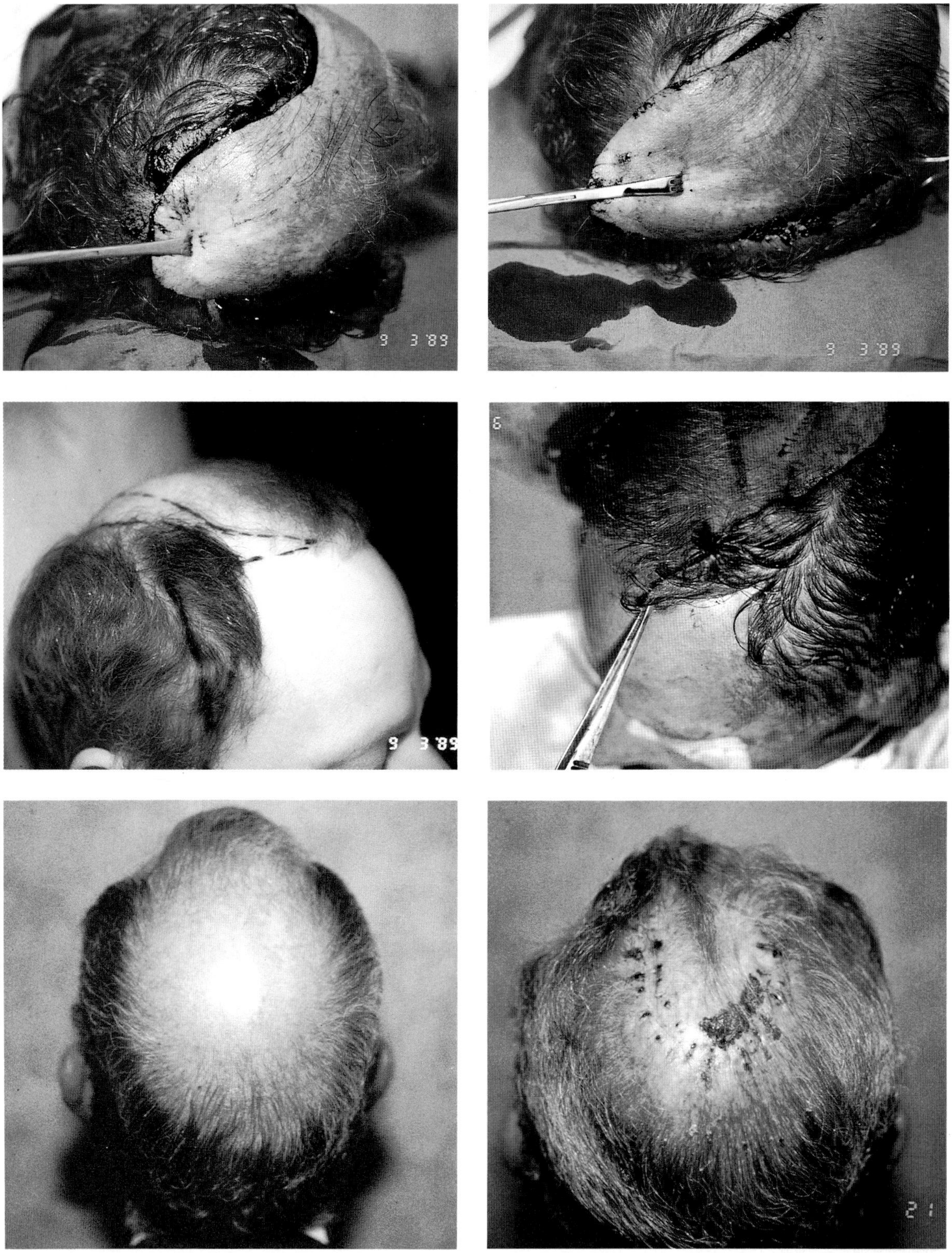

a b c d e f

Photo 18a–f.

Photo 18. a Ascension of vertex after classical stripping. **b** Ascension of vertex in same patient after lifting type of stripping of scalp. **c** Associated mini-flap. **d** Positioning of mini-flap. **e** Preoperative aspect. **f** Immediate postoperative result. **g** Excised specimen

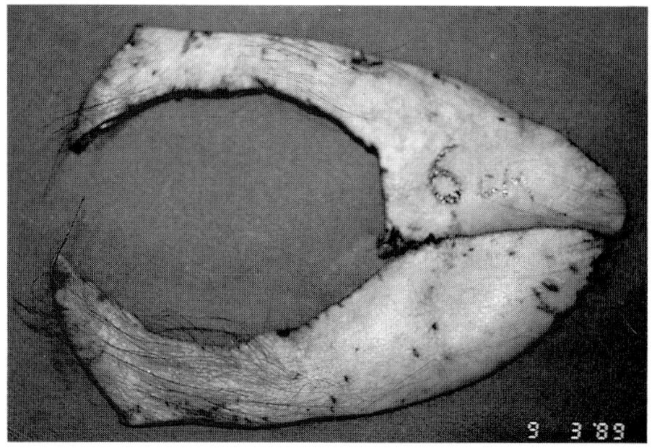
g

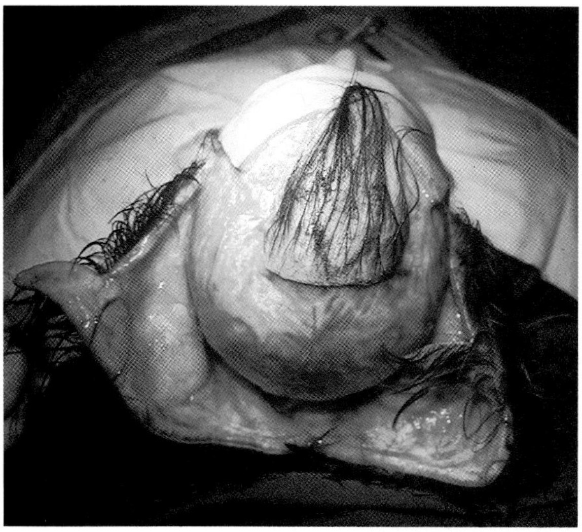
a

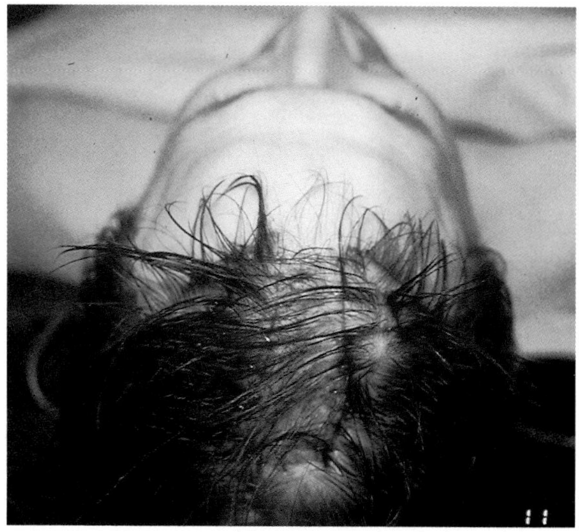
c

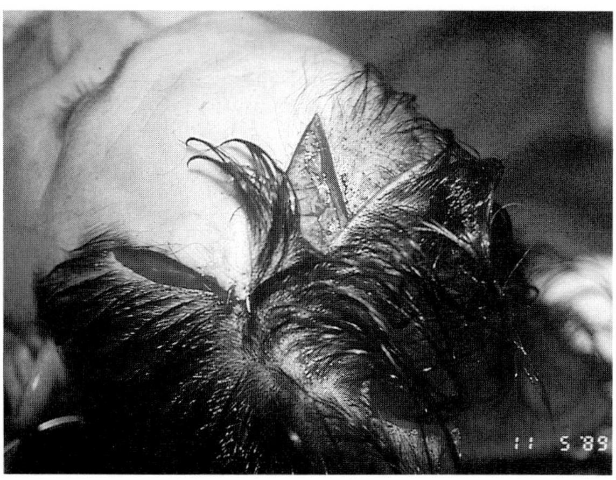
b

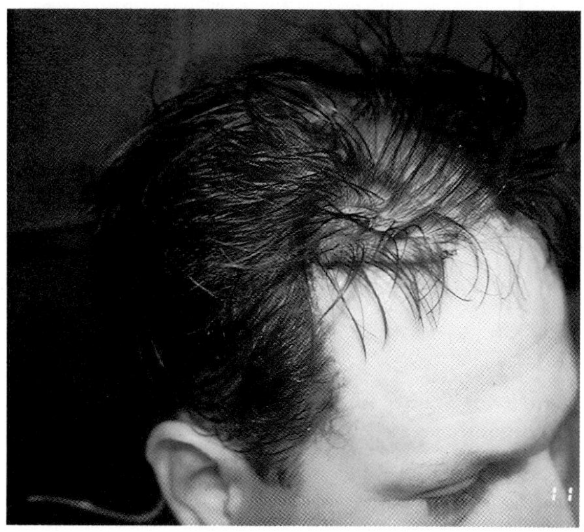
d

Photo 19. a Second lifting of scalp by peripheral route combined with two vertical mini-flaps in the same stage: incisions. **b** Closure of temporal line: the first flap raised is transposed inward, the second flap takes its place. **c,d** Transplantation completed: there is a clear view of the two flaps juxtaposed in the frontal region of either side, giving the equivalent of a 4 cm wide flap on each side

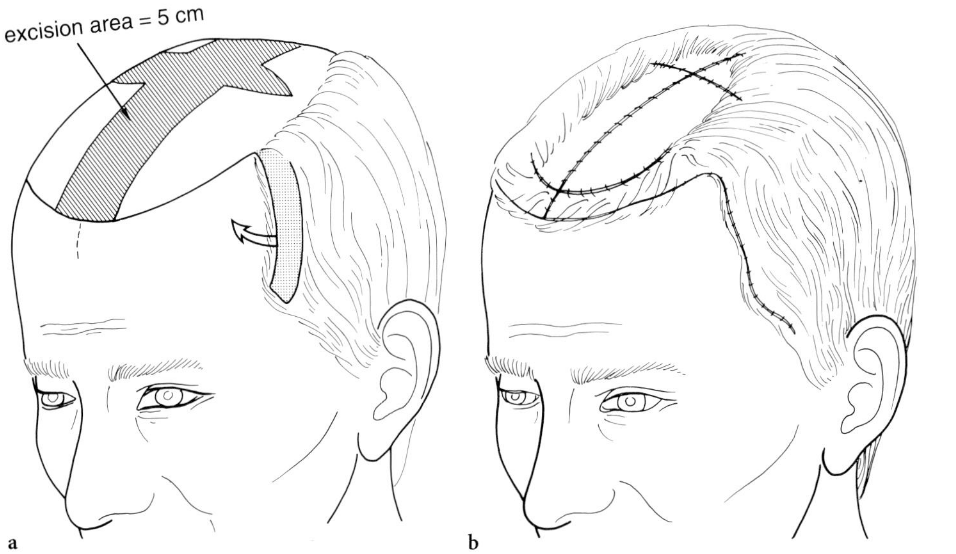

Fig. 15. **a** Lifting of scalp combined with two vertical flaps by the median sagittal route. **b** Result after first stage

of reductions, i.e. the impossibility of covering the frontal region. A long antero-posterior sagittal incision reaching the protuberance at the back is complemented by a marginal incision along the temporal line laterally and the future frontal line in front. An anterior temporal vertical mini-flap, identical to the previous one, is fashioned on each side in such a way that its superior pedicle is at least 2 cm below the future point G (base of the fronto-temporal recession). Stripping is then done over the entire scalp area, both laterally and at the back.

The lateral stripping allows excision of a median sagittal spindle 4–5 cm wide. The posterior stripping allows advancement of the scalp both medially and laterally, allowing the excision of a transverse spindle of 3–4 cm. Advancement of the temporal line then allows easy closure of the site of raising of the vertical flap on each side. Closure must be done beginning with the positioning and suture of the two frontal flaps. Then the sagittal spindle is excised and, lastly, after its closure, the transverse spindle is excised. It must be noted that, in this case, the two flaps must meet at the mid-line, which is why we make their ends square and not tapered.

After this first procedure the area of baldness is decreased by about half, as in the preceding technique. The two procedures differ essentially in the position of the scars. Some months later, the same procedure is made by excising another mid-line spindle and transposing two other vertical flaps in front of the first two, which are themselves transferred toward the middle part of the forehead. This creates the equivalent of a flap 4 cm wide on each side, which is enough to cover the frontal baldness, whereas the two reductions have covered the posterior baldness, sometimes leaving a median smooth spindle. This may be improved by the residual elasticity of a final reduction or by autografting.

Lifting of the Scalp by a Parasagittal Incision Combined with Two Vertical Mini-flaps

This technique (Fig. 16) is somewhat of a combination of the two preceding ones. The incision skirts the anterior temporal line on one side and then the upper border of the crown up to the mid-line, which it transgresses slightly. On the other side, it also skirts the anterior temporal line, but at its upper part it continues forward along the virtual anterior frontal line to reach the apex of the temporal line of the other side. It thus demarcates two asymmetric flaps, the first being represented solely by the hairy crown, the second comprising the hairy crown of the other side and the whole bald zone.

The dissection is the same as previously described and includes the entire hairy area and descends below the occipital pedicles, as far as the low posterior hairy margin. The two vertical flaps with their superior pedicles are then tilted and positioned. They should normally join at the mid-line. The positioning of these flaps produces ascension of the crown on each side, which will permit excision of a spindle of smooth skin if required. This excision is made from the front backwards. No tension is permitted at the front, so as not to cause ischaemia of the flaps; however, some tension is allowed at the back, as during a normal vertical reduction.

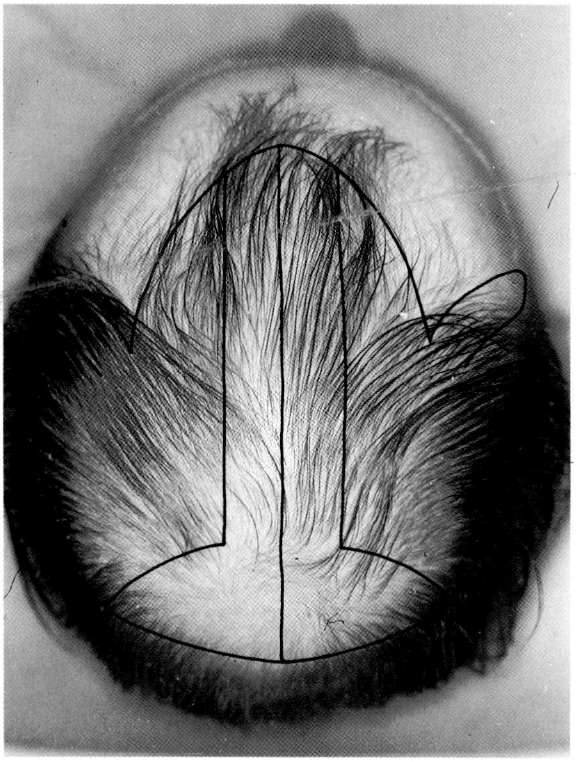
a

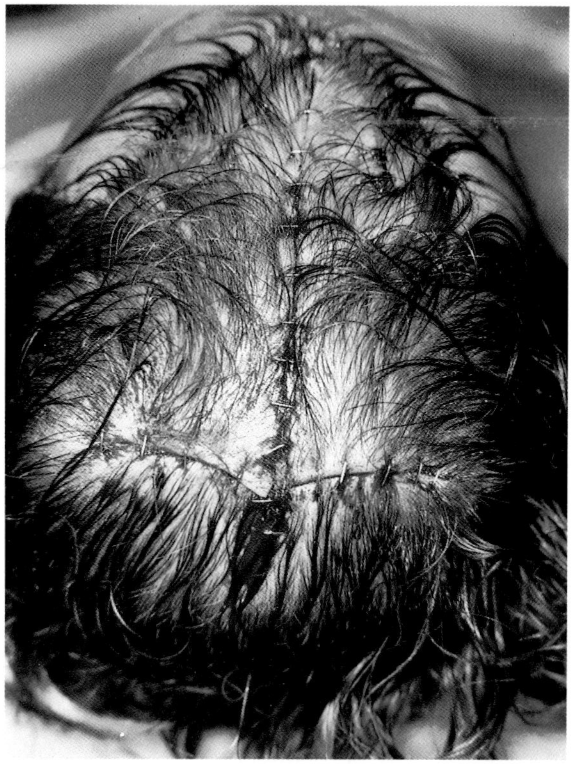
b

Photo 20a–e. Lifting by sagittal route combined with two vertical flaps. **a** Preoperative aspect and design of excision. **b** Immediate postoperative aspect. **c,d** Complete stripping and reflection of scalp. **e** Closure begun by placement of the two vertical flaps transposed in the frontal region

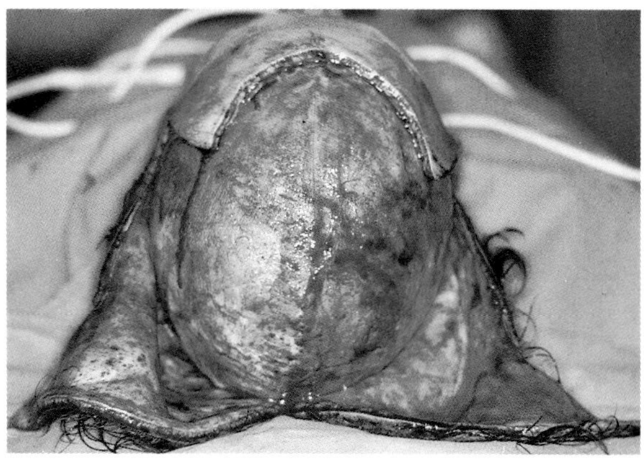
c

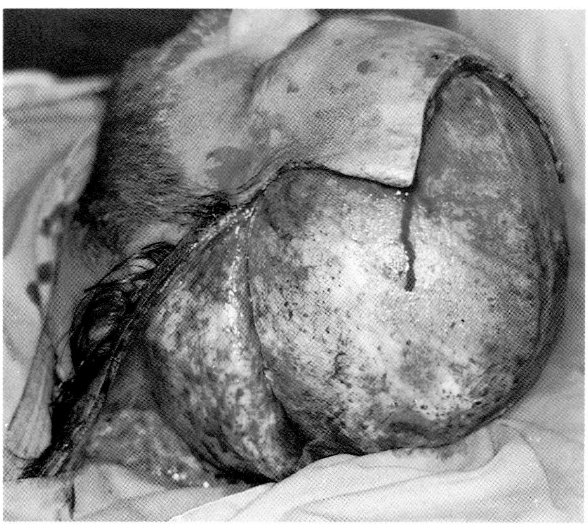
d

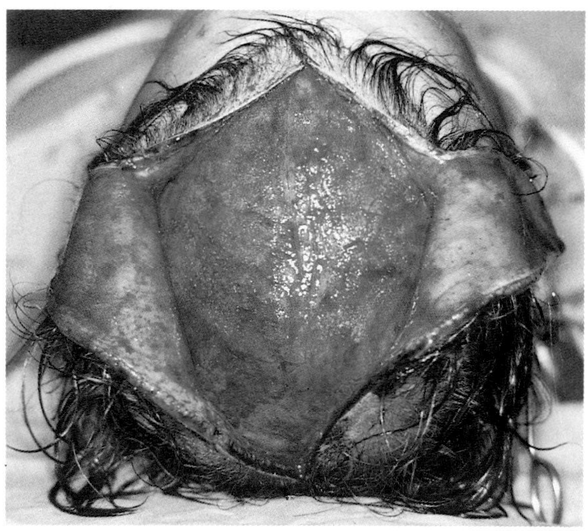
e

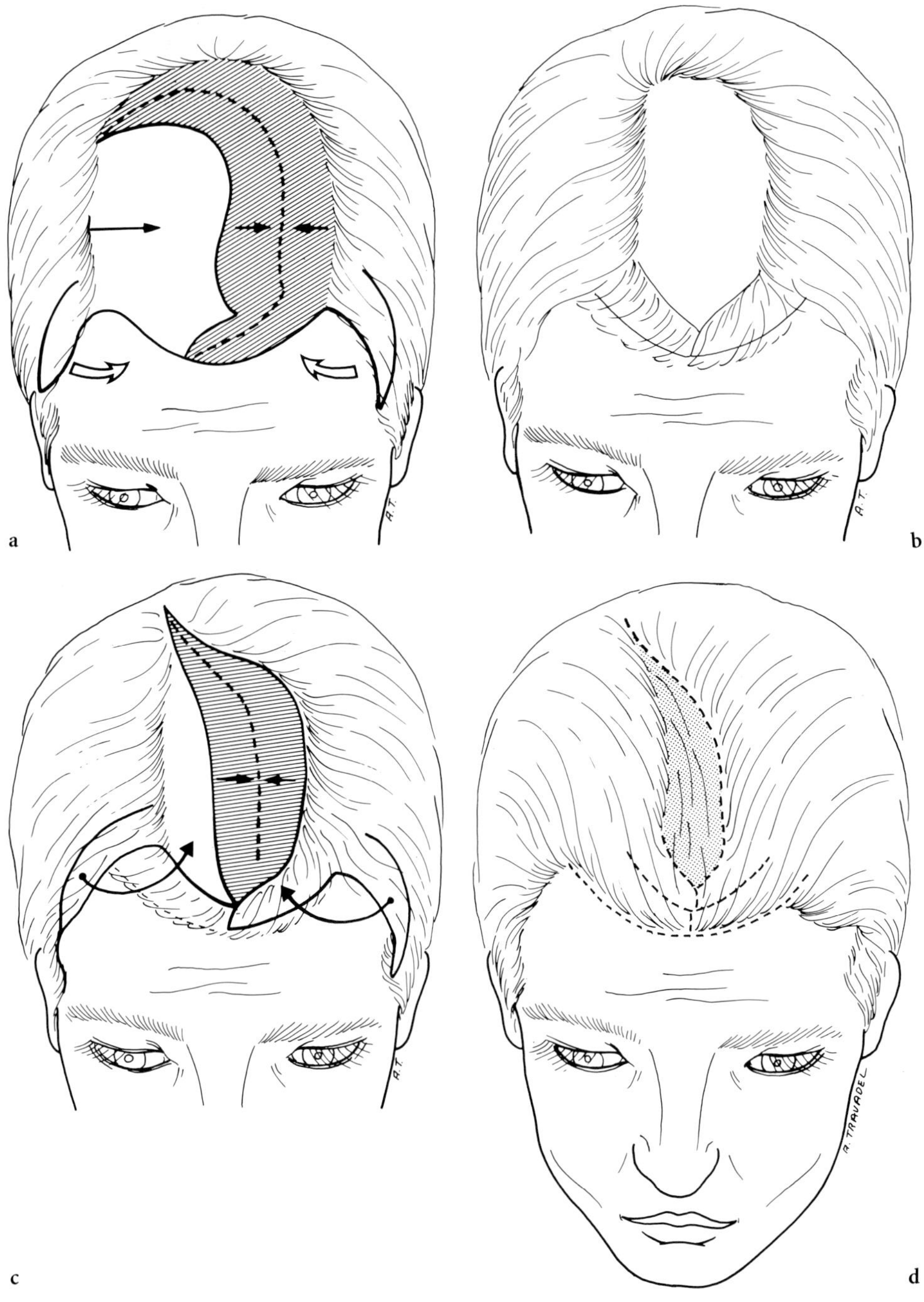

Fig. 16. **a** Lifting of scalp by parasagittal incision (*thick lines*), resected zone *hatched*. **b** Result after first procedure. **c** Parasagittal lifting. Second stage: incisions in *thick lines*, resected zone hatched. **d** Parasagittal lifting: result after second stage; a median smooth zone sometimes persists (*shaded*)

Thanks to the design of the incision employed, the result is a lateral ascension of the crown on each side and an antero-posterior ascension of the occipital part. The amount of smooth zone resected is always the same (around 5 cm), but the terminal scar at the summit of the cranium is shifted laterally compared with the preceding technique; since it skirts the upper border of the crown on one side it is less obvious.

During the second procedure, the incision follows the temporal line of the side of this scar to join it directly, thus dividing the pedicle of the first flap on this side. It then follows the same antero-posterior scar backwards. On the other side, the incision follows the anterior temporal line and then skirts the frontal line in front of the original flap as far as the mid-line. From this point it skirts the posterior scar of the opposite flap to reach the incision on the other side at the posterior part of the flap.

Complete stripping of the scalp is obligatory to allow sufficient ascension and advancement. Two new superior pedicle flaps are fashioned behind the temporal line and transposed to the frontal region. The design of the incisions implies that one of these flaps must be placed behind the original flap, which will not have been raised, whereas the other flap is positioned lateral to the original flap, which will have been raised and transposed inward. Thus, on one side the frontal scar of the first operation is preserved, safeguarding the patient from further submission to the usual cycle (Fig. 16). This design allows the excision of a second spindle of smooth skin of 3–5 cm depending on the elasticity of the scalp, thus correcting in two stages a bald area 8–10 cm wide, while the frontal region itself is covered by the four juxtaposed flaps.

Complications

Complications are relatively rare and usually without long-term consequences.

Haematoma

Haematoma is uncommon because of absence of major perforating vessels in the stripped zone and because of closure tension in the scalp, which is equivalent to a pressure dressing over a convex area. The only haematomas we have observed followed stripping of the low occipital region with section of the perforating branches of the occipital artery. Diathermy haemostasis may lead to secondary haemorrhage, in which case we advise haemostasis by ligature of the occipital arteries, which calls for good visual monitoring of the region and an adequate approach, as well as routine suction drainage.

Necrosis

Necrosis should, in theory, never be encountered, since a single temporal artery is enough to supply the entire scalp. Therefore there is always a predictable cause for necrosis after a reduction, which, as we have seen, may be one of the following:

- Excessive closing tension, which creates ischaemia of the margins and may lead to skin necrosis. This is favoured by two factors: careless incisions of the galea to permit greater stretching which damage the subcutaneous network and a history of smoking.
- Decrease of the subdermal network by grafting sessions preceding the reduction. This may consist of a necrosis of the scalp secondary to graft removal at the crown, usually at the occipital region. Obviously, in these cases giant reductions will be much more risky when they sacrifice the occipital arteries. There may also be a necrosis of the smooth vertical zone behind a grafted frontal area.
- Destruction of the subdermal plexus, secondary to stripping that is too superficial, particularly in the posterior cervical region.
- Absence of the temporal arteries after bilateral ligature or other procedures (such as a vertical preauricular flap) during a giant reduction.
- A major haematoma is a source of prolonged compression if it is not evacuated and drained early.

Alopecia

Following a reduction, a secondary patch of alopecia may appear towards the third week in part of the stripped zone (anagenic defluvium). We have seen that this phenomenon is due to temporary ischaemia of the follicles, caused in this case by tension and squeezing of the vessels. This rare phenomenon is always reversible after a classical reduction. However, it is much commoner in giant reductions if accompanied by sacrifice of the occipital arteries. The alopecia then always occurs below the superior occipital line, which confirms the fact that the large biparieto-temporal flap is supplied solely by one or two temporal arteries and that the supply from the cervical region is very reduced and exhausted at this level (Photo 21).

Further, it is in this region that very rare cases of localised necrosis have been reported, always in patients in whom too many grafts have been taken before the reduction in this vulnerable occipital region or during stripping that is too superficial. For this reason, we believe that it is essential with this giant reduction technique to stay well in contact with the perimysium after passage from the inferior

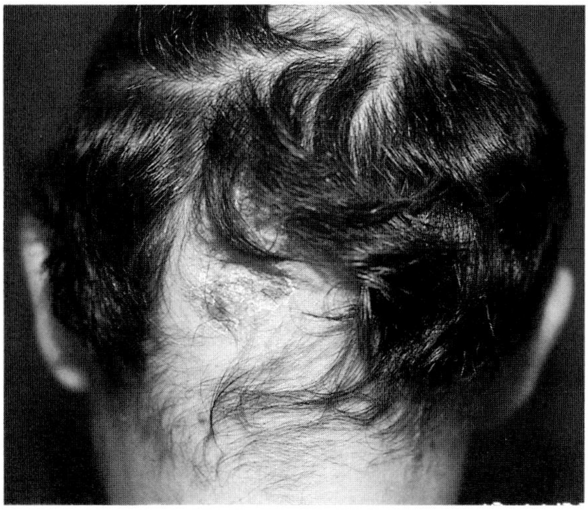

Photo 21. Complications of scalp lifting: transient low cervical alopecia

curved occipital line in traversing the occipital muscle.

Ugly Scars of Several Possible Causes

Ugly scars may have various causes:

1. Secondary broadening due to excessive closure tension:
   - Closure in two layers with a very firm suture does not prevent this complication.
   - Skin stitches add to the marginal ischaemia.
   - Closure in one layer by staples is much less traumatic and gives the best cosmetic results.
2. A poor position of the scar is sometimes the source of an unpleasant appearance, which is particularly the case with scars situated in a transition zone, i.e. when the hairs grow divergently on either side of the scar, forming an indelible parting. The only treatment consists of performing Z-plasties all along the scar to change the direction of the hairs.
3. Permanent alopecia along the margins of a secondary suture, also due to excessive closure tension.

Infection

Infection is uncommon after vertical reduction. Routine prophylactic antibiotic treatment seems not only unjustified, but even contraindicated insofar as it always carries a not inconsiderable risk of allergic reaction. Only the presence of an unevacuated haematoma involves a serious risk of infection. More common is mini-sepsis at stitch points and beneath crusts. The best treatment, both preventive and curative, is undeniably daily shampooing. Neglect of this type of sepsis leads to necrosis of the follicles near the scar margins and therefore to secondary alopecia around the scars.

Dehiscence of the Scars

In the days following the operation, dehiscence of the scars is usually due to an operative fault such as closure under excessive tension.

Conclusion

In our view, vertical reduction is an excellent technique because of the low complication rate, the rapidity of performance and of results and the quality of the cosmetic results obtained. On the other hand, it exhibits certain disadvantages:

- It cannot usually cover the frontal region, except in the cases which we have mentioned of scalp lifting combined with one or two vertical flaps.
- It is not very effective in subjects with poor scalp elasticity.
- It creates scars which may contraindicate subsequent flaps. When both techniques are indicated for the one patient, it is best to make the flap or flaps at a first stage and the reductions later. For the same security reasons we believe that it is preferable to carry out grafting, when predicted, after reduction. This emphasises the importance, in all cases, of planning the complete treatment of baldness right from the first consultation and of avoiding improvisations, which may subsequently prohibit the proper use of certain techniques.

References

1. Alt TH (1980) Scalp reduction as an adjunct to hair transplantation. J Dermatol Surg Oncol 6(2): 1011–1018
2. Alt TH (1981) Scalp reduction. J Cosmetic Surgery 1: 1–19
3. Bell ML (1982) Role of scalp reduction in the treatment of male pattern baldness. Plast Reconstr Surg 69(2): 272–277
4. Biemer E, Stock W, Wolfensberger C et al. (1979) Successful replantation of a totally avulsed scalp. Br J Plast Surg 32(1): 19–21

5. Blanchard G, Blanchard B (1976) La réduction tonsurale (détonsuration) – concept nouveau dans le traitement chirurgical de la calvitie. Rev Chir Esthet L 4: 5–10
6. Blanchard G, Blanchard B (1977) Obliteration of alopecia by hair lifting. A new concept and technique. J Natl Med Assoc 69: 639–641
7. Blanchard G, Blanchard B (1984) Proposition d'une approache topographique de la transplantation capillaire et de la réduction tonsurale. Ann Chir Plast Esthet 29(2): 152–161
8. Blanchard G, Blanchard B (1982) La réduction tonsurale, opération complémentaire de la transplantation dans la calvitie commune. Ann Chir Plast 27(1): 75–82
9. Bosley LL, Hope CR, Montroy RE (1979) Male pattern reduction (MPR) for surgical reduction of male pattern baldness. Curr Ther Res 25: 281–287
10. Bosley LL, Hope CR, Montroy RE, Straub PM (1980) Reduction of male pattern baldness in multiple stages: a restrospective study. J Dermatol Surg Oncol 6: 498–503
11. Brandy D (1986) The Brandy bitemporal flap. Cosmet Surg
12. Brandy D (1986) The bilateral occipito-parietal flap. J Dermatol Surg Oncol
13. Buncke HJ, Rose EH, Browstein MJ et al. (1978) Successful replantation of two avulsed scalp by micro-vascular anastomoses. Plast Reconstr Surg 61: 666
14. Dardour JC (1989) Les réduction de tonsure. Principles et innovation: le lifting du scalp. Ann Chir Plast Esthet 34(3): 234–242
15. Fleming J (1965) Surgery for baldness. a case report. Can J Surg 8: 400–403
16. Marzola M (1984) An alternative hair replacement method. In: O T Norwoord (ed) Hair transplant surgery, 2nd edn. Thomas, Springfield, pp 315–324
17. Miller GDH, Anstee EJ, Snell JA (1976) Successful replantation of an avulsed scalp by microvascular anastomoses. Plast Reconstr Surg 58: 133
18. Morestin H (1911) La mobilisation tégumentaire par décollements très étendus et ses applications en chirurgie réparatrice. J Chir (Paris) 8: 509–538
19. Morestin H (1968) La réduction graduelle des difformités tégumentaires. J Chir (Paris) 8: 509–511, reprinted in Plast Rec Surg 42: 163
20. Nahai F, Hurteau J, Vasconez LO (1978) Replantation of an entire scalp and ear by micro-vascular anastomoses of only one artery and one vein. Br J Plast Surg 31: 339
21. Nordstrom RE (1984) Stretch-back in scalp reductions for male pattern baldness. Plast Reconstr Surg 73: 422–426
22. Nordstrom RE (1984) La cinétique du cuir chevelu dans les opérations réductrices pour une alopécie masculine. Ann Chir Plast Esthet 29(3): 292
23. Norwood OT, Shiell RC (1984) Hair transplant surgery, 2nd edn. Thomas, Springfield
24. Norwood O'Tar (1983) Scalp reduction for baldness. Plast Reconstr Surg 71(1): 149
25. Norwood O'Tar (1975) Male pattern baldness: classification and incidence. South Med J 68(11): 1359–1364
26. Orticochea M (1969) Application de la technique des quatre lambeaux dans la rconstruction du front et des régions pariétales. Ann Chir Plast 14(2): 153–158
27. Orticochea M (1971) New three flap scalp reconstruction technique. Br J Plast Surg 24(2): 184–188
28. Real JP (1986) Le lambeau de scalp total: utilisation depuis 6 ans (1980–1985). Ann Chir Plast Esthet 31(4): 336–347
29. Unger MG, Unger WP (1978) Management of alopecia of the scalp by a combination of excision and transplantation. J Dermatol Surg Oncol 4: 670–672

Accessory Techniques

Pathogenic Procedures

In 1974, Maréchal [3] of Brussels suggested ligation of the six arteries supplying the scalp (temporal, occipital and posterior auricular) to check the progress of male baldness. This treatment was based on the empirical principle that testosterone acted on the target cells only after the local action of 5-alpha-reductase and that this was inhibited by hypoxia. Thus, ligation of the main arteries decreased blood-flow and replaced it by capillary flow, in this way decreasing the activity of 5-alpha-reductase and preventing the loss of hair.

The technique of ligation is simple and need not be described here. The superficial temporal arteries are located by palpation above the zygomatic arch just in front of the external auditory meatus; the occipital arteries are found at the occipital protuberance 2.5–3 cm from the mid-line; and the posterior auricular arteries are tied at the same level, but more laterally in the mastoid region at the junction of the smooth and hairy zones. Section of the vessels between two ligatures should ensure that patency cannot be re-established. Maréchal reported favourable results: 57% of his 303 cases were completely cured and 22% showed considerable improvement. The criteria of improvement were a reduction of the number of hairs lost daily from 65 to 40 on average and a decrease of the time of relubrication of the hair after shampooing.

Several aspects of this study seem open to criticism:

1. The chosen criterion of a decrease in the number of hairs lost daily seems unsatisfactory, in that it is not specified how long after the operation the study was made and over what period. Improvement could very well be transient or limited in time, which would deprive the technique of any value. Further, it is not stated whether seasonal factors were taken into account or not. Hair loss is known to be decreased in the spring, which might reproduce the same figures in an experiment, especially as the figures cited by the author lie within the average for normal hair loss in a healthy person.
2. Theoretically, we have seen that there is no reason to acknowledge that decreased vascularisation improves hair growth. The results obtained with minoxidil also contradict this theory in practice.
3. Patients who have sometimes had between 200 and 500 grafts exhibit a decrease of scalp vascularisation which is certainly much greater than after simple vascular ligature. No increase in growth rate or even any arrest of the progress of baldness has been noted in these patients.
4. In our technique with a pre-auricular flap, performed in over 500 patients, we routinely divide the superficial temporal artery. No patient has reported a decrease in hair loss; on the contrary, some of our patients have spontaneously reported a marked decrease in seborrhoea on the operated side. This proves irrefutably the effect of decreased blood-flow on seborrhoea, but also that there is no relationship between seborrhoea and hair loss and even more its regrowth.

Certain techniques of galeoplasty and galeotomy derive from the same prinicple and are open to the same criticisms. Section of the galea was advised by Polh Pincus [4], Schein [6], Young [9], Szacz and Robertson [7] and Brade [1]. Kessler peforms his galeotomy by a transverse frontal incision 2–5 cm long. Ponten [5] makes a transverse frontal skin incision and a galeal section of 7–11 cm. Feit [2] makes three incisions of 3–4 cm at the periphery of the smooth area and through these separates the galea from the periosteum with scissors and divides its attachments to the temporalis aponeurosis on both sides. Then he makes numerous sulci on the deep aspect of the galea with a curved scalpel and also divides the vessels and lymphatics of the superficial temporal, posterior auricular and occipital regions all around the galea with scissors.

Expansion

Principles of Technique

The procedure consists of stretching all or part of the donor site to achieve better distribution, by placing under the scalp a silicone balloon which is progressively inflated with normal saline via a one-way valve [4, 5, 24, 29]. The scalp is an ideal site because it is thick and firm. The expander is placed on an area firmly supported by the bony vault, so that expansion can only occur at the expense of the scalp. The possibilities of coverage may thus be considerably increased. This procedure is therefore much used in reconstructive surgery, but it has its constraints and a considerable risk of complications, which make its use in cosmetic surgery more difficult.

Description of Technique

The technique appears simple, but the rules for the various stages must be scrupulously observed according to a strict plan, so as to use the expansion to the full and to minimise the risk of complications.

Choice of Prosthesis and Planning of Expansion

There are numerous models, with the following features:

1. A particular volume, though over-inflation by 20%–50% is always possible. Thus the choice of size takes precedence over the choice of volume.
2. Shape: cubical, rectangular, cylindrical, hemicylindrical, spherical, crescent-shaped, banana-shaped or oval for differential expansion.
3. The filling valve is usually connected to the balloon by a tube, or else the valve is incorporated in the prosthesis.

The choice of prosthesis depends on:

- The hairy area available for expansion.
- The gain desired for coverage of the alopecic zone.
- The shape of the bald area considered as a loss of substance. It is possible in theory to predict the gain to be expected in terms of expansion of the flap (equal to the radius of a hemispherical prosthesis, twice the height of a rectangular expander). However, the different shapes of expander and various other factors (individual elasticity etc.) often modify such calculations. It is often necessary to choose an expander with the largest possible base of implantation so that the predicted gain is very large. The surface area of the expander is always more important than its volume.
- Lastly, the hairy zone chosen for expansion must always be of excellent quality, with adequate hair density, firm, thick and well-vascularised tissues (unscarred, no previous grafts, no previous radiotherapy) and without any inflammatory or septic conditions.

The patient must be prepared:

- Psychologically, for the constraint of progressive filling, surveillance, the need for two or three operations and especially for the deformation produced
- By preparation of the scalp, which must be perfectly clean and sterilised by the day of operation.

Initial Procedure

The initial procedure consists of judicious placement of the expander, which may be done under local or general anaesthesia. The incision necessary for stripping and then insertion of the prosthesis must not interfere with subsequent vascularisation of the flap; it should allow for any previous scars and always be performed in a zone of good quality; it should be as short as possible (usually 4–6 cm) and placed so as to be subjected to the least subsequent stretching, i.e. remote from the expanded zones and oriented radially in relation to the defect when an advancement–gliding flap is used. An approach parallel to the defect, and at the junction between the defect and the skin to be expanded, is inadvisable because of the risk of exposure [34].

Stripping

Stripping is always made in the subaponeurotic space of Merkel between galea and periosteum and is facilitated by preliminary injection of adrenalinised saline. It is sometimes difficult when it becomes distanced from the access route (needing long instruments, as in the occipital region, where there is a need for visual monitoring of the occipital vessels and change of plane to pass above the muscle and under the skin). The stripping must correspond to the dimensions of the base of the prosthesis or be very slightly in excess of this. A tunnel must be made for the filling valve to place it away from the prosthesis in a zone of good quality and easily located; in some cases it is possible to leave the valve in an external location. The filling tube is adjusted and positioned to avoid any kinking.

Insertion of the Expander

The insertion of the expander is preceded by haemostasis and careful irrigation of the stripped compartment with placement of a suction drain. The base of the expander is positioned to allow it to spread out properly. It is then inflated so that it spreads out and occupies the entire compartment and is then deflated to allow closure, which is made with a firm subcutaneous layer.

Inflation

Inflation may sometimes be begun during the initial procedure, which has the advantage of promoting haemostasis and proper unfolding of the prosthesis, especially when the incision is well away from the expander; 10% of the total volume is usual. Otherwise, it seems preferable to wait for at least 2–3 weeks. The best filling is theoretically continuous and progressive. In practice, the sessions are usually spaced out every 3–10 days, but the intervals and amounts are adapted to each case and observing the following criteria: pressure as experienced and palpable, pain experienced by the patient, aspect, skin colour and possible reactive alopecia. The distension uses normal saline injected slowly via a 23-gauge needle; depending on cases, distension may take 3 weeks to 3 months.

Second Procedure

The second procedure is done under local or general anaesthesia. When the desired volume is obtained (and this is measurable), the prosthesis is removed and coverage is made by the expanded flap. The incisions and choice of flap will have been planned at the first stage on insertion.To facilitate mobilisation of the expanded flap, cautious incision or incisions of the periprosthetic capsule may be made, but its excision is inadvisable, especially as it greatly contributes to the hypervascularisation of the flap. The flaps used are either simply those adjacent to the loss of substance, with a major advancement component, or else transposition flaps with closure of the donor area.

Advantages

The main advantage of the method is the considerably increased possibility of coverage by the hairy regions because of the gain in surface area. This allows the insertion of flaps with an area which often exceeds twice their initial extent and increase of the breadth of some transposition flaps, while allowing closure of the donor region. This is a positive gain and not just a borrowing; there is increased extensibility and stimulation of mitosis, and the transposed flap does not retract subsequently [7, 30]. The decreased hair density due to the expansion is not normally very apparent. The normal density is between 200 and 400 hairs per cm^2. In the extreme case where the scalp area is doubled, this density falls by half, which is far from obvious clinically except in extreme cases of very low density with very fine hair. However, we have shown that expansion of the scalp overlying a prosthesis is not uniform, the central portion at the apex being capable of undergoing stretching by up to five times its surface area, which leads to an equivalent reduction of density.

The skin supplied is of texture, sensibility, colour and mechanical properties comparable to those of normal skin, without deterioration in quality or in subequent hair growth [11, 28]. The procedure may also be repeated (if the balloon is left in place under the flap), provided one waits long enough (usually several weeks) before re-expansion and re-advancement of the flap. Lastly, there is known to be better vascularisation of the expanded flap [9,31–33], the reliability of expanded flaps being comparable to that of autonomised flaps.

Disadvantages and Complications

Disadvantages

There is a need for at least two procedures, and often three, which carry the strain of surveillance and progressive filling, although some patients can carry out the filling themselves or with the aid of another person. There is the cost of the treatment (i.e. of the prosthesis) and stretching is sometimes somewhat painful, especially after each inflation. Broadening of the scars is common and may require revision. The deformation produced, even if it is sometimes hidden by long hair and wearing suitable headgear, is the chief obstacle to current use of the procedure. The patient always has to stop work for 2–2½ months, which greatly restricts the indications for its use in cosmetic surgery. All this means that the expander can be used only in motivated patients who clearly understand the principle of the method and are well disciplined.

Complications

Complications are sometimes minor and do not prevent continuation of the expansion. In some cases the prosthesis has to be removed and the expansion discontinued. The incidence of complications (5%–30%) can be minimised by experience and strict observance of technique.

Haematoma

This calls for revision wth haemostasis, irrigation and reposition of the prosthesis with drainage. It occurs often enough to require routine drainage during insertion of the prosthesis and it often leads to other complications.

Deflation

In some cases, defects in the material are probably responsible; often, there are also technical errors (such as valve puncture by a stout needle, puncture of the prosthesis or tube) or external traumatism.

Skin Damage

Skin damage may be prevented by sufficiently spacing the inflation sessions and by regularly checking the tissue vitality, deflating if there is the least doubt. At the minimum it is evidenced by some degree of alopecia, usually transient, and at worst by skin necrosis with risk of exposure of the prosthesis and sepsis.

Infection

Infection should be prevented by strict asepsis during insertion; it is often secondary to haematoma. It calls for removal of the prosthesis and irrigation.

Effusions

Serous effusions may occur, especially after the second procedure.

Exposure of Prosthesis or Valve

Exposure of the prosthesis or valve is often due to placing the approach too close to the stretched zones or under vulnerable covering tissue, or to incautious inflation or to folds or ridges in the prosthesis. However, exposure does not always imply removal of the prosthesis, and one may sometimes perform several inflation sessions before the second procedure. Exteriorisation of the valve and the filling tube often permits continuation of inflation, but increases the risk of sepsis.

Indications

Reconstructive Surgery [13, 15, 17]

Indications in reconstructive surgery include the following:

- The most current indications are for cicatricial alopecia [13, 15, 17] after burns (with increased risk of infection), after injuries such as scalp avulsion and postoperatively, usually to deal with a loss of substance initially grafted, or for the graft donor zone of a flap, i.e. remote from an excision (usually for a benign or malignant lesion) [18]. More rarely, it is done for post-irradiation lesions, though there are risks in expanding an irradiated zone, or for the sequelae of certain dermatological disorders, but well away from any inflammatory lesions.
- For certain extensive benign lesions such as giant nevi of the scalp.
- More rarely in young children, for aplasias or even the separation of Siamese twins [36].
- On the whole, the use of the expander is an elective procedure, devoid of urgency (because of the risk of sepsis or exposure), in the absence of all infective or inflammatory lesions, and when any oncological problems have been resolved. Also, in reconstructive surgery of the scalp, the use of the expander must be reserved for cases where simpler procedures are not capable of yielding an equivalent result.

Cosmetic Surgery

Use of expanded skin may be made in different ways by still employing the principle of reductions or flaps. Numerous techniques have been and will be described. Here, we shall mention four.

Technique of Manders [14–18]

Manders' technique has been used by the author since 1984, usually for severe alopecia. The principle is one of bilateral expansion of the remaining crown to suppress the baldness by sliding the residual hair-bearing scalp upward and forward. The author uses two special prostheses, one right and one left. Their usual volume is 600 ml and their shape sigmoid, so as to follow the supra-auricular curved line of hair attachment. They can be differentially expanded, allowing expansion further forward where baldness is greater, so as to be able to reconstitute the frontal line.

The initial procedure is usually made under local anaesthesia with a peripheral ring block. The 5-cm incision is in the occipital region, mid-line vertical and at ear level. Stripping is pursued under the residual hair-bearing crown and laterally in the occipital region and then the supra-auricular temporal region up to the anterior temporal line. The prosthesis and drains are inserted and inflation is begun 2 weeks after operation and ceases when the extent of scalp gained (measured by the distance between the ears before and after expansion) exceeds by 1–2 cm that of the original bald area (usually 3–4 months).

The second procedure is preceded by preoperative marking-out of several possible levels for the frontal line. It begins with a superior mid-line incision in the smooth zone, with stripping toward the periphery so as to reach the expanded zones (with removal of the expanders). Ablation of the bald area is made progressively from the back forwards, thus adjusting the tension before any excision), progressively ascending the two lateral flaps attached to the mid-line to the level of the anterior frontal line. Differential expansion permits greater mobilisation inward and forward, with a final T-shaped scar.

Advantages. The considerable provision of residual hair-bearing areas allows coverage of certain cases of very extensive baldness, up to 12 or even 13 cm in breadth. The procedure does not divide any main blood supply and can even be repeated if the baldness progresses.

Disadvantages. These include those of the expansion (strain, deformation) and the fact that the mid-line scar is often a little obvious. Residual anterolateral dog-ears may exist, though they greatly lessen with time. The frontal line often appears too straight and unnatural, with absence of deep fronto-temporal areas of recession, and in particular the lateral growth of hair does not hide the anterior scar, which often obliges the surgeon to fill in this region with several grafting sessions. However, we have noted the difficulty of taking cylindrical grafts on these stretched zones and recommend the taking of strips, which are cut up into micrografts. Lastly, progress of the baldness may make the scars very obvious.

Expansion of Temporo-parieto-occipital Flaps

The expansion of temporo-parieto-occipital flaps (Juri type) [1, 2, 21, 26] has been described by Anderson et al. [2]. It consists of placing two expanders in a crescent in the remaining temporo-parieto-occipital hair-bearing zones, with a parietal incision in the smooth zone a little above the future upper limit of the flap. The expansion usually lasts 8 weeks, sometimes more, and then allows mobilisation of a temporo-parieto-occipital flap of the Juri type, 6–8 cm long, to reconstruct the frontal line. The contralateral expansion allows either mobilisation of another Juri flap transposed behind the foregoing, leaving a smooth zone between them, or the performance of a mobilisation of the contralateral expanded scalp in a vertical type of reduction.

Advantages. Only two procedures are required, including a stage of autonomisation of the Juri flap, using a large enough flap.

Disadvantages. These include those of expansion in general and also those of the Juri flap, in which hair growth is directed backward.

Dardour's Technique (Photos 1, 2)

Dardour's technique combines expansion of a vertical flap with a superior pedicle intended for the frontal line and mobilisation of the contralateral scalp by a Fleming-type paramedian reduction. The first operation based on this technique was performed in 1984 [10].

Two banana-shaped or rectangular expanders 18–20 × 7–8 cm in size are placed at the hippocratic crown, using either a mid-line sagittal incision or, as we now prefer, two retro-auricular incisions, which allow control of the occipital vessels when the stripping has to be carried below their emergence. Moreover, a mid-line incision involves subcutaneous stripping of the vertex, and this often allows secondary shift of the prosthesis upward and therefore the expansion of a useless part. Inflation is begun at the 15th day and lasts about 2 months, the injections being made once or twice a week, when possible. The amount of saline injected each time into each prosthesis varies from 30 to 100 ml, according to the elasticity of the scalp and the period of inflation. The final injections are always less than the first. It is not rare to reach 800–1000 ml per expander at the end of the second month.

The second procedure is performed under local or general anaesthesia, as the patient wishes. The designs are made in indelible ink before infiltration. On one side, usually the left, a pre-auricular flap is designed with a superior pedicle concave towards the front, as previously described; because of the skin expansion, this flap will be wider than the classical flap of between 5 and 7 cm at the level of this pedicle. The average length of the flap will be 18 cm, more if possible, such that, when it is in place, it reaches at least to the mid-frontal line or beyond it for 1–3 cm. On the other side, the design is that of a reduction, similar to that performed in giant reductions, skirting the anterior temporal line and then the upper limit of the hippocratic crown. For safety reasons as regards closure of the donor zone of the flap, we first make the incision of the anterior margin of the flap. The underlying expander is then removed and the width of the flap is then easily obtained by overlapping its margins. The flap is then completely cut out and positioned after closure of the donor site, which must be without any tension. The paramedian reduction is then made on the other side, with care not to cut the pedicle of the flap, which leaves a considerable dog-ear in some cases and always some extent of smooth skin at the periphery of the pedicle.

A third stage is always necessary to remove this dog-ear. When it is minimal, and the residual smooth zone considerable, it is right to wait 3 months before this last procedure, as this will allow performance of another reduction at the same time. In contrast, if the dog-ear is large, and the residual smooth area minimal, it is more useful to perform simple resection of the former earlier, which involves section of the pedicle of the flap; this can be done 15–21 days after the previous operation.

This technique allows virtually total correction of major baldness, but may however leave a median smooth zone of 4–5 cm in very extensive cases, when the height of the crown (HC) is 8 cm (stage VI of Hamilton's classification). We currently prefer a somewhat different technique which consists of making two symmetric superior pedicle flaps to meet at the mid-line at the second stage. Each flap has a straight anterior border and a curved posterior border. The anterior borders of both flaps should meet at the mid-line to leave a sagittal scar, while the lateral margins will form the anterior frontal line and extend over the upper part of the crown. Of course, a dog-ear persists at the vertex in a bald area and is excised 3 weeks later (Fig. 1, Photos 1, 2). This technique has the advantage of transposing to the vertex hairs that are directed strictly forward and of creating an absolutely perfect frontal line.

Technique of Ozun [27]

Used since 1986, Ozun's technique has much the same principle as the previous one. It combines a wide vertical flap on one side with a paramedian type of reduction on the other [27]. The expanders are inserted by a straight bilateral retro-auricular approach, 7–8 cm long. We use two rectangular expanders of 20×10×6 cm with a lateral valve. Inflation is begun around the 15th day and lasts for some 2 months, reaching 800–1000 ml on either side.

Placement of the flap is carried out by making a very wide (10–12 cm) vertical flap with a superior pedicle on one side, combined with ascension of the opposite crown (Fig. 2). During this procedure, the second, now empty, expander is inserted in the postero-right region without removal of its valve, which is left in place and slightly inflated. The expander is slightly inflated at intervals from the 12th day.

The last stage is performed at the 15th–20th day, when the dog-ear is widely excised like the quarter of an orange, simultaneously removing all the residual zone of baldness. The second expander, now empty, is removed. A posterior Z-plasty gives a better direction of the hairs, which otherwise are somewhat divergent and leave a visible scar. Another possibility for this last stage is to move a second transposition flap into the posterior region. On the whole, this technique seems attractive, as it allows total coverage of the baldness with hairs oriented in the right direction and a minimal terminal scar.

Conclusions

Each of the techniques described above has its advantages and disadvantages. Generally speaking, the better the final cosmetic result, the more difficult the technique, and vice versa. However, all these tech-

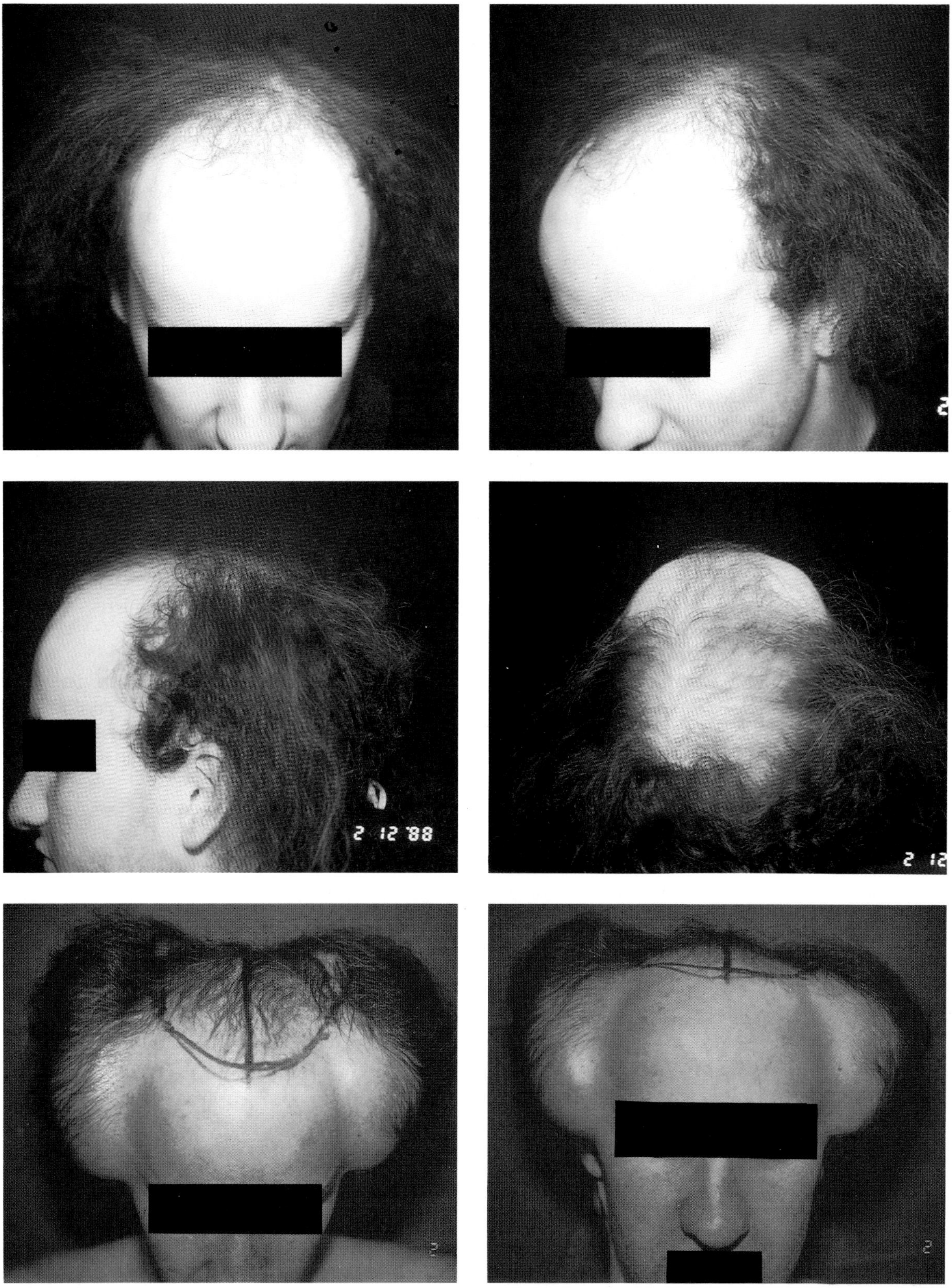

a b c d e f

Photo 1a–f

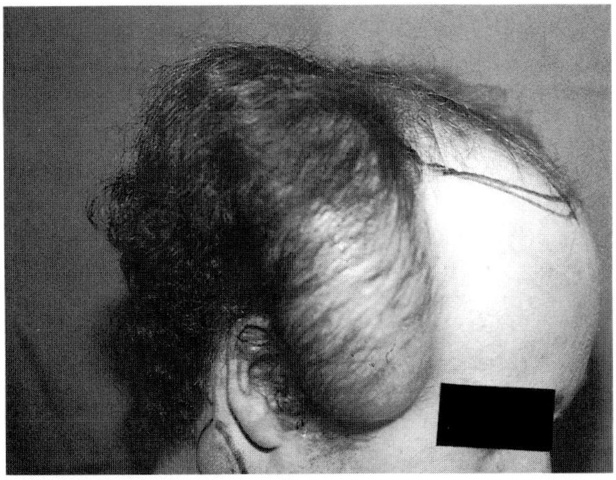

g

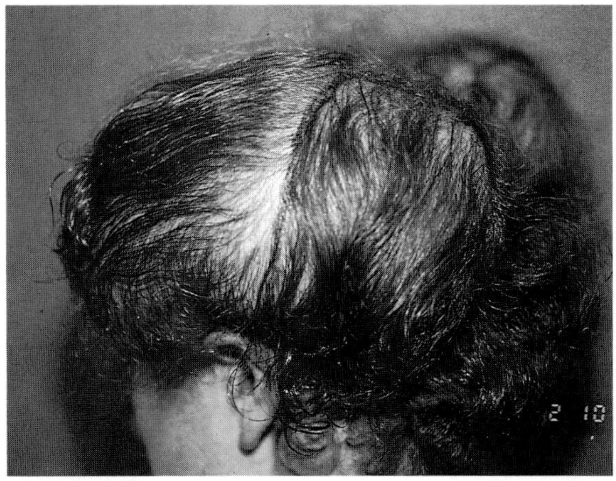

h

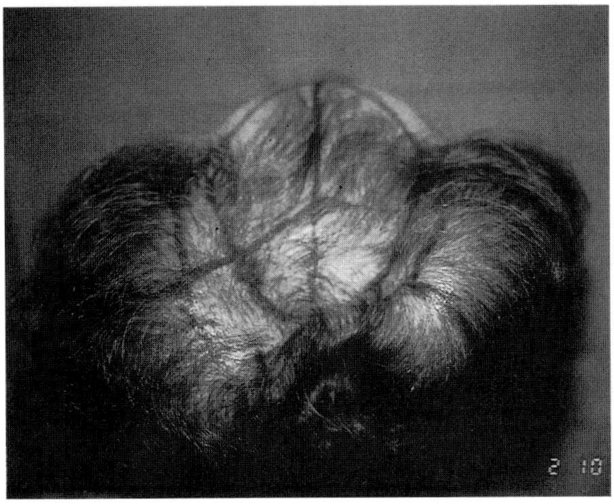

i

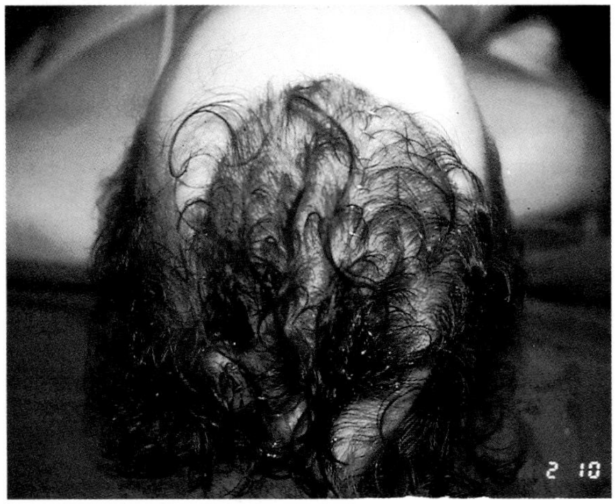

j

Photo 1. a–d Major baldness in a young subject. **e–g** Aspect obtained after inflation of two banana-shaped expanders of 20× 9 cm inflated to 700 ml. **h,i** Design of flaps with excision of upper part of crown. **j** Final aspect with complete coverage of baldness

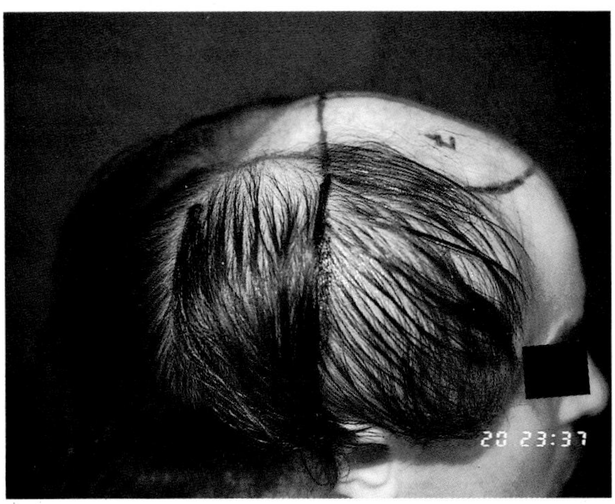

a

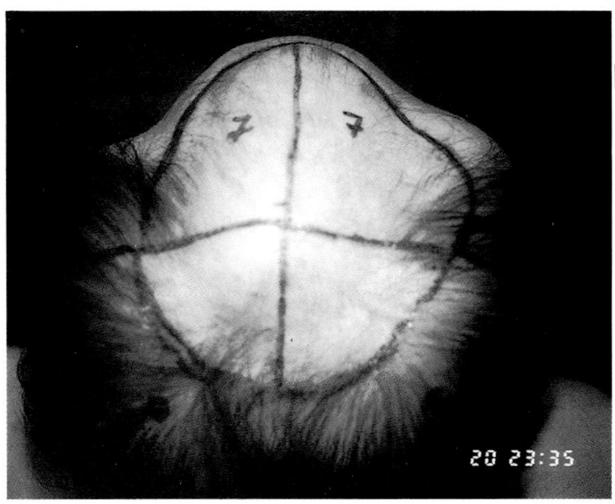

b

Photo 2a,b. Design of flap

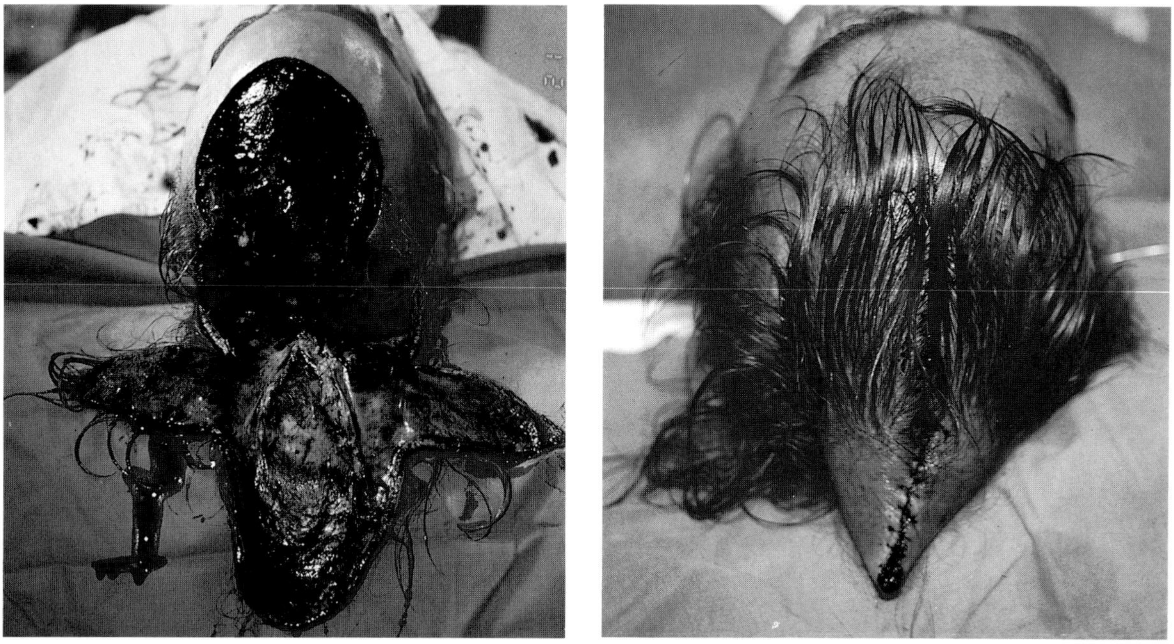

c d

Photo 2. **c** Residual dog-ear after procedure, to be resected after 3 weeks. **d** Perioperative aspect showing both lateral flaps and the smooth median zone which will be resected

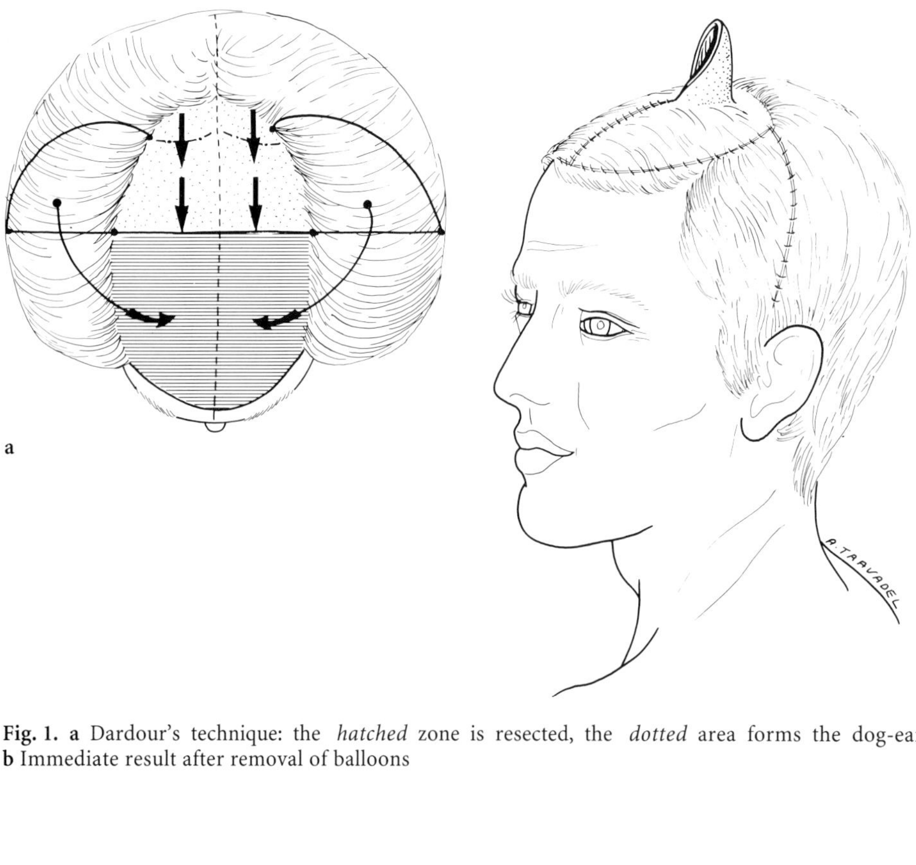

a b

Fig. 1. **a** Dardour's technique: the *hatched* zone is resected, the *dotted* area forms the dog-ear subsequently resected. **b** Immediate result after removal of balloons

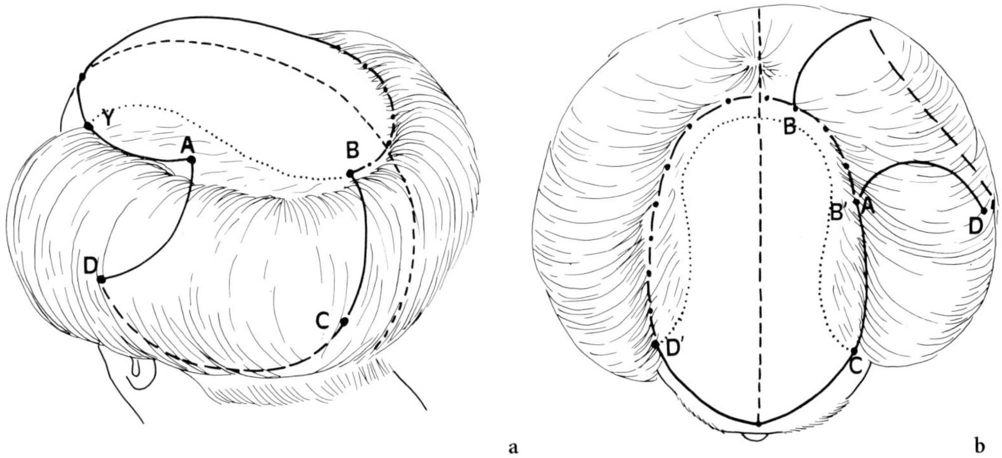

Fig. 2a,b. Ozun's technique

niques have a major disadvantage, which is the considerable deformation; this compels cessation of work and often withdrawal from social life for at least 2 months, which is unacceptable for most patients, especially since this is a cosmetic and not a reconstructive procedure.

The major advantage of these techniques, which considerably stretch the residual hair-bearing zones, is that they can treat major baldness where the height of the hippocratic crown is 8 cm or less, whereas until now only partial – though not inconsiderable – coverage has been obtainable in these extreme cases.

The second indication for expanders is in patients where elasticity of the scalp is nil and where no flap or reduction is possible. In such cases we readily use a crescent-shaped expander of 15–18 cm, placed in the temporo-parietal region, which allows construction of a vertical pre-auricular flap with a superior pedicle of the Dardour type and which may be supplemented by a giant reduction or by multiple grafts. The deformation obtained by such an expander of moderate size is more compatible with a social life.

Generally speaking, we believe that skin expansion is difficult to use in cosmetic surgery and has not clearly demonstrated its superiority.

Synthetic Hair

Various procedures for implantation of synthetic hair have been suggested for androgenic or even cicatricial baldness. Whatever the artificial hair chosen, and however well tolerated, it is inevitably rejected after a variably short period. It is therefore essential to have a good understanding of the different materials proposed by manufacturers (usually Japanese or American). The surgeon must seek the synthetic fibre closest to natural hair in calibre, colour and laxity, the most reliable and durable and the best tolerated. Although they are usually minimal, the existence of side-effects and often irksome preventive treatments (shampooing, antiseptic and anti-inflammatory lotions) calls for careful weighing up of the indications.

Different Types of Synthetic Hair

Different types of synthetic hair have been proposed for many years by American, Japanese and Italian laboratories. Nearly all have been abandoned by most experts because of the extent of side-effects. A schematic table [5] gives a morphological comparison of the different types of fibres and of the knots and needles required for their implantation. The material most often used is polyester fibre of 80–100 mm in diameter. The colour of the fibre can be determined by dyes or inorganic pigments. The needle diameter for implantation varies between 230 and 1070 m. The root or knot of the synthetic hair may be of very varied appearance, with a monofibre knot or one joining several fibres. The scalp area destroyed around each implant varies from 0.05 to 0.9 mm^2 depending on the procedure used.

Experimental Study of Nido Synthetic Hair

Monitoring of Toxicity

Studies made by the Japanese Food and Drug Administration have confirmed the safety of Nido fibre for implantation in the human body. Chemical, biological and oncological tests have been carried out [12].

Histological Study [12]

Histological sections examined from successive biopsies during the progress of implanted hair have shown:

- Day 0: minor haemorrhagic foci, infiltration of neutrophils, lymphocytes and some fibroblasts over small areas.
- Days 7–15: presence around the fibre of fibroblasts, histiocytes and some multinucleate giant cells, complete epidermisation of implantation orifices.
- Days 30–60: few significant changes from preceding section. A cuff of fibroblasts and collagen surrounds the fibre and the inflammatory infiltration has greatly diminished.
- Days 150–600: the epidermis surrounds the fibre and invaginates toward the dermis. The cellular infiltration continues to decrease. The connective tissue proliferation surrounds and penetrates the knot.

As to durability, a study by Taniguchi [12] on the implantation of Nido synthetic hair in 95 cases over 18 months showed the percentage of residual hairs to be 88.7% at 6 months, 78.7% at 12 months and 74.6% at 18 months.

Macrophotographic Study

Bouhanna carried out a similar study on 16 selected patients implanted with some 60 Japanese Nido synthetic hairs. Clinical and macrophotographic follow-up of the four small areas was continued for 6 months. This study was made more in the context of an investigation than of practical use of the method (Photos 3–5).

Material and Methods

The polyester fibres and implantation needles were supplied by Nido. The fibre is made of polyethylene terephthalate 3 and is 0.09 mm in diameter, with an alpha-type loop at its end (Photo 3). This fibre was implanted on the galea after traversing the epidermis, dermis and hypodermis with a special 0.23-mm needle (Photo 4) in 16 healthy men and women aged 20–45 years. Thirteen of these had androgenic alopecia of types III and IV in Hamilton's classification, and three had a non-progressive cicatricial alopecia. Examination of the scalp gave a clinical grading of 0–3 for seborrhoea, pruritus, dandruff, thickness and laxity. The synthetic hairs were implanted on four areas of 0.25 cm^2 localised by tattooing in each of the 16 patients (Photo 5). They were counted in three successive macrophotographs on days 0, 90 and 180 (Photo 6). Tolerance was assessed as poor, moderate, good or excellent. Complications

3
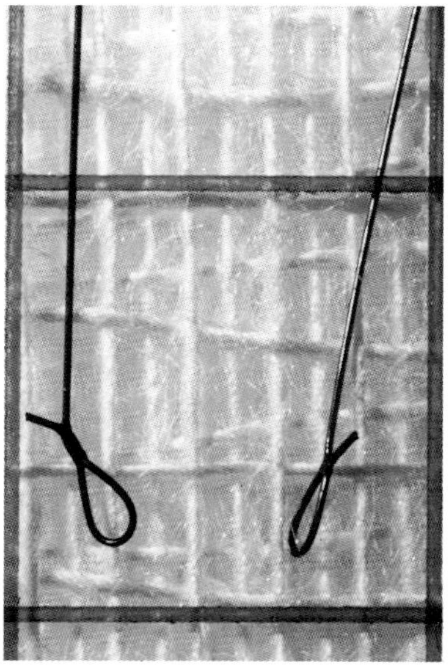
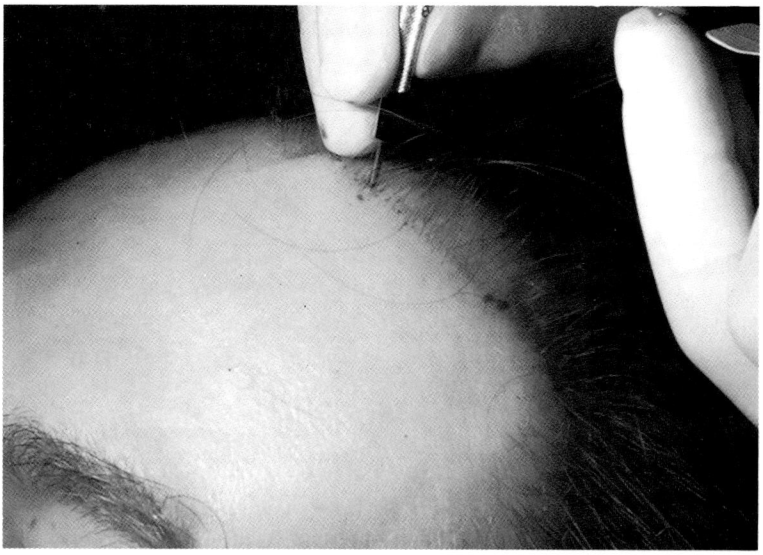
4

Photo 3. Synthetic hair with a loop to allow retention

Photo 4. Technique of implantation of synthetic hairs one by one

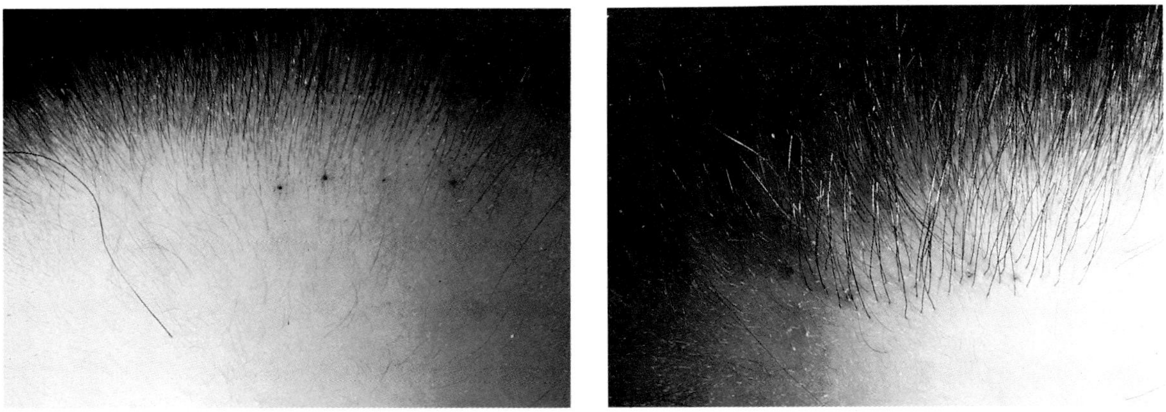

a b

Photo 5. **a** Bald zone located by four micro-tattooings. **b** Same zone 1 month after implantation of 50 synthetic hairs

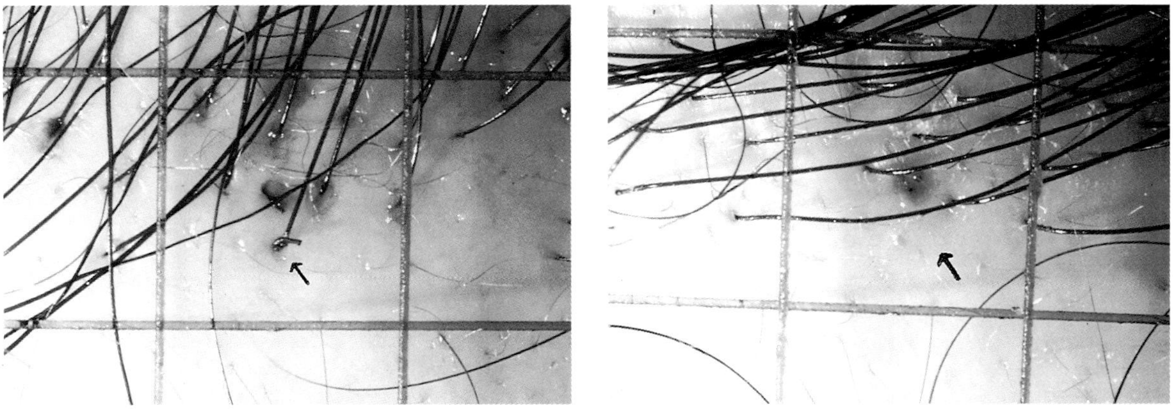

a b

Photo 6. **a** Perioperative macrophotograph of implantation of synthetic hairs and spontaneous extrusion of one hair. **b** Same area identified by micro-tattooing and macrophotography 1 month after implantation

such as folliculitis, seborrhoeic dermatitis, follicular seborrhoeic deposits and scar pits were also assessed.

Results

Our results after implantation gave rates of fixation rather different from those of the Japanese studies:

- A mean density per cm^2 of implanted hairs varying from 137.48 at day 0 to 116.64 at day 90 and 90.5 at day 180
- A mean percentage of fixation of 84.84% at 2 months and 65.82% at 6 months as against Taniguchi's 88.7%
- A mean incidence of complications of 31.25% for folliculitis, 6.25% for seborrhoeic dermatitis, 6.25% for scar pitting and 43.7% for follicular seborrhoeic deposits, due essentially to inadequately repeated local care using shampoo (Photo 7)

The mean percentage of tolerance was excellent in 31.25% of cases, good in 25% and moderate in 43.75%; there were no bad results. During the 6 months' surveillance of this study, no foreign body granulomatous reactions were found. The study was too short to provide a complete assessment of this procedure, as we have reported certain complications outside this series (Photos 8, 9).

According to Di Gregorio [2, 10], Hanke [4], Lepaw [6–9] and Schwartz [11], different synthetic hairs gave different degrees of complications after implantation: foreign body granulomas, secondary infective pustules, residual scars etc. (Photo 10).

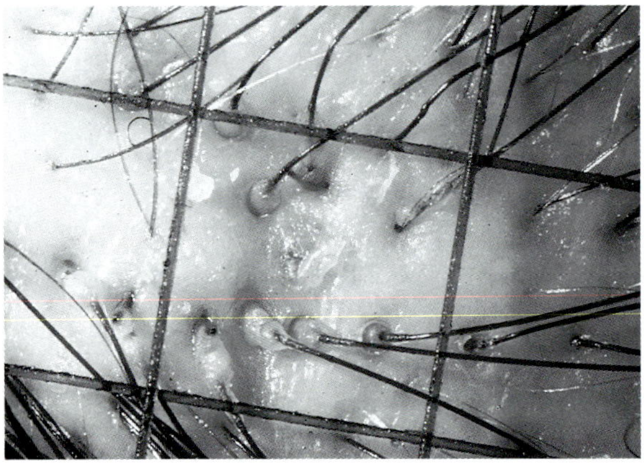

Photo 7. Seborrhoeic reaction and epidermal pits provoking extrusion of synthetic hairs and leaving scar pits

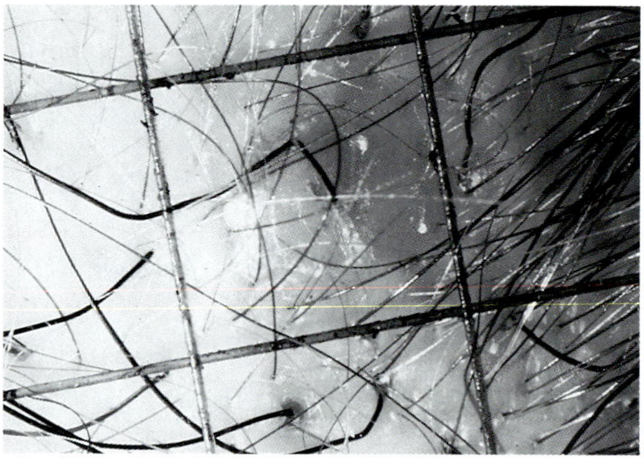

Photo 8. Inflammatory granulomatous reaction after implantation of synthetic hairs

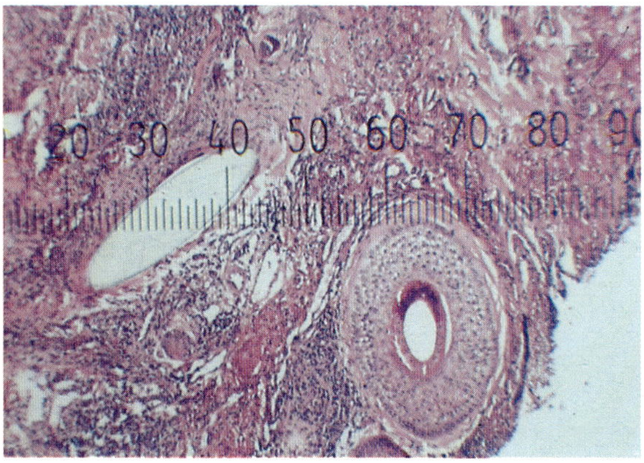

Photo 9. Histological section showing foreign body granuloma: a synthetic hair on the left and a normal hair on the right

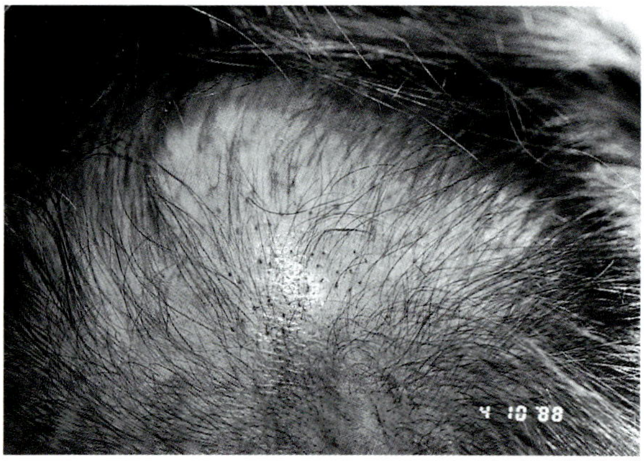

Photo 10. Artificial hairs broken flush with the scalp several months after implantation

Discussion

The implantation of Nido synthetic hairs must adhere to very strict criteria as regards choice of patients: on the one hand, absence of major seborrhoea, dandruff, pruritus; on the other, adequate laxity and thickness of the scalp. The patient should be informed of the absolute necessity for daily care of the scalp with specific lotions and shampoos. This capillary hygiene should make it possible to avoid or attenuate the development of parakeratotic and pruritic states, follicular seborrhoeic deposits, scar pits or extrusion of synthetic hairs. Folliculitis is treated by local and systemic antibioitics similar to those advised for acne. For recurrent folliculitis, the synthetic hair responsible is removed with forceps, grasping it near its emergence.

The patient should never wear a compressive head covering such as a hat, bathing cap, wig etc., in order to avoid tugging and breakage of the shafts of the synthetic hairs and thus the formation of foreign body granulomas (Photo 10).

Apart from the local and general contraindications to this treatment, we advise a preliminary test with 60 synthetic hairs over a monitoring period of 3–6 months.

Conclusion

Synthetic hairs are of variable reliability, durability and tolerance depending on the procedure chosen. Very strict selection is essential in the choice of fibre and the implantation procedure. Two to 3000 hairs are needed for preliminary baldness and 10000 for

Photo 11. a Immediate aspect after implantation of 500 synthetic hairs. b After 1000 synthetic hairs. c After 2000 synthetic hairs. d Same patient a year later

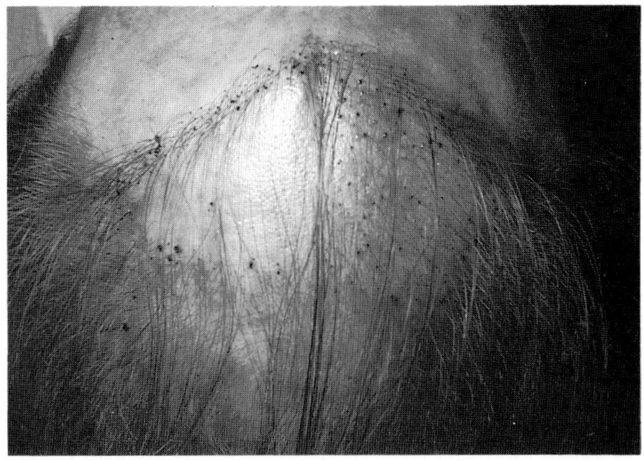

a

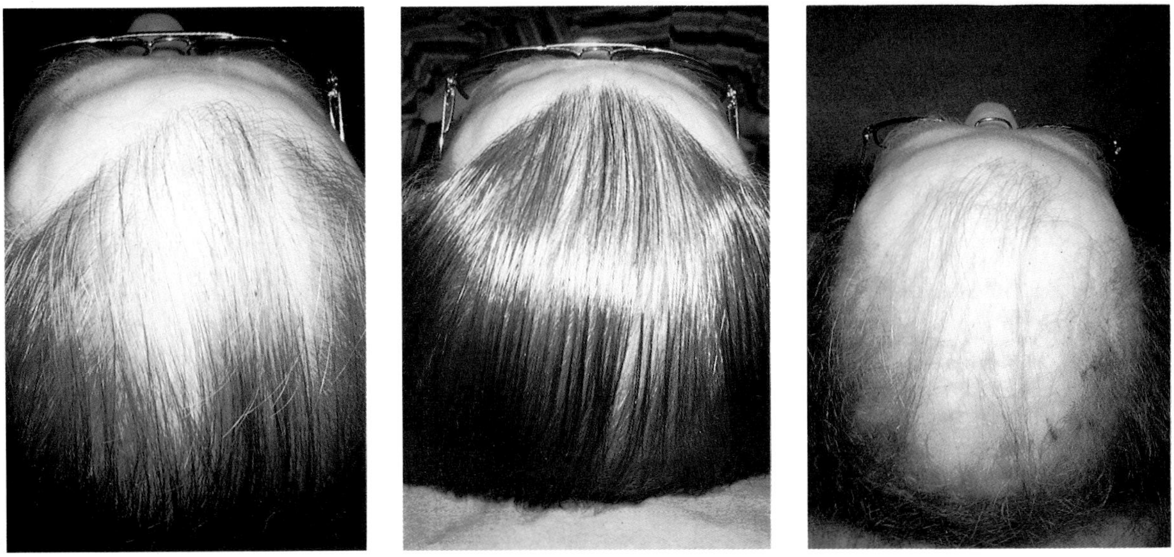

b c,d

major baldness. Actually, the indication for this treatment seems to consist only of the contraindications to surgical techniques using the patient's own hair, which alone guarantees a definitive and unconstrained result. The patient applying for this treatment must be told of the different possible complications and of the inevitable rejection of the implanted synthetic hairs in the more or less long term (Photo 11a–d).

References

(Ligation)

1. Brade S (1960) Surgical treatment of baldness (subcutaneous frontalotomy and occipitalotomy). Z Arztl Fortbild (Jena) 54: 1037–1038
2. Feit LJ (1969) Pathogenic classification of male pattern baldness: new innovations in surgical techniques. Int Surg 51(1): 58–67
3. Marechal R (1972) Alopécies séborrhéiques – traitement par ligature des arteres. Presse Med 4: 257–259
4. Polh Pincus J (1950) Cited in Szasz TS, Robertson WM. Arch Dermatol 61: 34–48
5. Ponten B (1963) The results of frontal galeotomies for losses of hair. Acta Chir Scand 126(5): 406–413
6. Schein M (1903) Uber die Entstehund der Glatze. Wien Klin Wochenschor 40: 1862–1864
7. Szasz TS, Robertson WH (1950) A theory of the pathogenesis of ordinary human baldness. Arch Dermatol Syph 61: 34–48
8. Unger WP (1978) Hair translplantation. Dekker, New York
9. Young MW (1948) Anatomical and pathological factors in senile alopecia. Anat Rec 100: 728

(Expansion)

1. Adson MH, Anderson R, Argenta LC (1987) Scalp expansion in the treatment of male pattern baldness. Plast Reconstr Surg 79 (6): 907–914
2. Anderson RD (1987) Expansion assisted treatment of male pattern baldness. Clin Plast Surg 14 (3): 477–479
3. Argenta LC, Marks MJ, Grabb WC (1983) The use of tissue expansion in head and neck reconstruction. Ann Plast Surg 11: 31
4. Argenta LC (1985) Advances in tissue expansion. Clin Plast Surg 12 (2): 159–171

5. Argenta LC (1984) Controlled tissue expansion in reconstructive surgery. Br J Plast Surg 37: 502–529
6. Argenta LC, Dingman RO (1986) Total reconstruction of aplasia cutis congenita involving scalp, skull and dura. Plast Reconstr Surg 77: 650
7. Austad EA, Thomas SB, Pasyk K (1986) Tissue expansion dividend or loan. Plast Reconstr Surg 78 (1): 63–67
8. Chang TS, Jin YT (1986) Application of tissue expansion in the treatment of post burn skin contractures and alopecia. Eur J Plast Surg 9: 7–12
9. Cherry GW, Austad ED, Pasyk KA (1983) Increased survival and vascularity of random skin flaps elevated in controlled expanded skin. Plast Reconstr Surg 72: 680
10. Dardour JC (1988) Utilisation d'une prothèse d'expansion dans le traitement de la calvitie masculine. Ann Chir Plast Esthet 23 (4): 347–349
11. Johnson PE, Kernahan DA, Bauer BS (1988) Dermal and epidermal response to soft tissue expansion in pig. Plast Reconstr Surg 81(3): 390–395
12. Leighton WD, Johnson ML, Friedland JA (1986) Use of the temporary soft tissue expandeur in post traumatic alopecia. Plast Reconstr Surg 77(5): 737–743
13. Leonard AG, Small JO (1986) Tissue expansion in treatment of alopecia. Br J Plast Surg 39: 42–56
14. Manders EK (1983) Reconstruction of the scalp by tissue expansion. Symposium on tissue expansion, Ann Arbor
15. Manders EK (1982) Scalp reconstruction utilizing soft tissue expansion in reconstructive surgery. Symposium, Ann Arbor
16. Manders EK, Friedman M (1985) The treatment of male pattern baldness utilizing a differential expander. Annual meeting ASAPS, Boston
17. Manders EK, Graham WP (1984) Alopecia reconstruction by scalp expansion. J Dermatol Surg Oncol 10: 967
18. Manders EK, Graham WP, Schenders MJ et al. (1984) Skin expansion to eliminate large scalp defects. Ann Plast Surg 12: 305
19. Manders EK, Schenden MJ, Furrey JA (1984) Soft tissue expansion concepts and complications. Plast Reconstr Surg 74: 493
20. Manders EK, Wong RKM (1986) Flap design in soft tissue expansion. Tissue expansion today. Symposium, Hershey
21. Manders EK, A VK, Wong RKM (1987) Scalp expansion for male pattern baldness. Clin Plast Surg 14(3): 469–475
22. Marion R (1985) Expanders for male pattern baldness. Plast Reconstr Surg 76: 797
23. Masser MR (1988) A twin tissue expander used in the elimination of alopecia. Plast Reconstr Surg 81 (3): 444–449
24. Neumann CG (1957) The expansion of an area of skin by progressive distension of a subcutaneous balloon. Plast Reconstr Surg 19: 124–128
25. Nordstrom REA (1985) Scalp stretching with a tissue expander for closure of scalp defects. Plast Reconstr Surg 75: 578
26. Nordstrom R (1988) Tissue expansion and flaps for surgical correction of male pattern baldness. Br J Plast Surg 41: 154–159
27. Ozun G (1986) Traitement de la calvitie par expansion cutanée. 31st national congress SFCPRE
28. Pasyk KA, Nostad ED, Argenta LC (1987) Histopathology of human expanded tissue. Clin Plast Surg, 14–3 July
29. Radovan C (1984) Tissue expansion in soft-tissue reconstruction. Plast Reconstr Surg 74(3): 482–492
30. Rappard JHA et al. (1988) Surface-area increase in tissue expansion. Plast Reconstr Surg 82(5): 833–839
31. Sasaki GH (1982) Vascular changes during tissue expansion. PSEF Symposium on soft tissue expansion, Ann Arbor
32. Sasaki GH, Pang GY (1984) Pathophysiology of skin flaps raised on expanded pig skin. Plast Reconstr Surg 74: 59
33. Sasaki GH, Krisek TJ. Functional blood flow and skin viability in random skin flaps constructed on expanded skin phenomenon in action. Plastic Surgery Research Council, Durham
34. Sasaki GH, Jurkiewicz MR, Krizek TJ, Mathes MJ, Ariyan S (1986) Refinements of tissue expansion. Plast Surg
35. Schneider et al. (1988) The tensiometric properties of expanded guinea pig skin. Plast Reconstr Surg 81(3): 398–405
36. Shively RE, Bermant MA, Buchjolz RD (1985) Separation of craniopagus twins utilising tissue expanders (case report). Plast Reconstr Surg 76(5): 765–773

(Synthetic Hair)

1. Bouhanna P (1989) Clinical and macrophotographic study of the percutaneous implantation of synthetic hair (Nido shi) In: Van Neste D, Lachapelle JM, Antoine JL (eds) Trends in human hair growth and alopecia research. Kluwer, Boston, pp 257–263
2. Di Gregorio VR, Rauscher G (1981) Experience with the complications of synthetic hair transplantations. Plast Reconstr Surg 68 (4): 498–504
3. Hanke CW, Bergfeld WF (1981) Hair implant complication. JAMA 245: 1345
4. Hanke CW, Bergfeld WF (1981) Fiber implantation for pattern baldness. J Am Acad Dermatol 4: 278–283
5. Kobayashi T, Kamiyama G, Akagawa T, Akamatsu T (1980) Research and investigation of artificial implantation. JSAPS 3: 12–40
6. Lepaw MI (1972) Hair implant complications. Cutis 9: 304
7. Lepaw MI (1980) Therapy and histopathology of complications from synthetic fiber implants for hair replacement. J Am Acad Dermatol 3(3): 195–204
8. Lepaw MI (1979) Complications of implantation of synthetic fibers into scalps for "hair" replacement. J Dermatol Surg Oncol 5: 201–204
9. Lepaw MI (1982) Synthetic fibers and processed human hair implants for the correction of male pattern alopecia. In: Epstein E and Epstein E Jr (eds) Skin surgery, 5th edn. Thomas, Springfield, pp 586–592
10. Rauscher GE, Di Gregorio VR (1981) Surgical treatment of fiber-implanted scalps. Plast Reconstr Surg 67(4): 449–452
11. Schwartz RS, Down Ham TF (1980) Dangers of synthetic fiber implantation for male pattern baldness. Cutis 25: 491–492
12. Taniguchi (1984) Histopathological study of the percutaneous implantation of polyester fibers. Aesthetic Plast Surg 8: 67–74

Operative Indications

The surgical techniques available for cosmetic correction of baldness are so numerous that the surgeon needs to evaluate them carefully, guided by the features of the classification and by the cosmetic wishes of the patient, particularly for design of the frontotemporal line. The operation is planned to obtain both an immediate or short-term result and an assessment of the supplementary surgery required in the future to cover any persistent bareness. Whatever technique is used, the surgeon will always be confronted with a number of problems, which will now be discussed:

- The limits of operable baldness and variant factors
- Assessment of the position of the frontal and temporal lines
- Actual operative indications allowing for various factors, including assessment of progress of the baldness and its place in definitive planning, the problem of sparse hair which may or may not fall out depending on its site and the problem of progressive baldness.

Limits of Operable Baldness and Variant Factors

When Does Baldness Become Inoperable?

The question of when baldness becomes inoperable has already been answered in the chapter on "Male Baldness" (p. 29ff.). In theory, we have seen that it is possible to decrease the density of the hair by half, leaving a satisfactory clinical aspect. This implies a doubling of the hair-bearing skin area, which is theoretically possible today thanks to skin expansion; this corresponds to a bald area of 300–350 cm^2 for an equivalent donor zone, i.e. a crown height (HC, as defined at the level of the ear) of 8 cm and a breadth of vertex of the order of 13–14 cm. In practice, these figures must be corrected slightly because of the impossibility of stretching all the remaining area.

It should be stressed that two techniques have extended the limits of operability:

- Thus extreme cases (Hamilton's stage VII or, in our classification, HC=7–9 cm; width of vertex, 14–16 cm; antero-posterior length, HT=24 cm) may benefit from a uniform distribution of micro- and minigrafts (see chapter on "Autografts", p. 92f.).
- Less extensive baldness (Hamilton's stage VI, our HC=8–10 cm; width of vertex, 12–14 cm; antero-posterior length, HT=22 cm) may be capable of treatment by use of skin expansion. Apart from use of these techniques, we have fixed the normal limit of treatment of major baldness at around 200 cm^2 for the bald zone and 400 cm^2 for the donor area (2 cm^2 of hair-bearing zone is needed to cover 1 cm^2 of bald zone). In practice, this corresponds to a crown height (HC) of 10 cm and a vertical width of 10–11 cm, with an antero-posterior length of around 22 cm. In practice, our everyday experience confirms these limits, which correspond to stage V of Hamilton's classification. Certain factors may sensibly alter these limits. The most important of these is the elasticity of the scalp. When this is graded 1 in our classification, the height HC may be 9 cm (minimum). In contrast, when it is graded 3 or 4, HC can reach at least 12 cm, in the knowledge that only a narrow flap and grafts can be used to the exclusion of any other technique, with the obvious exception of expanders, for which this is one of the best indications.

The patient's age may be a limiting factor in the sense that one would hesitate to propose too large a series of procedures for a subject above a certain age. One would also be more cautious in the use of flaps. However, we are less restrictive as regards one or two sessions of minigrafting. Other factors are less important, though not altogether negligible. They are more involved in the final quality of the result.

Favourable Factors

Favourable factors for the presence of a certain residual frontal or vertical density (F2 or T2) include:

- Thick hair (E1)
- Frizzy hair whose covering power is better
- Dense hair
- Crinkly hair
- Fair or greying hair
- Hair that can grow long

Unfavourable Factors

Poor density of the donor zone (C3) is unfavourable; factors influencing this include:

- Very fine stiff hair (E3) (except for micrografts)
- Black hair on a white skin (except for micrografts)
- Sparse hair
- Poor rate of hair growth

Position of the Fronto-temporal Line

The design of the frontal line, which is reconstructed allowing for the position of the temporal line, is the primary stage before any procedure. This fronto-temporal line, and especially the junction point between the two parts (called point G in our classification) or base of the fronto-temporal recession, has been described by Walter Unger [12]: in a frontal view, a vertical line from this point passes through the outer canthus. In white subjects, when the baldness sets in and develops, this point recedes but the vertical projection to the outer canthus remains the same (Fig. 1a). We would add that a horizontal line from this point defines a crown height (HC) of 10 cm.

According to W. Unger, the two frontal and temporal lines evolve symmetrically, the one upward and the other backward, while the temporal triangle tends to open out (Fig. 1b). Our belief is that the evolution of the position of these two lines, which figure in our classification as *f* and *t* is not necessarily symmetric. Thus, the frontal line ascends more often than the temporal line recedes; it is also not uncommon to see in some patients a total absence of hair in the frontal region, while the temporal line remains in an anterior position. This explains the dissociation in our classification between the gradings of the position of the temporal lines as 1, 2 or 3, depending on whether they are in the normal position, slightly receded or very receded (Fig. 2a,b). Usually, the aim of surgical treatment is to reconstruct a normal frontal line with an area of fronto-temporal recession of reduced depth but still present.

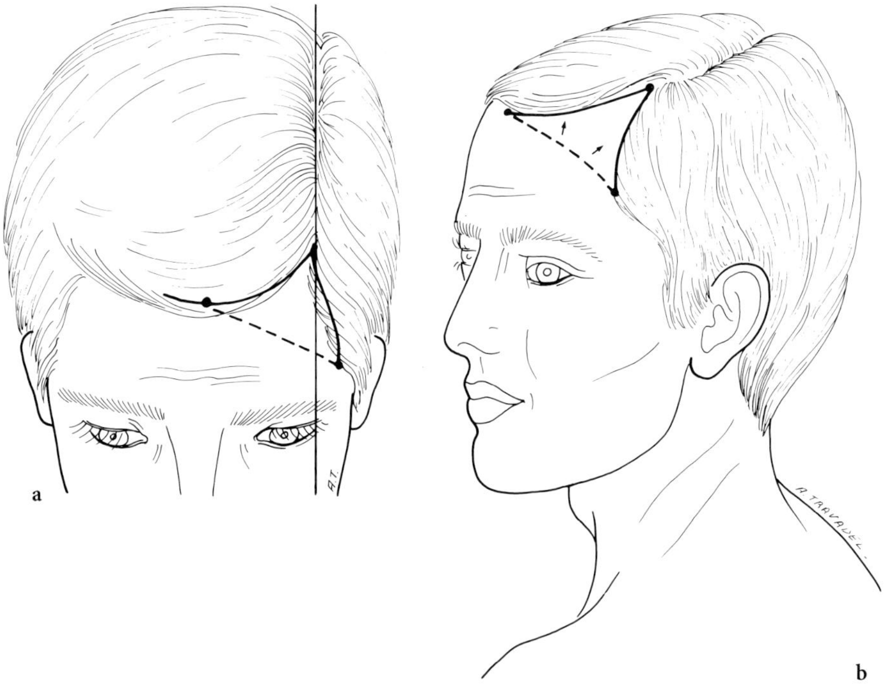

Fig. 1. **a** Projection of point G at level of outer canthus. **b** Recession of frontal and temporal lines (Unger)

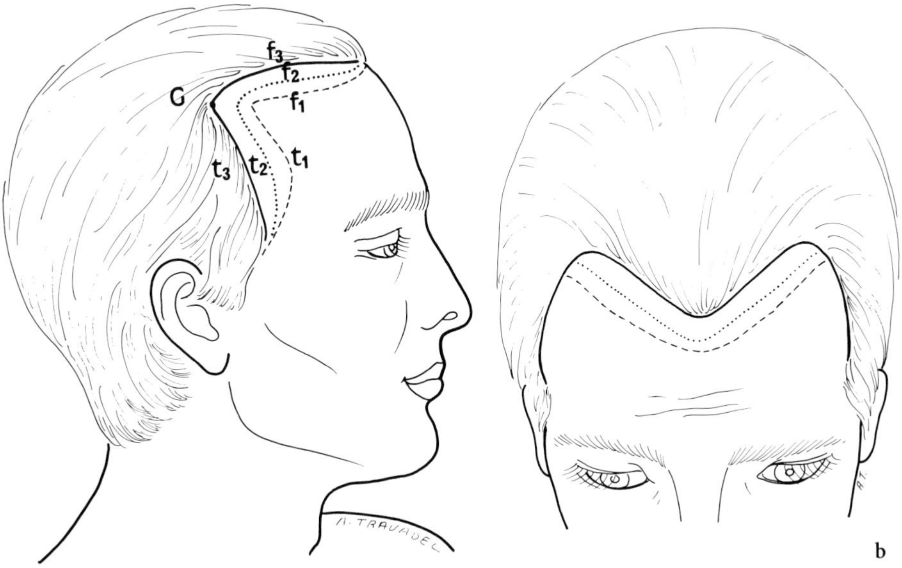

Fig. 2. **a** Position of frontal and temporal lines and determination of point G. **b** Isolated recession of frontal line

The hairs situated on the frontal line are normally oriented forward, whereas those of the temporal region grow downward, sometimes slightly forward as well. All the recommended techniques must, for cosmetic reasons, absolutely ensure entry to the fronto-temporal recession and an emergence of hair directed forward (grafts, micrografts, vertical flaps); nevertheless, it should be noted that reconstruction of the frontal line by a vertical pre-auricular flap gives the result which best meets all requirements. However, taking a flap in this region tends to move the anterior temporal line back by ½–1 cm. This is usually quite tolerable, except in cases where this line is in too posterior a position from the outset (*t*3, G3). This is, in our view, an indication for a retro-auricular flap, which does not move back the temporal line during closure of the donor site, but which requires three operative procedures (Photo 1).

Usually, advancement of the temporal line is not indicated, since its recession is not troublesome cosmetically. Moreover, its reconstruction by grafts always gives a poor result, as the hairs in this region are very fine and sparse in front. Furthermore, no flap technique is available that is capable of reconstructing this line. If this were to respect the normal direction of hair implantation, it would have to be taken at the frontal region, i.e. in a zone destined to become bald. However, it is possible, if really necessary, to advance the temporal line by performing a very large rotation flap with an inferior pedicle. The incision for this flap begins below at the sideburn, skirts the anterior border of the temporal line up to the deepest point of the fronto-temporal recession and then extends transversely backwards. In major baldness, this last incision skirts the upper border of the crown. The best results are obtained in the context of reductions of the Marzola or Brandy type, as posterior stripping of the occipital region allows very considerable advancement of the temporal region as well as ascension of the crown. In this case, the greater the ascension of the crown, the less one can advance the temporal line, and vice versa (Photo 2).

To reconstruct the frontal line, the median frontal point must be positioned. We normally locate this at four fingerbreadths above the glabella or slightly higher. In practice, it is often easy, on careful examination of the frontal region, to identify a fine down which marks the original limit of the patient's hair before he became bald. Lastly, if the frontal muscle is contracted, there is always a mobile zone and an adherent zone whose boundary forms the frontal line, which is then easy to trace.

Quite often, during the consultation the patient requests a frontal line which is too low or complete filling of the fronto-temporal recession. This request must be formally denied, as the cosmetic aspect obtained is never natural for a middle-aged man and risks attracting attention. Absence of fronto-temporal recession is normal only in the young child and in women. However, it may also exist, though with some degree of recession, in certain negroid or mongolian subjects.

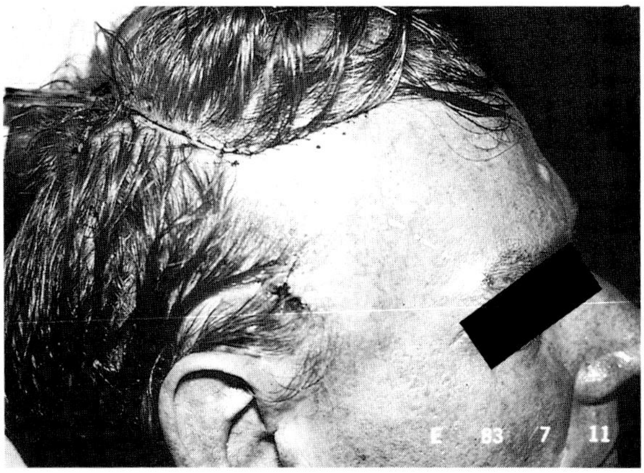

a

Photo 1. **a** Recession undergone by point G and line *t* after a Dardour-type pre-auricular flap. **b,c** Recession of temporal line by 1 cm after pre-auricular flap

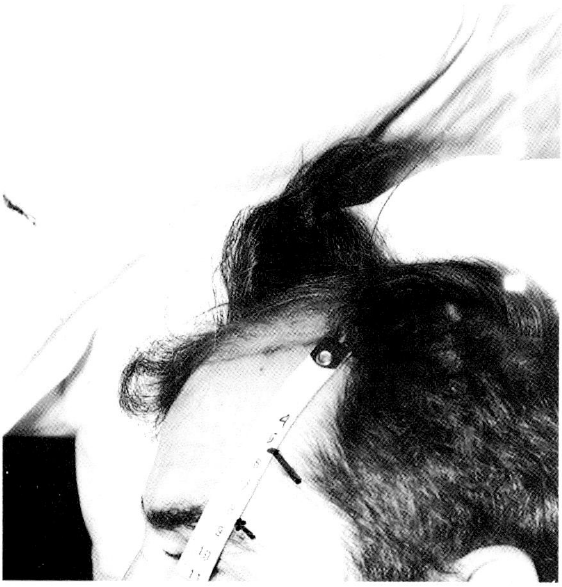

b

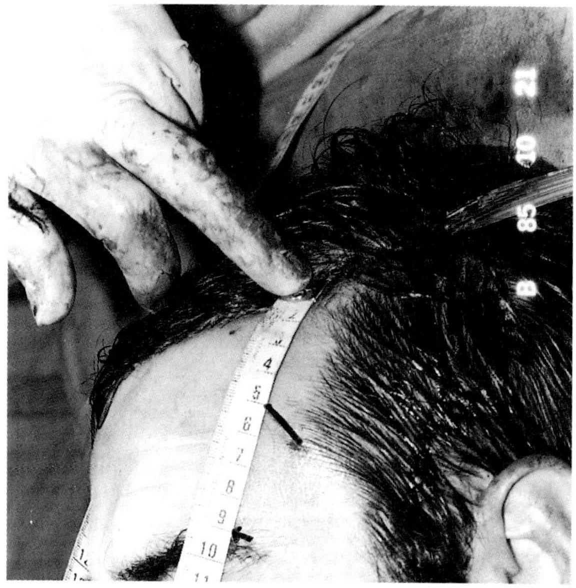

c

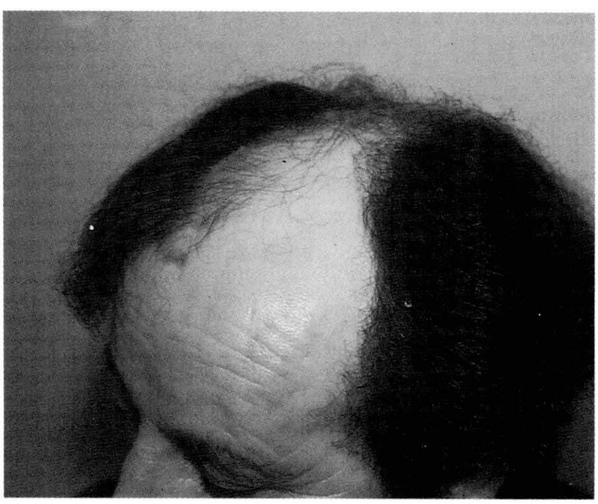

a

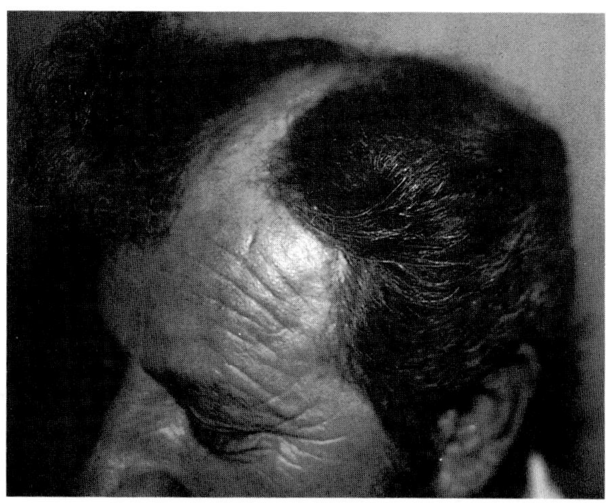

b

Photo 2a,b. Advancement of anterior temporal line after operation for lifting the scalp

Operative Indications

The operative indications in the surgery of baldness are very difficult to define, since a great number of parameters, which we shall try to analyse, are involved in the choice of strategy. For major baldness, multiple repeated techniques are always essential. For minor and moderate baldness, one to three stages may suffice (vertical flaps, reductions, grafts).

When To Operate: Assessment of the Progress of Baldness

Before going into detail, we must deal with an accepted and common idea which consists of treating only stabilised baldness, as it is otherwise impossible to say how far it may progress. Our belief is that the history, clinical findings and paraclinical investigations currently provide us with sufficient evidence for very rapid assessment of the prognosis. Nevertheless, it seems wiser to lay down an operative plan which allows for maximal progress in the long term. We have already seen that even major baldness, of Hamilton's stage VII, with a crown height (HC) less than 8 cm, does not pose an insoluble surgical problem (use of micrografts and expanders). Furthermore, when a patient has major baldness, we must necessarily propose several successive procedures which, by their proximity in time, risk producing major traumatism and especially a prolonged handicap (if only cosmetic). In particular, the first operative stages often give cosmetic results that are temporarily very ugly, except for micrografts.

In contrast, early interventions, provided they are well planned, have the advantage of being very spaced out in time, thus increasing the surgical possibilities because of the return of better scalp laxity. In addition, the traces left by each of these procedures will be minimised by the presence of consistent peripheral hair, which conceals the temporary unaesthetic traces of each procedure. Lastly, this saves the patient from having been completely bald, since the baldness will have been corrected as required from its onset.

The whole problem actually rests in the planning of the procedures. It is no longer a matter of suggesting to the patient a particular operation to begin with and then improvising as one goes along. An overall plan must be laid down and proposed, predicting the order, number and succession of procedures. An unfortunate session of grafting or reduction may sometimes exclude any future possibility of a flap. This fundamental fact must always be properly assessed before any surgery of the scalp, whether cosmetic or reconstructive in intent.

If all three techniques must be used in the same patient, in general, and for technical security reasons, it is preferable to perform first the flaps (whose pedicles must be free from scars), then the reductions and finally the grafts. In some cases, it is possible to do alternate grafting and reductions.

What to Do

In the preceding chapters the different techniques for the surgical treatment of baldness have been described with their risks and complications; however, a dangerous technique should not be confused with a difficult one that requires real competence on the part of the surgeon. Quite often, one technique is described with a stress on the complications of others or (something which amounts to the same thing) by comparing the bad results of one technique, due to a poor indication or an inexperienced surgeon, with the good results of another where the indication had been correct and the surgeon competent. The result of a bad flap should not be compared with that of good grafting, or vice versa.

We believe that it has been amply demonstrated that the different techniques, when properly carried out with good indications, allow every surgeon to achieve similar cosmetic results. This is certainly what makes the operative indications so difficult and the results so impressive. For the same baldness, they can vary radically in terms of the desires of the patient (the time at his disposal, his occupation and character) and especially in terms of the competence of the surgeon himself.

It must be realised that until now, in the main works dealing with the surgery of baldness, the indications are laid down with primary attention to the possibilities offered by grafts, leaving only the contraindications to the other techniques. We believe that today it is essential to reconsider these very slanted indications, which are rather out of date, so as to utilise the advantages offered by each technique, whether old or recent. We shall first review the advantages and disadvantages of each technique and then the indications related to the stage of baldness, modified in terms of the numerous other parameters we have already discussed.

Ligation

We mention, only to exclude them, ligations of the temporal and occipital arteries, which have not proved to be effective, and the surgical fixation of hair-pieces, which results in far too many complications.

Artificial Hair

The use of artificial hair may be a technique of the future, but not of the present. While, with certain types of hair, the short-term infections are few, the incidence of long-term infections is completely unknown, as are the true percentages of secondary hair loss in the short and long term (35% at 6 months in our study). Lastly, the permanent care required to prevent infection and the time lost in sessions of hair re-implantation every year constitute constraints that seem dissuasive. Actually, this is the only technique that guarantees the patient that he will have hair on his head on leaving hospital; but there is absolutely no guarantee that it will still be there 6 months later.

Grafts

The use of grafts [9, 11, 12] is the oldest technique and the one most performed up to now. It is also one of apparent simplicity. In fact, this is rather a technique whose principal complication [1], i.e. non-regrowth or feeble regrowth of hair, is not spectacular or dramatic for the patient, insofar as it may be qualified as a "chronic" complication rather than an "acute" one such as is represented by necrosis of a flap.

This technique does not require any profound degree of surgical knowledge, and the conditions of asepsis required during its performance are so minimal that it can easily be performed under local anaesthesia in the consulting room. However, both the equipment and the minutiae of the surgical procedure must be perfect, which therefore implies very great patience, something which not every practitioner has. The apparent ease of the method means that it is often performed by practitioners without adequate experience.

Regardless of the area to be covered, at least three or four sessions are required for the same receptor site, each leaving an unaesthetic appearance for around 3 months. This handicap can be camouflaged when the grafted zone is situated behind a well-furnished zone, but it always remains very obvious in the frontal region. Furthermore, if the patient changes his mind after one or two procedures, he cannot stop without suffering the penalty of a very ugly cosmetic result. On the other hand, this technique allows distribution of the hair more or less uniformly and spread over the receptor site, which may be very useful for patients affected by major baldness and with very poor elasticity of the scalp.

Reduction Procedures

Reduction procedures [4, 7] represent without doubt the safest method; complications and bad results are rare. It is also the most cosmetically successful method, since the smooth zone treated is reduced in a perfectly uniform manner. Lastly, it gives immediate results; the patient can see the outcome as soon as the first dressing is removed.

However, reductions have two major disadvantages: they give disappointing results when the elasticity of the scalp is very poor, and in particular they do not usually allow reconstruction of a suitable frontal line. Moreover, reductions create scars in the region of the vertex, which may contraindicate subsequent flaps. When both techniques are indicated in the same patient, the flap(s) must be performed before the reductions. According to Dardour, the technique of "lifting" the scalp seems to be a considerable step forward from this point of view. This technique, while retaining the advantages of reductions (operative security and uniformity of the zone covered), eliminates the two disadvantages of classical reductions mentioned above.

We have seen that this technique allows major skin resections, even when scalp elasticity is poor, and that it allows satisfactory coverage of the frontal region during the same procedure. According to Dardour, lifting of the scalp is bound to occupy an increasingly important place in the future in the surgical treatment of major baldness. However, this technique usually requires general anaesthesia and 4–8 days absence from work, but two procedures may suffice for the treatment of extensive baldness.

Flaps

The use of flaps [3, 6, 8] is undeniably more difficult and, unlike the others, can only be mastered by a trained and competent surgeon. This is often the real reason why some authors object to this technique, claiming that it is dangerous. In one way they are right, since it is certain that the surgeon's degree of experience affects the risks involved. The two chief complications of flaps are partial necrosis of the end of the flap and alopecia of the donor area. These acute complications are often experienced by the patient as dramatic, but it has been shown that their incidence becomes negligible with a skilled operator. Moreover, it is always astonishing to note how, in the long term, the effect of these complications is usually minimal and is easily corrected either by implantation of some grafts at the necrosed area of the flap or by simple revision of the scar at the donor zone. In fact, quite often a patient who has had a flap with terminal necrosis requiring secondary grafting is cosmetically satisfactory after a period of 6 months, whereas if only the grafting technique had been performed 9–12 months would have been necessary.

The main advantage of flaps is indeed the rapidity with which they allow the achievement of a satisfactory cosmetic result, especially at the frontal zone. Quite often, a single procedure allows immediate achievement of this result, so that, with his hair styled, the patient is no longer bald. Reductions or grafting can then be done posteriorly, where the transient unaesthetic result is masked by a very thick lock of hair situated in front and judiciously arranged. Lastly, the flap is a technique which provides the maximum density at the grafted site, well superior to grafts, something which once again is particularly valuable at the frontal region.

We have noted the advantages and disadvantages of different types of flaps in a previous chapter and stated the reasons why we prefer vertical flaps with a superior pedicle, whether pre- or post-auricular, depending on the case.

Skin Expansion

Whether skin expansion is combined with reduction or with flaps, it may allow the correction of major baldness in a few months, with only two or three visits to the operating room, but at the price of a temporary but very considerable deformation which obliges the patient to withdraw from social life for at least 2 months; this greatly limits the indications for this technique.

Generally speaking, the ideal indication for the patient is that which will give the best cosmetic result in the minimum time and with the least possible procedures and the fewest possible risks. This is why all the techniques reviewed, far from being mutually exclusive, should rather be combined to arrive at the indication which best suits the individual patient. We shall first look at the indications in terms of the clinical stage of baldness and then at their modifications in terms of the patient, of certain local factors and of the technical competence of the surgeon.

Indications Related to the Clinical Stage of Baldness and to the Surgeon

There is certainly a degree of subjectivity as regards operative indications, as each author will favour particular parameters among the numerous ones that exist. Therefore, we have chosen to discuss the operative indications as seen by each of the two authors of this book in succession. The final quality of the result is of course essential, but we have seen that it may often be much the same with different techniques, provided these have been properly performed. We believe that the second criterion must be the rapidity of achievement of a particular result and the number of operative procedures required for this. This is why, quite often, we prefer reductions and flaps rather than grafts, the results of which are more delayed.

Indications (Bouhanna)

The classification of Bouhanna is used here (1976) (Fig. 3).

Minor Baldness (Stage I)

Stage IA

If the patient wants restoration of his original frontal line, the possibilities include:

- Two small pre-auricular flaps transposed in one or two sessions if the laxity of the donor zone suffices (Fig. 4, Photo 3a–g)
- Two strip grafts with long hairs transplanted at one session, combined with transplantation of minigrafts behind these (Fig. 5, Photo 4a–d)

If the patient desires simple thickening of the fronto-temporal recession, 200–400 minigrafts and micrografts transplanted in one or two sessions often prove adequate (Photo 5a,b).

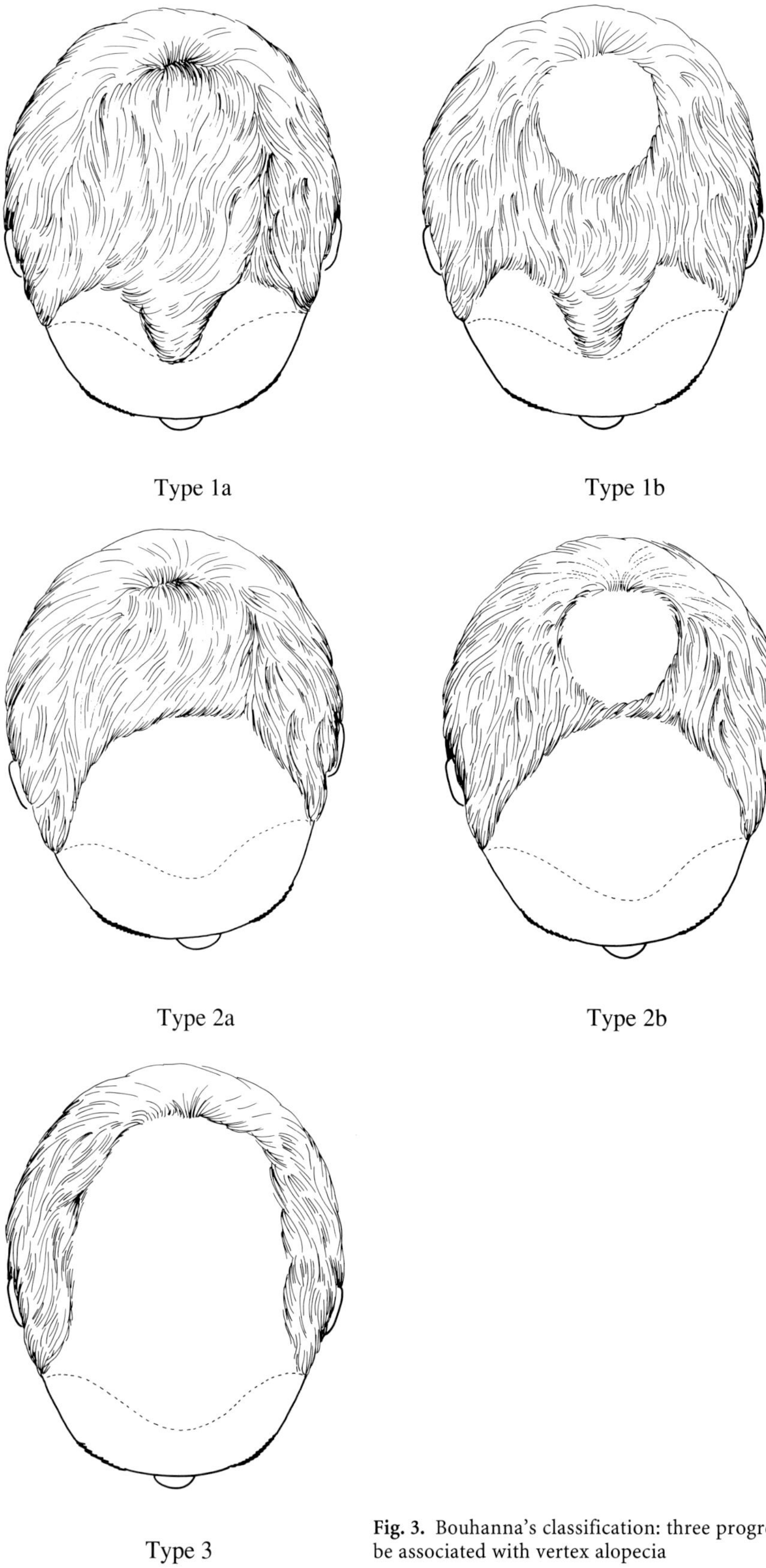

Fig. 3. Bouhanna's classification: three progressive stages, which may or may not be associated with vertex alopecia

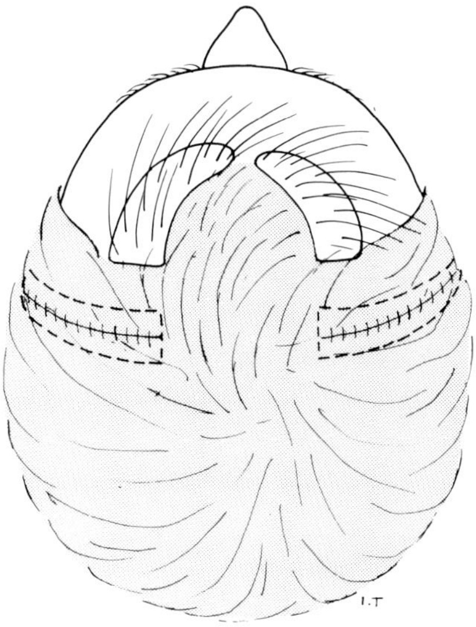

Fig. 4. Simultaneous transposition of two small pre-auricular flaps allowing immediate correction of both areas of fronto-temporal recession at one session

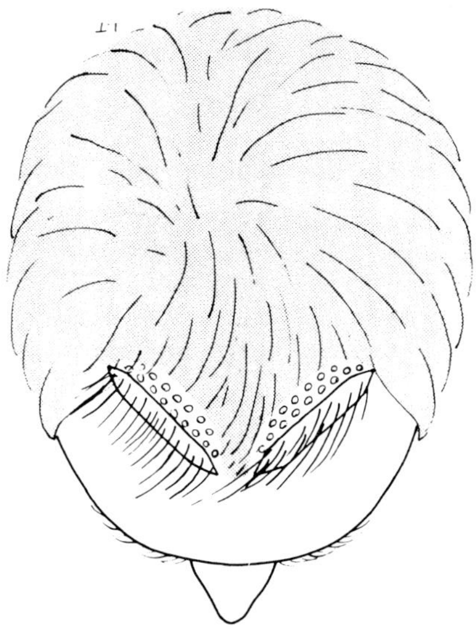

Fig. 5. Simultaneous transplantation at one session of two long-haired fusiform grafts, possibly supplemented by a session of minigrafting at a second session for correction of frontal recession

Stage IB

The patient presents with an isolated vertex, or one associated with frontal baldness. If the vertex and its periphery are lax, possible treatments are the following:

- Simple, single or repeated reduction complemented by one or two sessions of minigrafts arranged in a spiral (Photo 6a–c)
- Transposition of one or two flaps, complemented by one or two sessions of excision of the residual bald zones (Fig. 6a,b, Photo 7a–d).

If the vertical and perivertical scalp is taut and rigid, 300–400 minigrafts are transplanted in one or two sessions arranged like the spokes of a wheel. For final tidying-up, micrografts are arranged at the centre of this spiral (Photo 8).

Moderate Baldness (Stage II)

Stage IIA

The patient has baldness of the entire frontal region.

1. Patients with Dark, Stiff or Wavy Hair. If the laxity is satisfactory (S1 or S2), two pre-auricular flaps are transposed in one or two sessions. This is combined with a concave flap of the Dardour type and a second straight flap (Bouhanna). The residual bald area between these flaps may be excised by a sagittal reduction (Fig. 7, Photo 9a–f), or it may be filled by one or two minigraft sessions, e.g. 150–200 fragments (Photo 10a–d). Flaps are often indicated for the frontal baldness of Asiatics.

If laxity is nil (S4), transplantation of 500–800 minigrafts of three to four hairs in two sessions with completion of the anterior frontal line by micrografts may be suggested (Photo 11a–c).

2. Patients with Dark, Curly or Crinkly Hair or Patients with Fair Hair. Here, the indications are the same as in the preceding paragraph but, in the case of minigrafts, the finishing touches at the anterior frontal line prove less essential (Photo 12a,b).

For frontal baldness we recommend either 300–500 minigrafts transplanted in two sessions or transposition of two vertical pre-auricular flaps, possibly complemented by a session of 100–200 minigrafts (Figs. 7, 8, Photo 13a–g).

In Black patients we find the indication for minigrafts as acceptable as that for flaps. However, the latter procedure provides a more immediate result, with denser hair cover.

In any case, two preliminary conditions seem essential: height of the temporal crown of 10 cm or more and adequate laxity (HC=10 cm and S1 or S2).

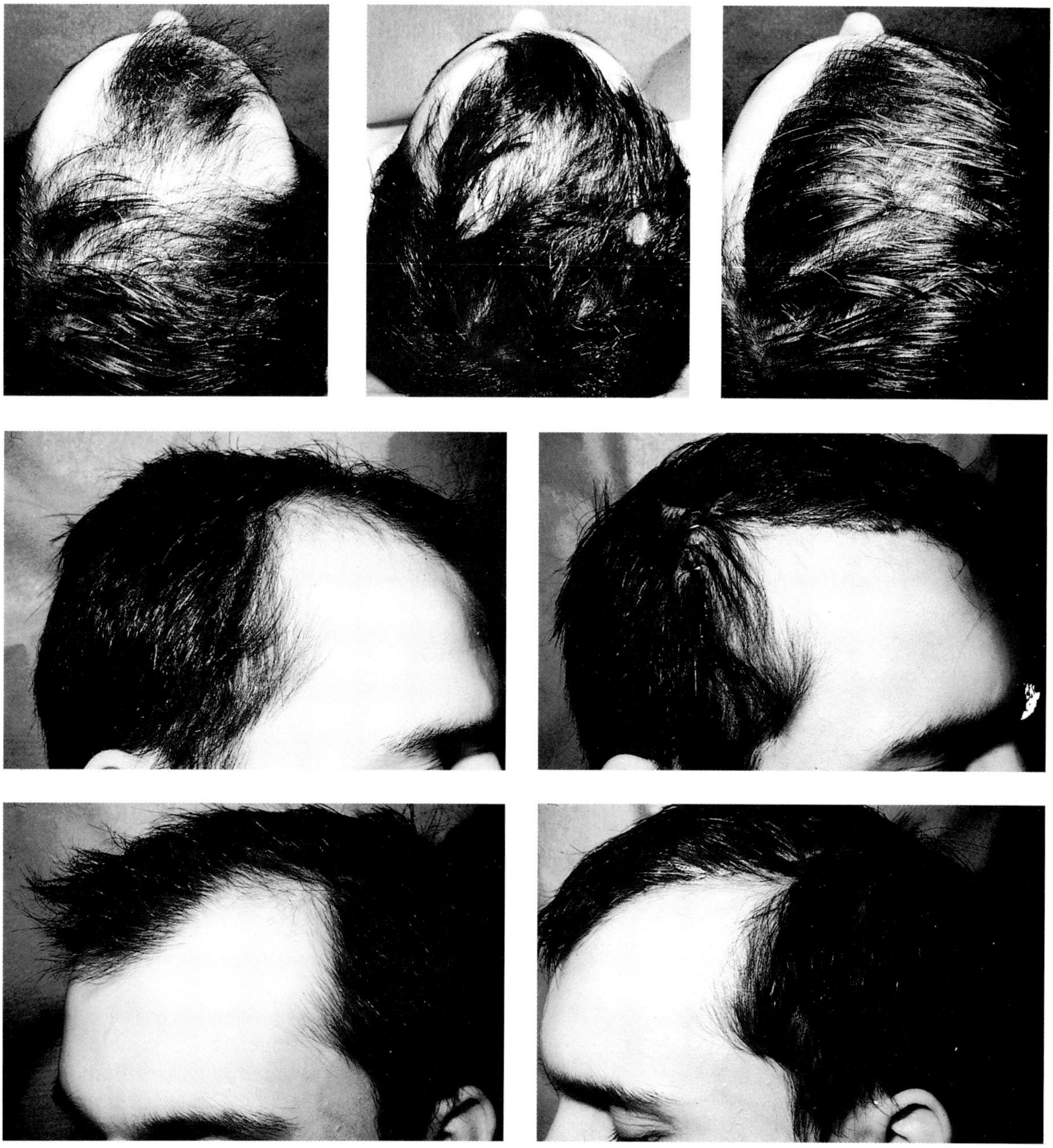

Photo 3a–g. Simultaneous transposition of two small pre-auricular flaps: pre-, peri- and postoperative aspects. **b,c** Note presence of dog-ears at the time of the operation and their disappearance by the seventh day

Stage IIB

There is vertical and occipital thinning combined with frontal alopecia.

If laxity is adequate and the temporal and occipital crown heights exceed 10 cm (HC<10 cm and HO>10 cm), the appropriate treatment is successive transposition of two, three or four superior pedicled, non-autonomised flaps. The bald area between these flaps is either excised (Photo 14a–c) or filled by transplantation of minigrafts in one or two sessions (Photos 15a–g, 16a–f).

If laxity is adequate and the temporal and occipital heights are less than 10 cm but more than 9 cm (10 cm>HC>9 cm), treatments consists of transposition in three stages of a large retro-auricular flap (Fig. 9, Photo 17a–d). The residual bald area may be decreased by one or two successive reductions and possibly by transposition of a contralateral retroauricular flap (Fig. 9, Photo 18a,b). Here too, some finishing touches using minigrafts are often needed.

If laxity is inadequate and the temporal and occipital heights exceed 10 cm (HC>10 cm), the placement of two expanders is followed after 2 months by transposition of two large flaps at successive sessions with a 1-month interval.

If laxity is inadequate and the temporal and occipital heights are less than 10 cm (HC<10 cm), 800–1500 minigrafts of four hairs each on average can be implanted in two to three successive sessions. If the hairs are frizzy, their covering effect in situ requires an average transplant of 3000 hairs in two sessions. If the hairs are stiff, an average transplant of 4000–6000 hairs in two or three sessions will provide adequate hair coverage (Fig. 10, Photo 19a–f). The use of long-haired grafts [2] gives an immediate but transient result while awaiting the usual regrowth at the second or third month. Sometimes, a simple session of 100 minigrafts may provide a good cosmetic outcome despite the small amount of hair transplanted.

Severe Baldness (Stage III)

The indications in severe baldness are identical with those advised for the correction of type IIB baldness (Fig. 9).

Conclusion

We believe that a judicious choice from among all the available techniques will allow satisfactory cosmetic correction in most types of baldness. This choice is guided by the reliability, cosmetic efficiency and simplicity of each procedure. For most cases of baldness, our primary choice is for the transfer of vertical flaps. Mini- and micrografts may be chosen if the patient does not require very dense hair

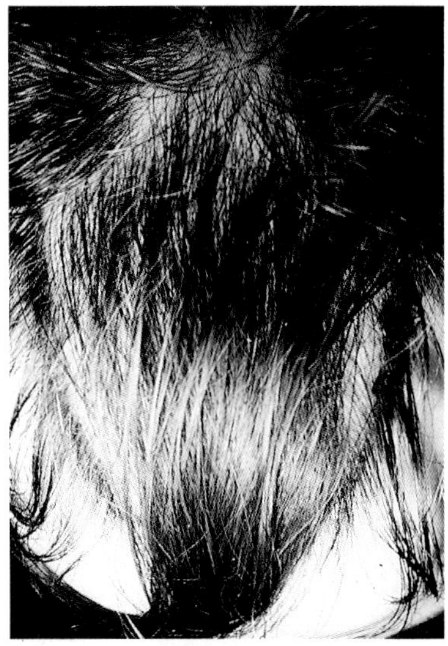
a

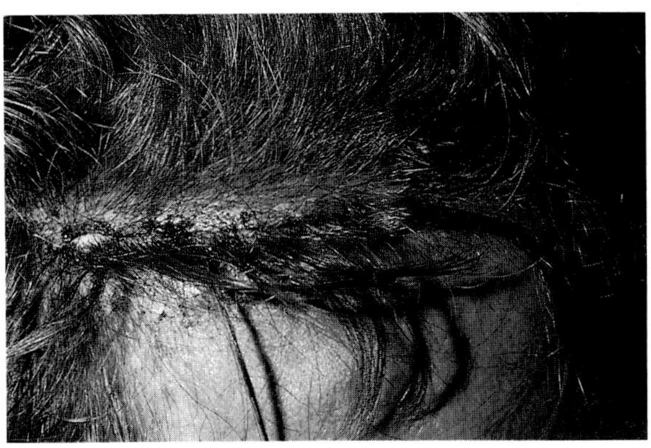
b

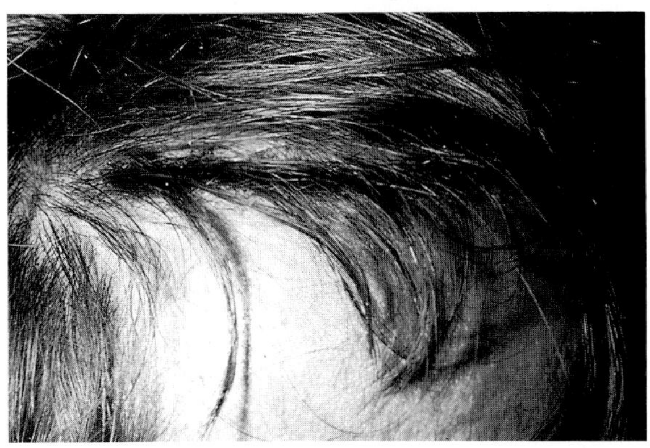
c

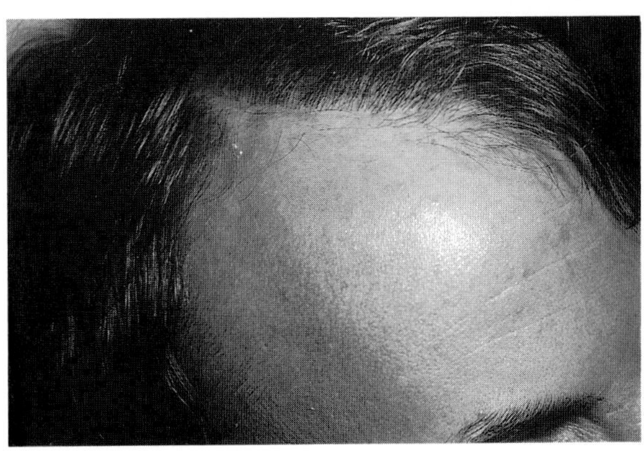
d

Photo 4a–d. Simultaneous transplantation of two strip grafts with long hair: peri- and postoperative aspects (seventh day)

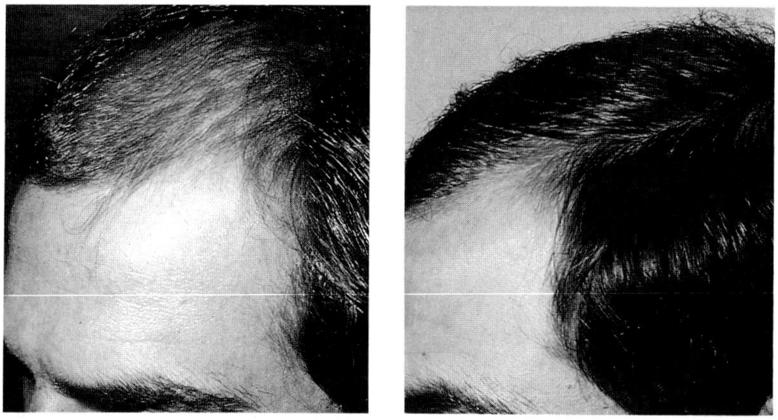
a b

Photo 5a,b. Transplantation of 140 minigrafts in two sessions. (Photo 5b was taken 10 years after transplantation and shows persistence of grafted hair and also progress of alopecia behind the transplanted zone)

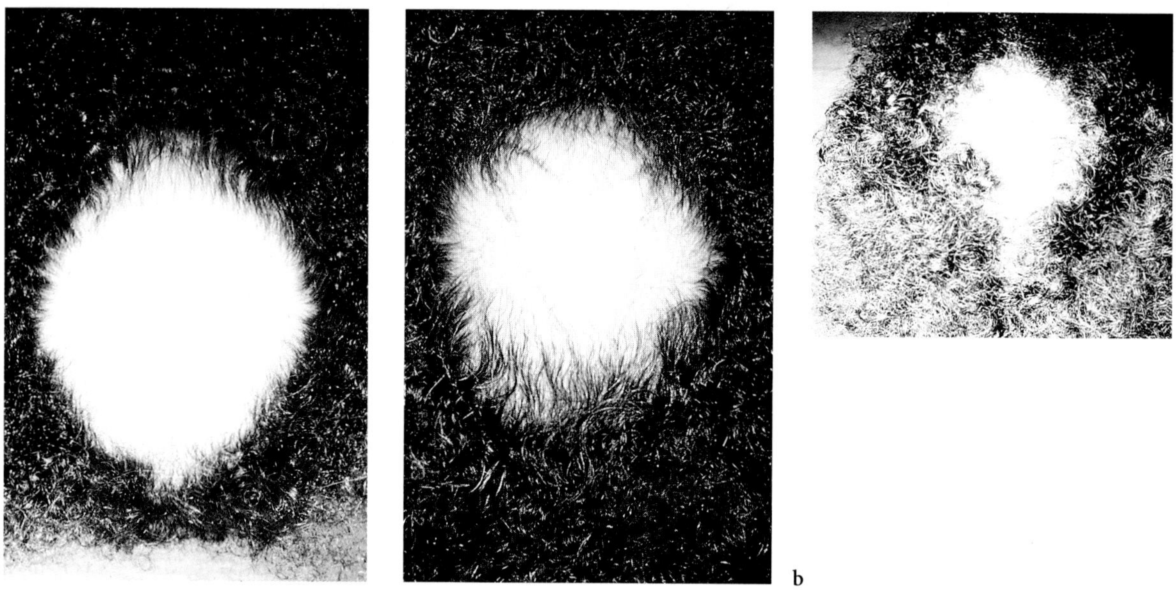
a b c

Photo 6a–c. Aspect of vertical alopecia after one reduction (procedure type "VY")

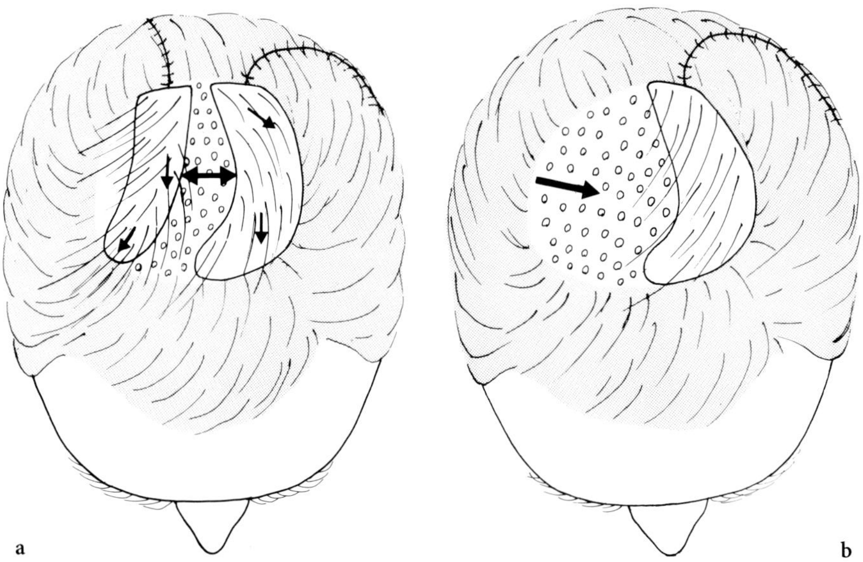
a b

Fig. 6. **a** Treatment of vertical alopecia by mixed left occipital flap combined with a reduction and one session of minigrafting. **b** Treatment of vertical alopecia by mixed flap and a straight flap, combined with a reduction and a session of minigrafting

Photo 7a–d. Correction of vertical alopecia in three sessions: successive transposition of two superior pedicle flaps and intermediate reduction

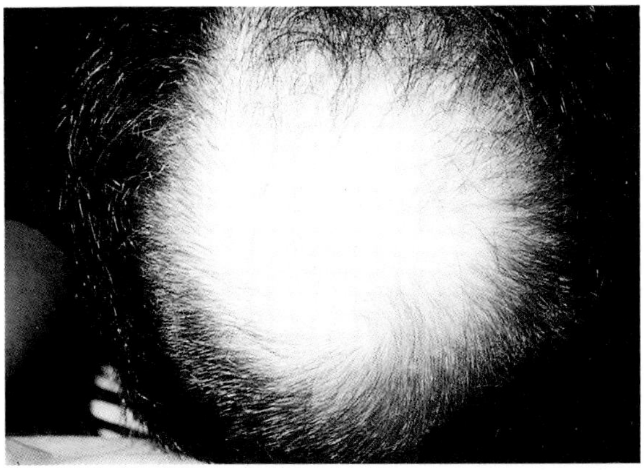

a

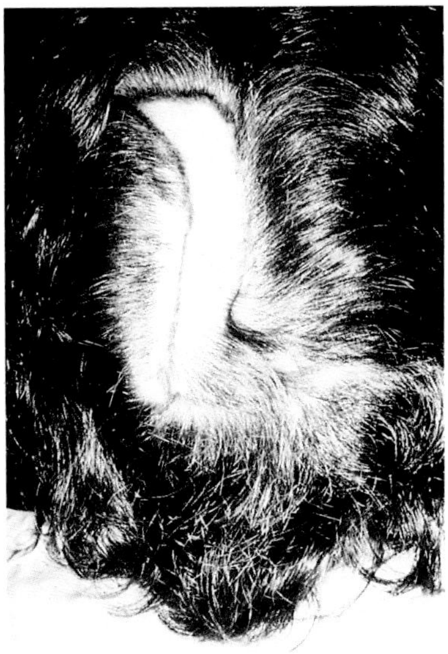

b

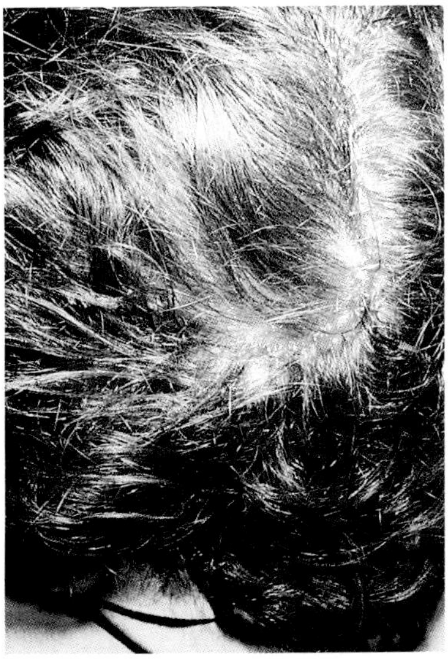

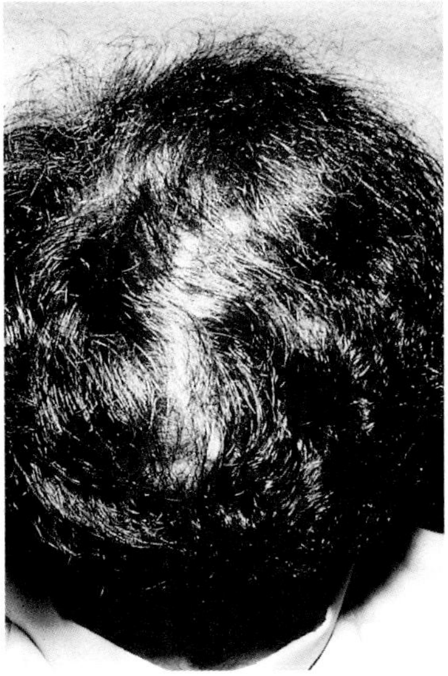

c,d

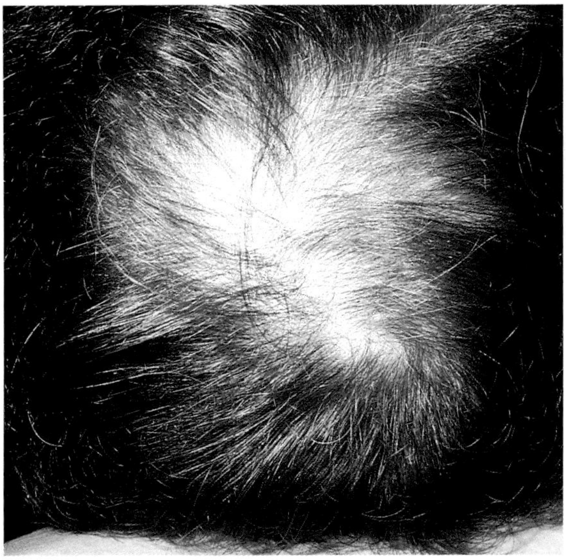

a

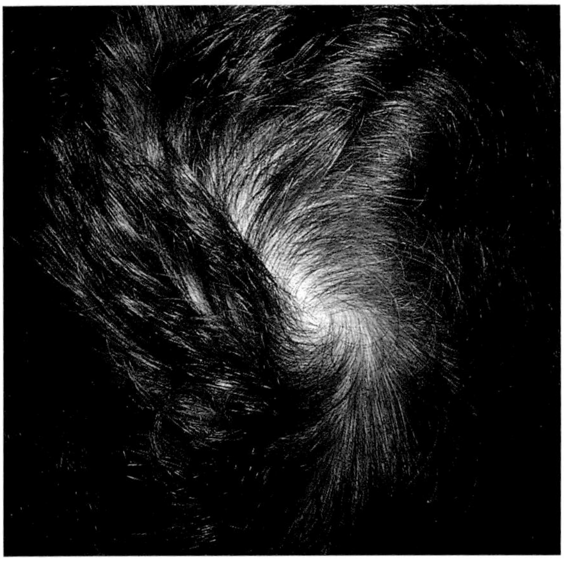

b

Photo 8a,b. Correction of vertical alopecia by transplantation of minigrafts

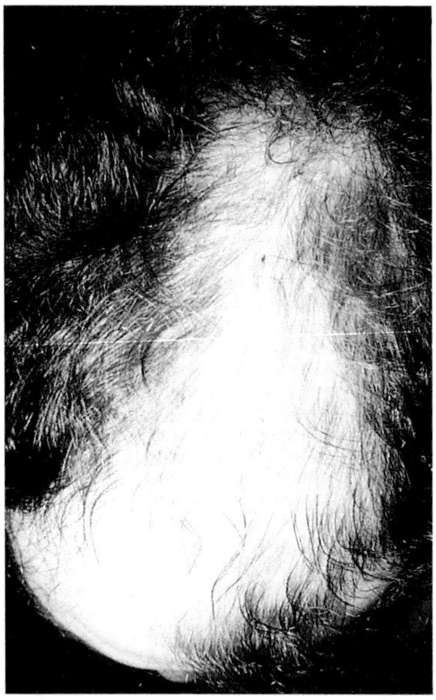

a

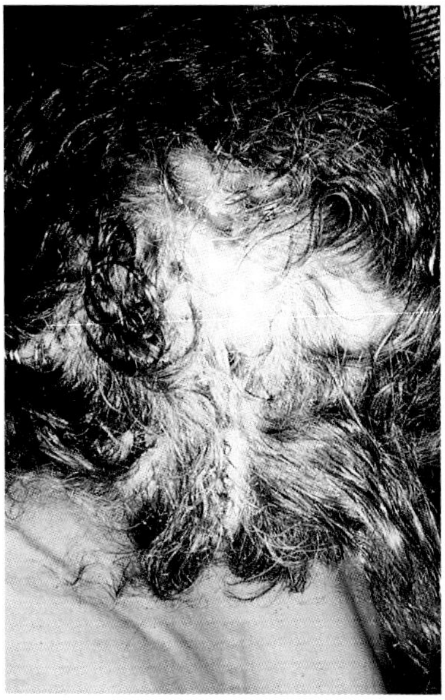

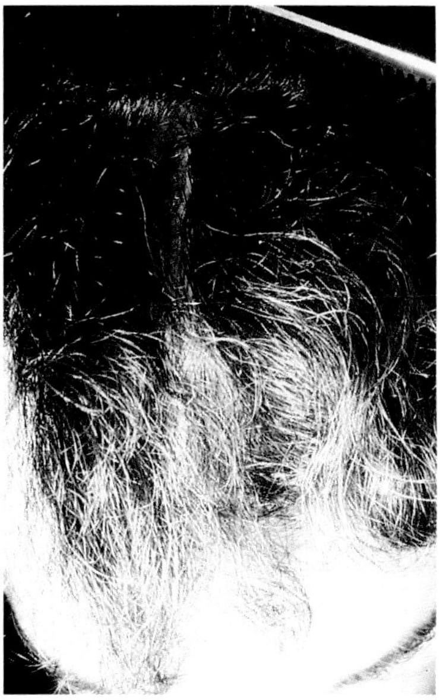

b,c

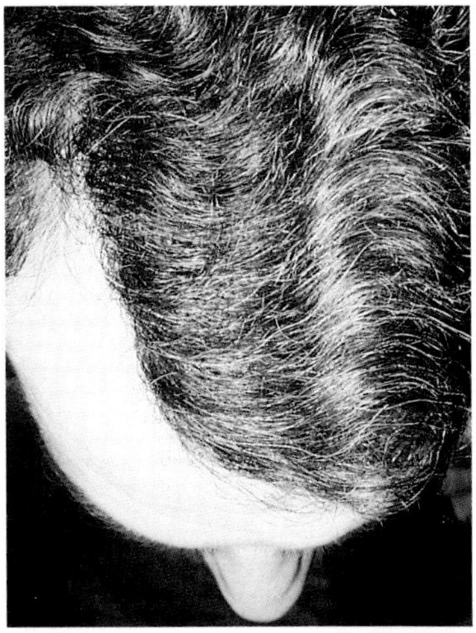

d

Photo 9a–f. Transposition of two pre-auricular flaps complemented by intermediate reduction. Complete correction in three sessions with pre-, peri- and postoperative aspects. Note the result with the hair not styled (**c**) and with the hair combed (**d**)

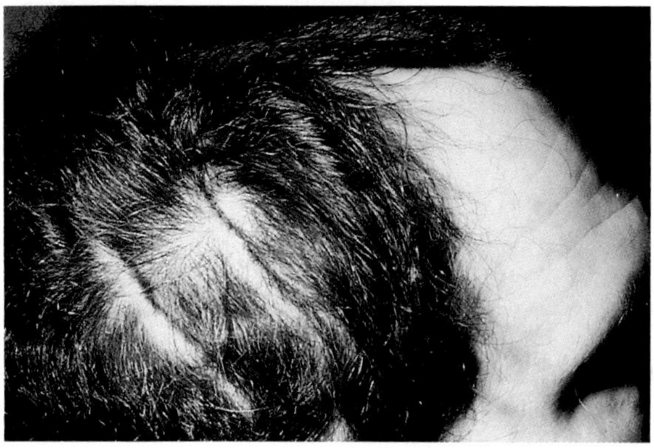

e

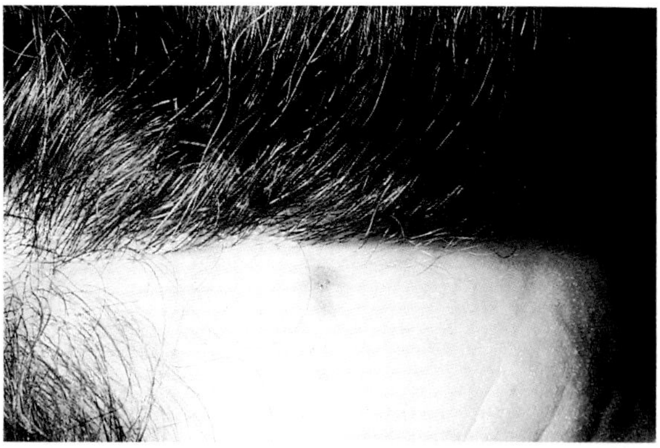

f

Fig. 7. Patient with long hair and side parting: transposition of two flaps (convex on left, straight on right) combined with reduction of bald intermediate zone and/or densification by minigrafts

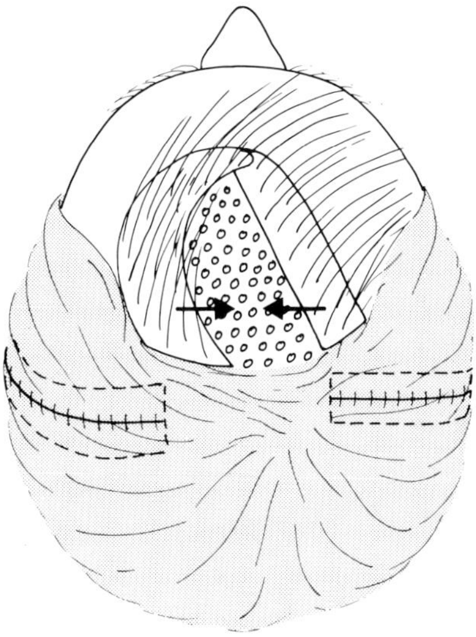

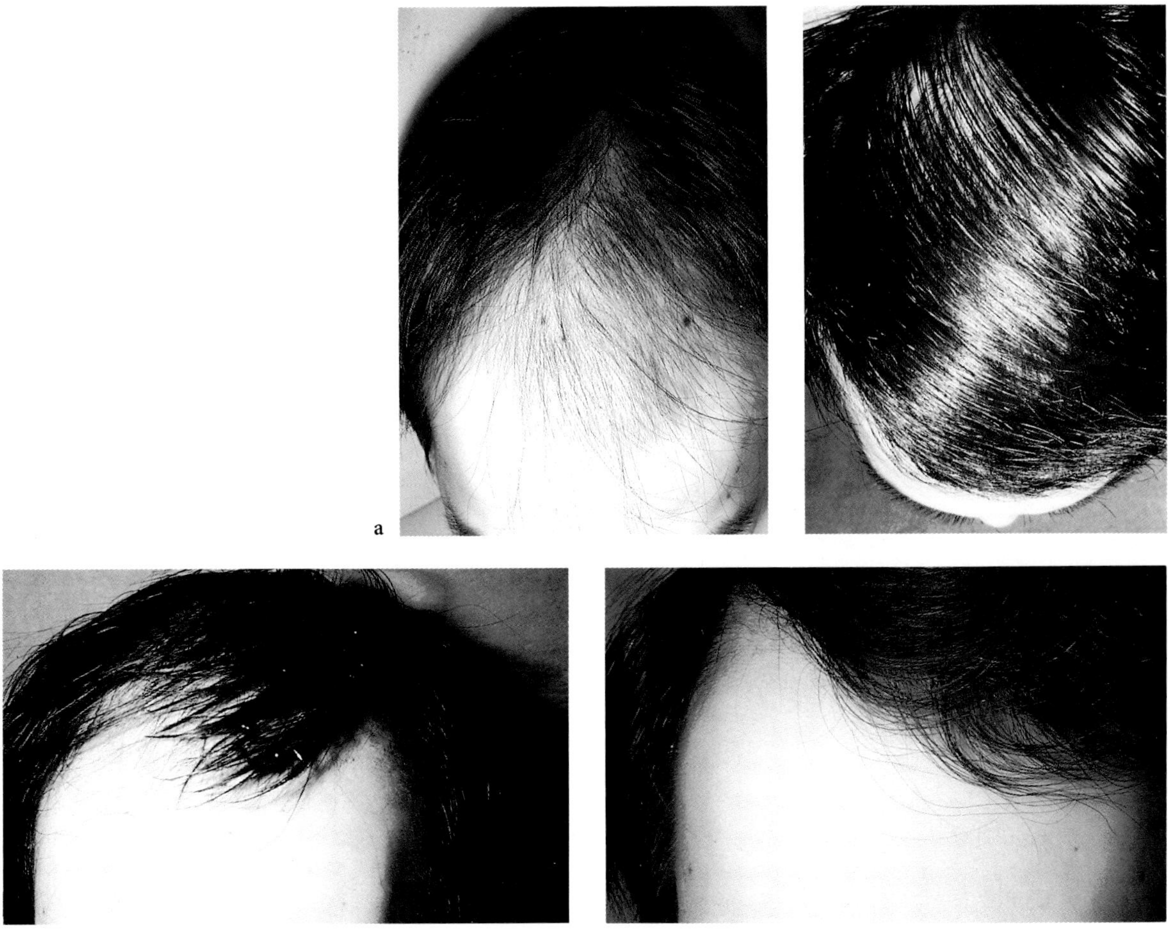

a c b d

Photo 10a–d. Asiatic patient before and after correction in three sessions by transposition of two pre-auricular flaps and intermediate transplantation of minigrafts: pre-, peri- and postoperative aspects (6 months later)

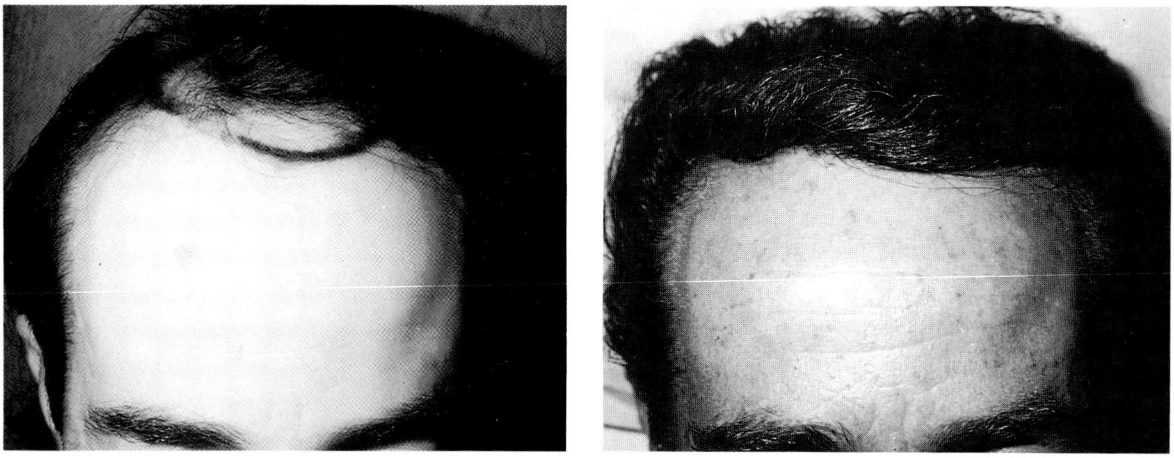

Photo 11a,b. Transplantation of 200 minigrafts in two successive sessions for correction of frontal alopecia: pre- and postoperative aspects (6 months later)

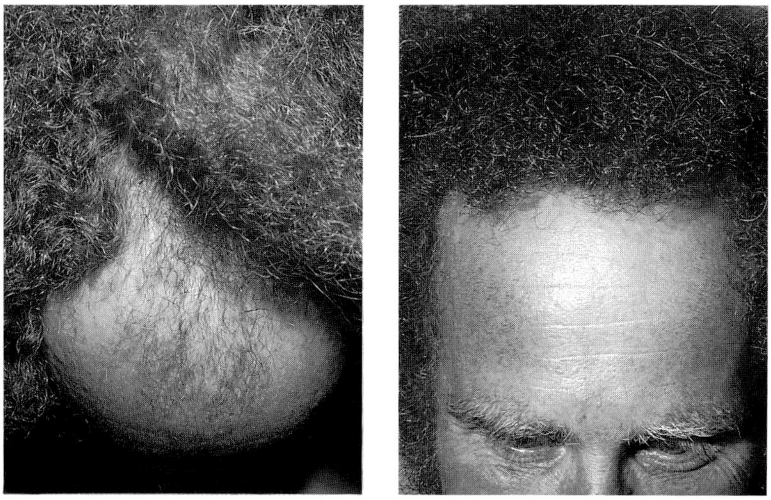

Photo 12a,b. Patient with frizzy, blond hair: correction by transplantation of 70 grafts to frontal region in one session. The patient was sufficiently satisfied not to require a session for supplementary densification

cover and in the case of severe baldness before any other surgical possibilities. Reductions are essentially supplementary techniques [10].

Indications (Dardour)

For a better understanding of the principles of operative indications, which cannot be discussed in detail for each particular case, they are first considered for major baldness, remembering that every patient is potentially seriously bald and that the first procedures must never destroy the bridges for those that follow.

Severe Baldness (Stage 3)

For severe baldness – C1 T4 (T3) F4 (F3) – the indications are simple:

1. If HC is 10 cm (stage VI of Norwood or Hamilton), S is 1 or 2 and *t* is 1 or 2, two procedures are available:
   a) Pre-auricular flap plus giant reduction [7, 8]. The first stage is a vertical pre-auricular flap as already described, in one stage if possible, which rapidly restores the frontal line on one side and allows the creation of a large lock of hair which, when dressed, conceals the tempo-

Fig. 8. Patient with long hair dressed backwards for either frizzy or crinkly hair: transposition of two convex flaps combined with reduction of intermediate bald area and/or densification by minigrafts

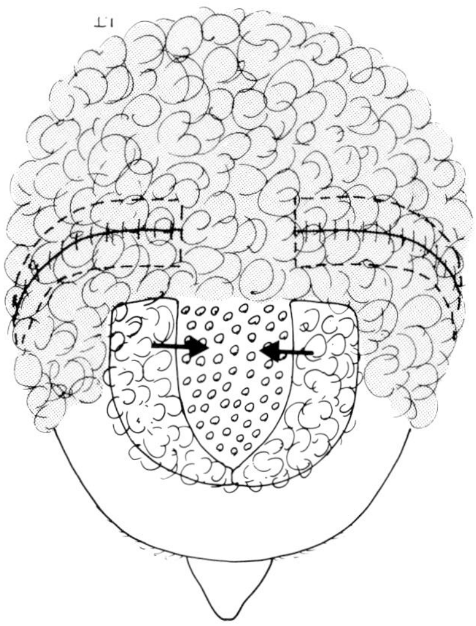

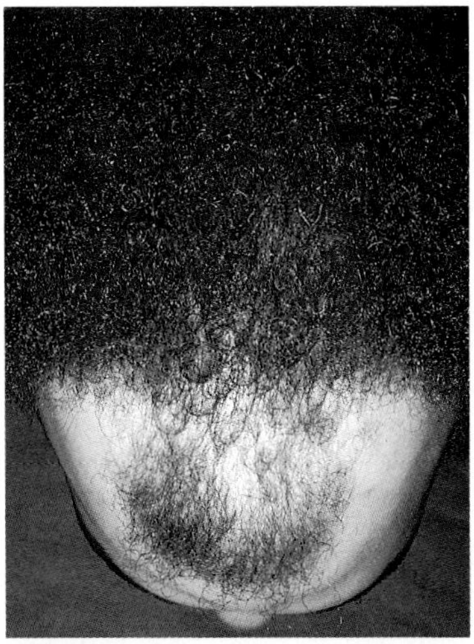

a

Photo 13a–g. Black patient with crinkly hair: correction by successive transposition of two flaps, supplemented by one grafting session: pre- and postoperative aspects (1 and 3 months later)

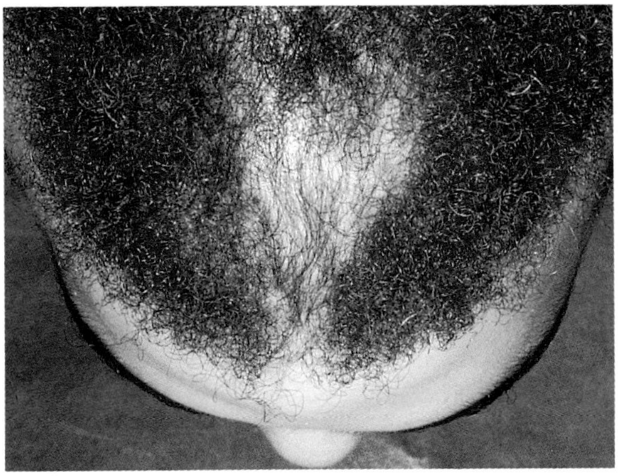

b

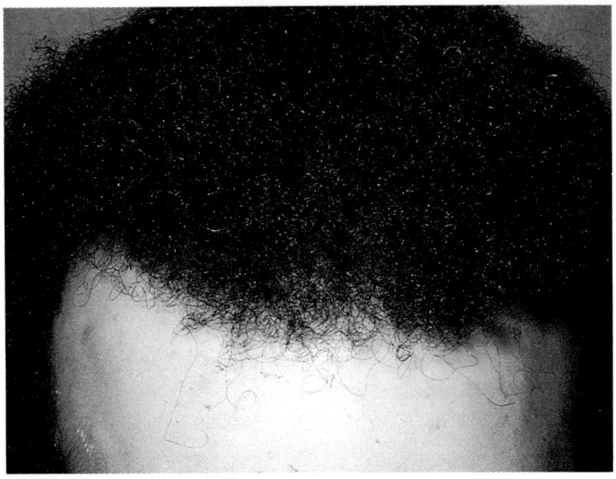

c

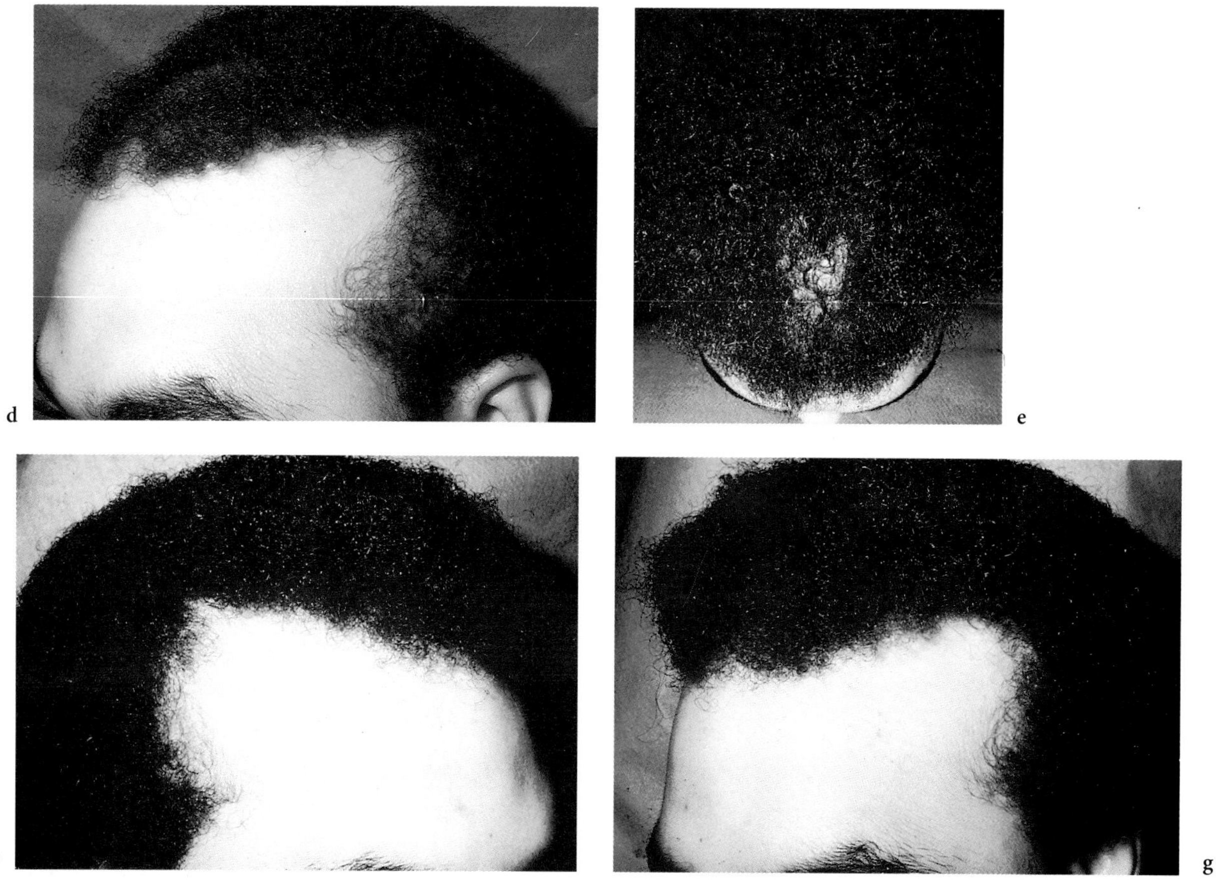

Photo 13d–g.

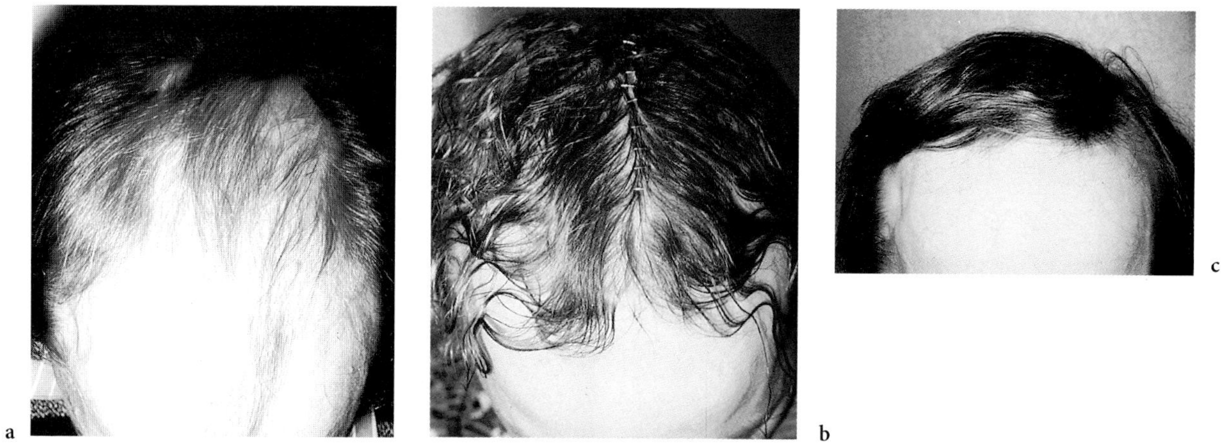

Photo 14a–c. Baldness type IIIb with satisfactory scalp laxity: correction by successive transposition of two retro-auricular flaps and intermediate reduction: pre-, peri- and postoperative aspects (15th day)

rary uncosmetic effect of the following procedures (Photo 20).

The second stage is a giant contralateral reduction (lifting of the scalp), which, as we have seen, can ascend the crown by 3 cm laterally and 6 cm at the back. It also allows advancement of the anterior temporal line (*t*) when necessary. When this line is already in an advanced position (*t*1 or *t*2), it has been shown that it is possible, at the same time, to

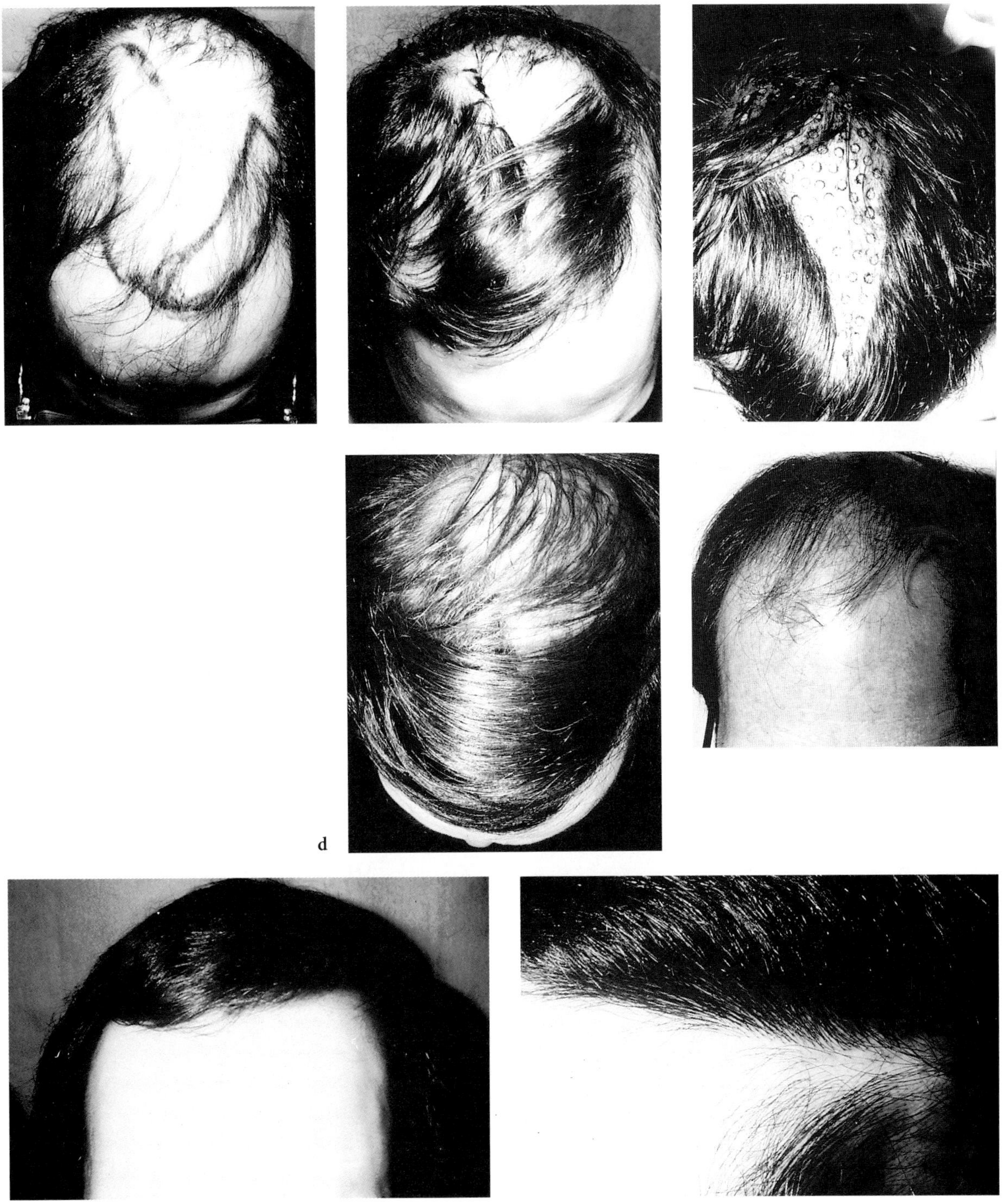

Photo 15a–g. Baldness type IIb: correction by successive transposition of two vertical flaps and transplantation of grafts to bald region between flaps. Pre-, peri- and postoperative aspects (3 and 6 months later)

construct a vertical mini-flap intended to complete the anterior hair line (Photo 21). The incision, which skirts the upper border of the crown, will cut the pedicle of the first flap, which permits the spread of any dog-ear, and then descends along the scar of the donor area, which can also be corrected if of poor quality.

After this second procedure, there remains a median smooth strip of 5–6 cm at most,

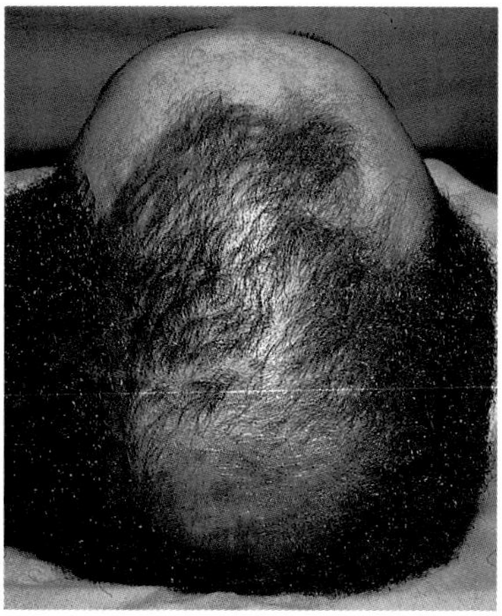
a
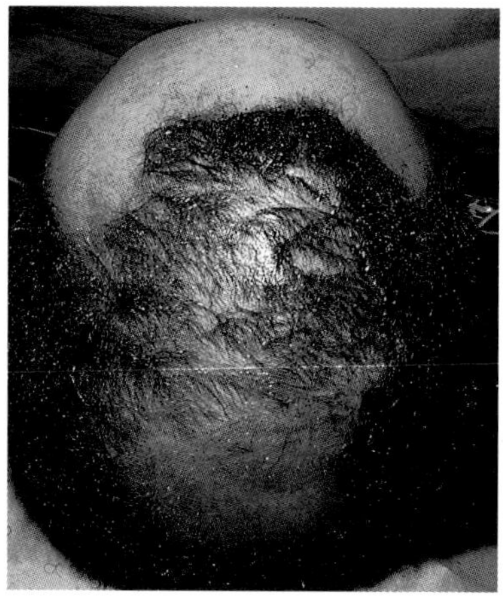
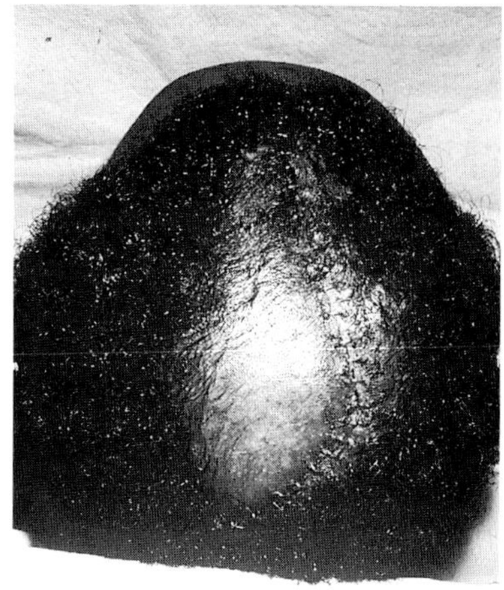
b,c

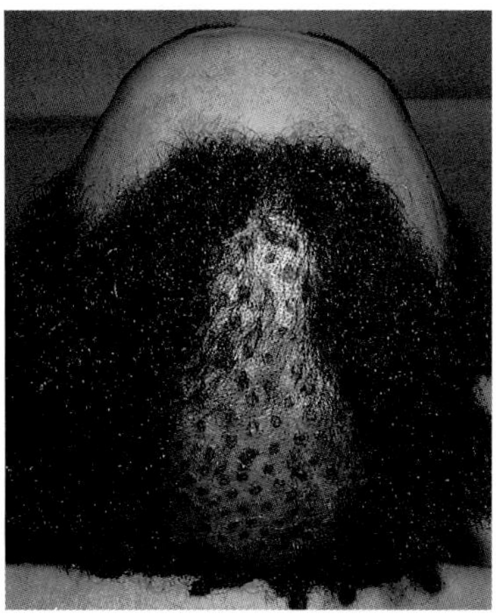
d

Photo 16a–f. Baldness in a black patient with crinkly hair: correction by successive transposition of two flaps and intermediate reduction. Aspect before and immediately afterwards, supplemented by grafting

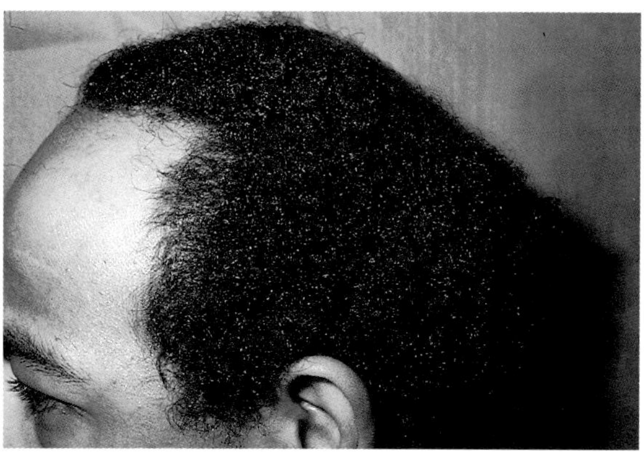
e
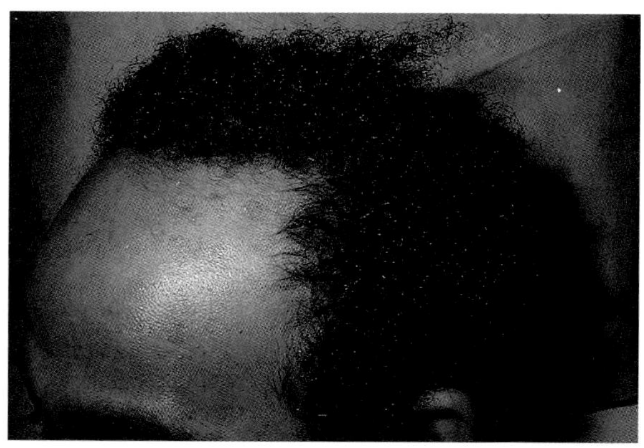
f

which allows with suitable styling can be easily covered (Fig. 11, Photo 21). Thus the last stage or stages will consist of one or two paramedian reductions and two or three sessions of grafting on the residual zone. In fact, if S is 1, the breadth of this residual smooth zone may only be 1–2 cm after a single reduction (Photo 22). Thus this original sequence, advised by us for major baldness, comprises four procedures at most (and usually only three), whereas coverage by autografts alone or combined with classical reductions comprises at least eight to ten [12]. Moreover, after the second operation the cosmetic appearance is very satisfactory. Some patients will be satisfied enough to stop treatment; this is not the case with the other techniques, where the patient has to continue to the end of the programme or suffer an unac-

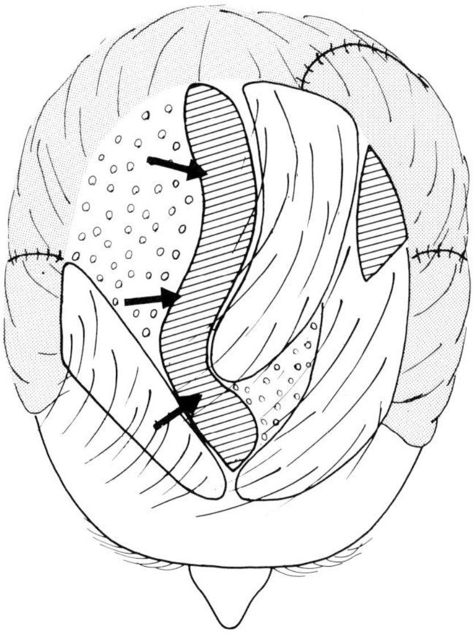

Fig. 9. Treatment of major baldness in five sessions combining transposition of three flaps, one reduction and finishing off with minigrafts

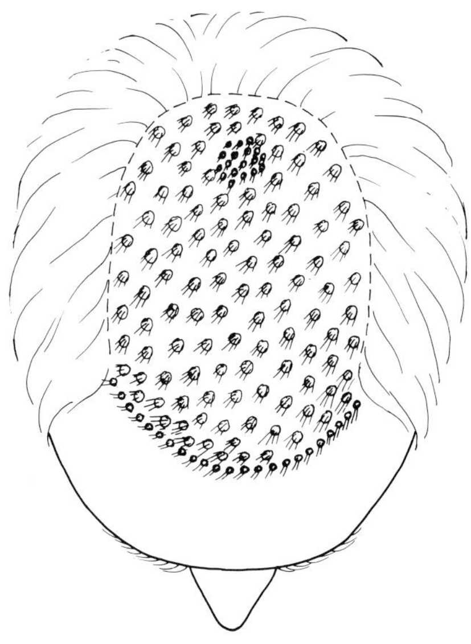

Fig. 10. Transplantation of 100–600 minigrafts at one to three sessions with finishing touches by micrografts

ceptable cosmetic defect. This is the major disadvantage of the grafting techniques. In contrast, with our technique, if we decide to cover the residual smooth zone with grafts, their temporary unaesthetic appearance is masked by the primary flap.

b) Repeated lifting of the scalp combined with two vertical flaps. This is another possible technique, just as rapid and with very similar results.

When a small central hair-bearing zone persists, the operation must be performed by a peripheral route (Photo 23). The two flaps then end at 2 cm from the mid-line, leaving an anterior skin bridge 4 cm wide, necessary for vascularisation of the residual zone at the vertex (Fig. 12). At the second operation, 4 months later, the two flaps previously positioned are raised again while a new lifting of the scalp is performed. Two other vertical flaps are then raised which, after rotation through 90°, take the place of the previous ones to form the frontal line. The two former flaps then spontaneously take up positions within and in front of the new ones; they now reach the mid-line and thus, after the second procedure, there are two flaps 4 cm wide in the frontal region, while the upper limit of the crown is ascended by 4–5 cm on either side and by 8–10 cm at the back (Figs. 13, 14).

When the vertex is completely bald, we perform the same procedure by a sagittal route or, more often, parasagittally. The skin resection in this case is at the summit of the cranium. It is combined with resection of a posterior transverse spindle intended to ascend the occipital crown. In this case it is now possible to join the first two flaps at the mid-line at the outset (Photo 24). The second stage procedure is also made by a sagittal or parasagittal route and also consists of placement of two new vertical mini-flaps. Usually, this second lifting of the scalp comprises only a sagittal resection which ends behind in a Z-plasty to conceal the posterior part of the scar (Figs. 15, 16, Photo 25). The sagittal incision is also very useful when the upper limit of the crown is not clearly demarcated and there exists a zone of intermediate hair of 1–2 cm which one hesitates to sacrifice at the outset (Photo 26) or when the distance HO is less than 15 cm.

The repeated lifting of the scalp as we have described seems an excellent alternative to the sequence pre-auricular flap plus lifting of the scalp, as it avoids the hazards, however minimal, of a flap. However, it transposes forward the hairs of the most anterior temporal region, which are sometimes less abundant than those of the parietal region and are capable of subsequently undergoing partial thinning.

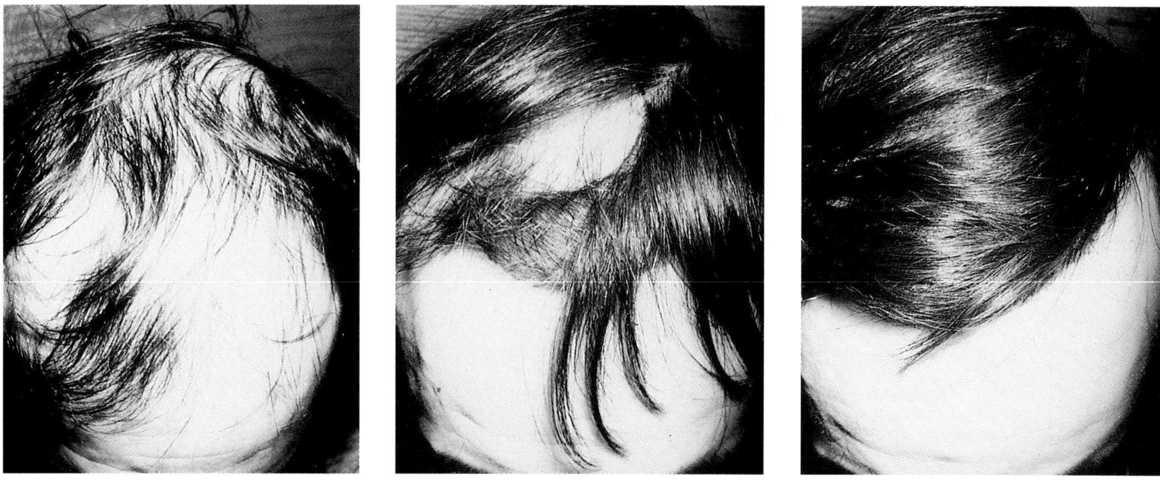

a b,c

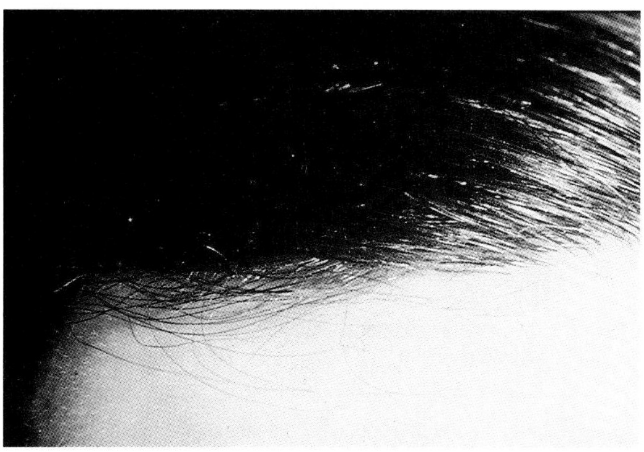

d

Photo 17a–d. Baldness before and 24 h after transposition of a large, vertical, autonomised flap: aspect with and without hair-styling the following day and aspect of frontal line 2 months later

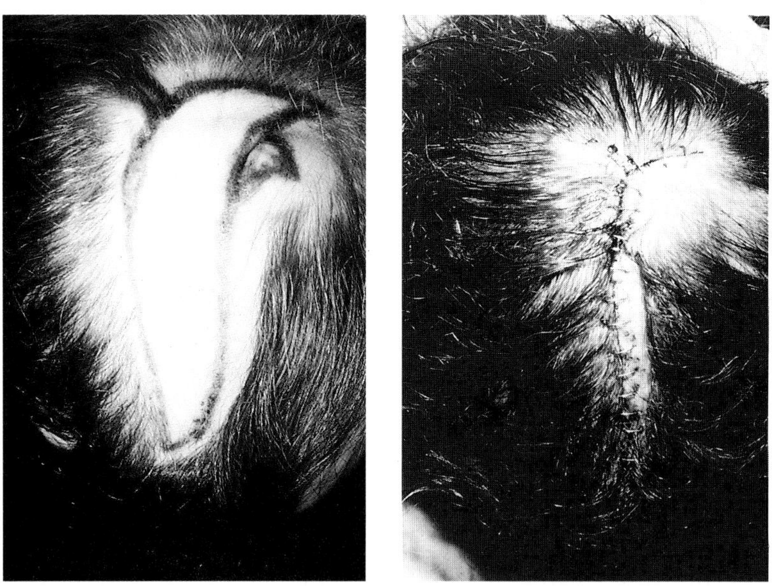

a b

Photo 18a,b. Aspect after transposition of two large vertical flaps and before reduction between the flaps and excision of the two residual "dog-ears"

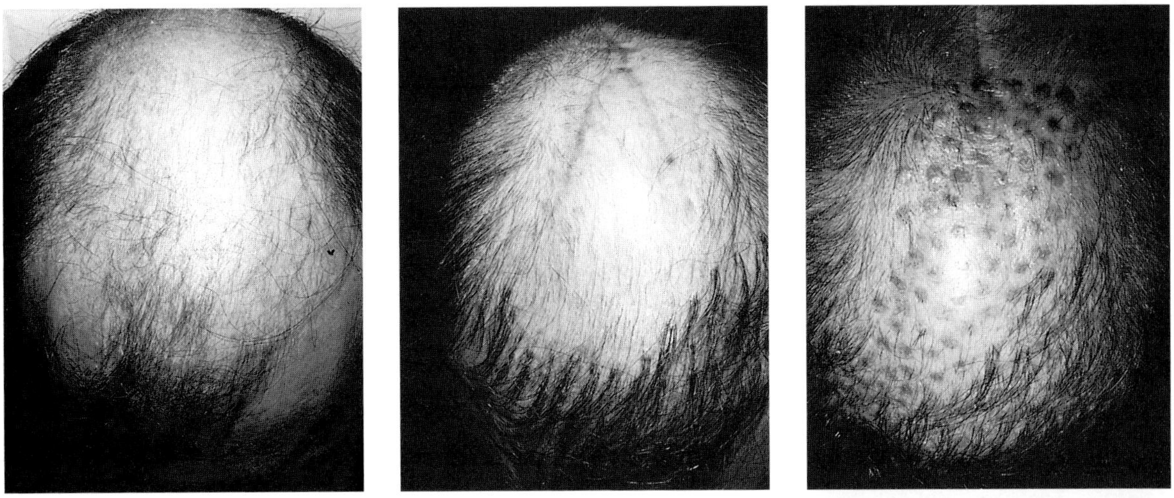
a b,c

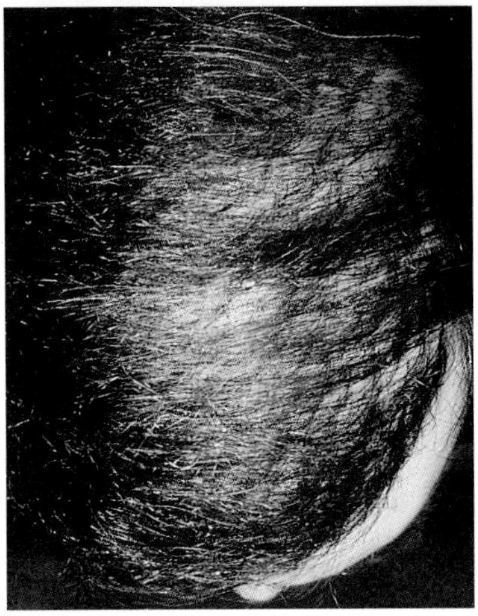
d

Photo 19a–f. Correction of extensive baldness by transplantation of 350 cylindrical grafts in four sessions and supplementary reduction: pre- and postoperative aspects (after 6, 12 and 18 months)

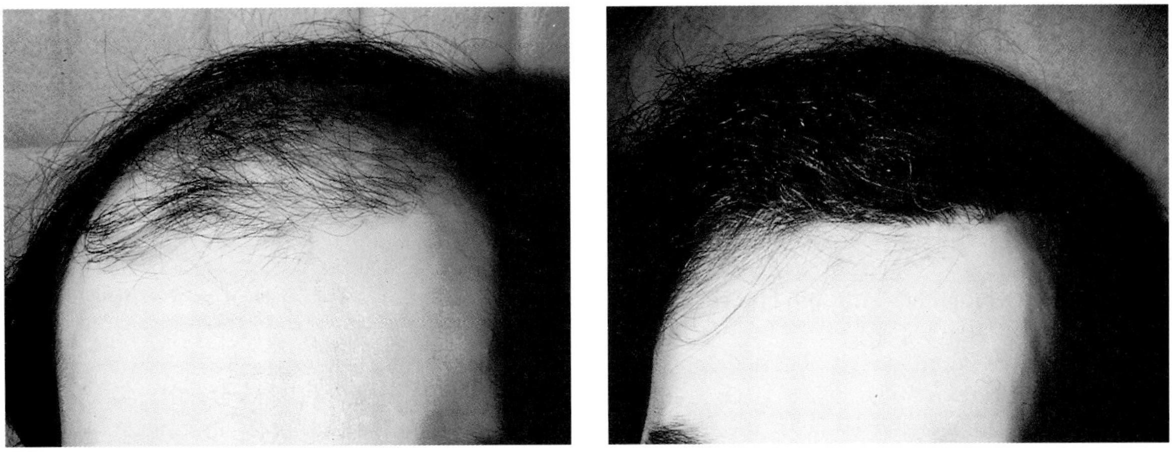
e f

2. If HC is 10 cm and *t* is 3 (temporal line very posterior; Photo 27), the pre-auricular flap is replaced by a retro-auricular flap, which has the advantage of not moving back the temporal line, but which has to be made in two or three stages and usually leaves a dog-ear at its origin until the second stage of giant reduction.
3. In patients with this degree of baldness, i.e. C1 T4 (T3) F4 (F3) and HC=10 cm, in whom the scalp elasticity is very poor (S=4), the operative

a 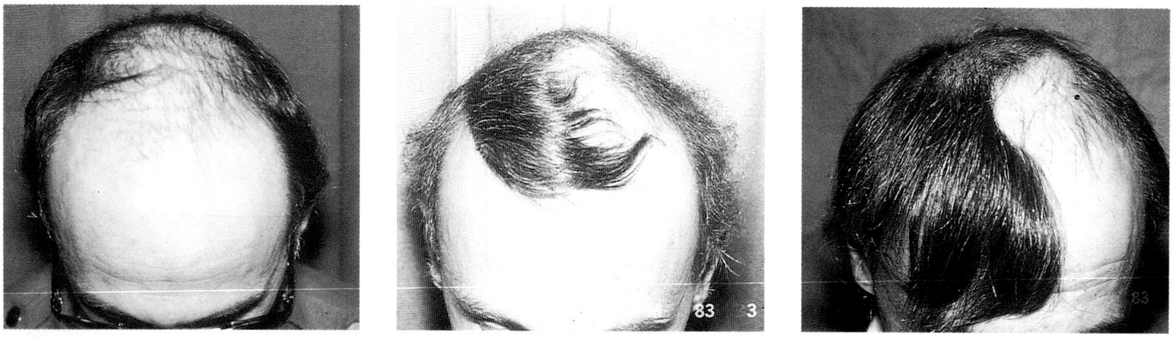 b,c

d 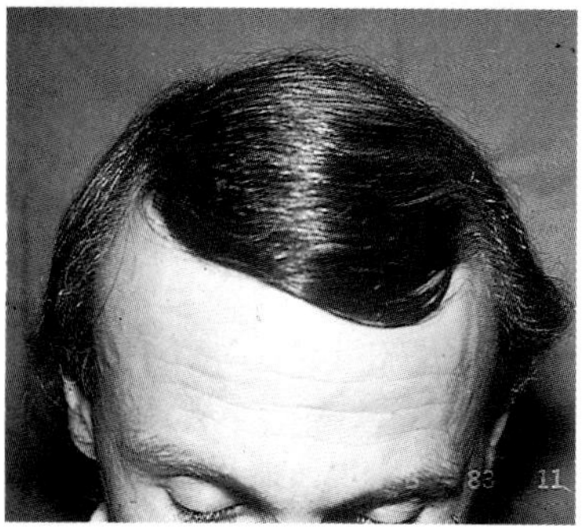

Photo 20. **a** Very extensive baldness. **b** Immediate result after a Dardour-type retro-auricular flap. **c,d** Same patient after some months: the hair has grown and conceals all the bald area when combed, allowing easy completion of treatment by other techniques

plan must be modified. Three options are possible:

a) First stage: a pre-auricular or retro-auricular flap (if *t*=3). The flap can sometimes be made after placement of a small expander (Photo 28). The subsequent stages are a matter of choice: three or four autografting sessions, a giant reduction followed by autografts or a reduction after skin expansion.
b) Use of a technique with skin expansion, preferably by the technique of Ozun or Dardour. These two techniques are the only ones allowing provision of hair in the frontal region and of hair that grows forward.
c) Transplantation of cylindrical grafts, supplemented by minigrafts at the frontal line, or of fusiform grafts. When the patient has curly, crinkly or blond hair, finishing touches prove less essential.

4. If the height of the crown (HC) lies between 8 and 10 cm and if the occipital height (HO) is of the order of 10 cm, we advise one of the following treatments:
   - A dispersion of 600–1000 minigrafts if the patient accepts very sparse hair cover
   - A technique of skin expansion
   - If S is 1, even repeated lifting procedures which, if they are possible, give a very acceptable result

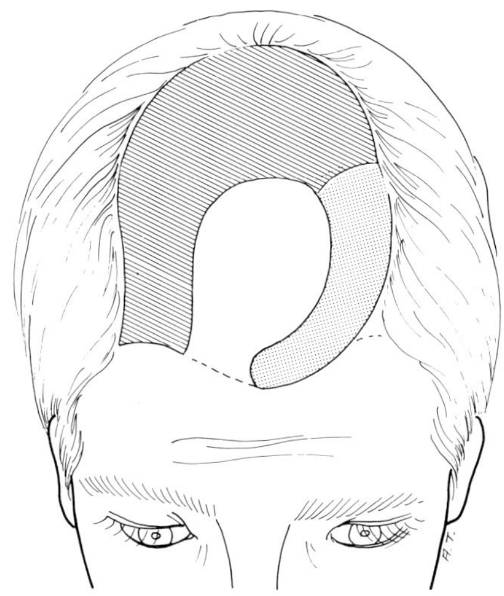

Fig. 11. Baldness C1 T4 F4, height of crown (HC)=10 cm, treated by a pre-auricular flap and secondary giant reduction

5. The indications do not change if HC is less than 12 cm but greater than 10 cm (Hamilton's stages Va, III vertex, and IV). Two plans of treatment are available:
   a) First stage: pre-auricular flap (if *t*=1 or 2) or retro-auricular flap (if *t*=3). Second stage: lifting of scalp; here the residual smooth zone is smaller (3–4 cm) and may therefore either be ignored or subsequently eliminated by a sagit-

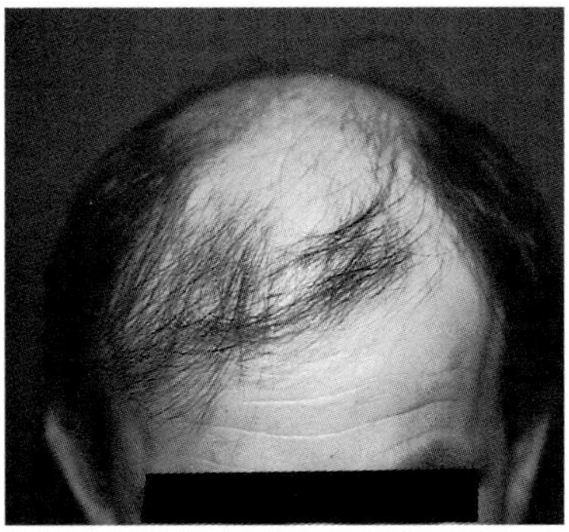
a

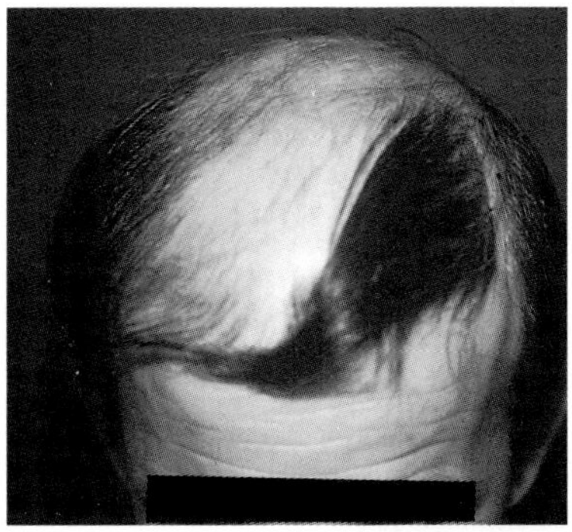

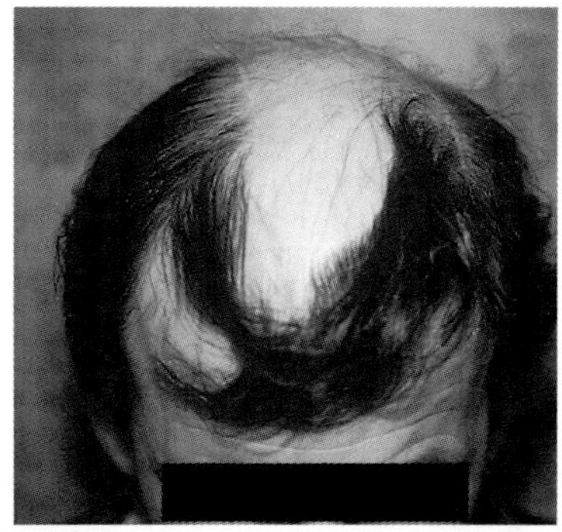
b,c

Photo 21. **a** Major baldness stage 3: preoperative condition. **b** Aspect after vertical pre-auricular flap of the Dardour type. **c** Aspect after left pre-auricular flap and scalp lifting combined with right vertical mini-flap, all in one stage. **d–f** Result after second scalp lifting combined with a second right vertical pre-auricular flap: patient with and without hair-styling. **g** Same patient, superior view, after left pre-auricular flap. **h** After first scalp lift. **i** After second scalp lift

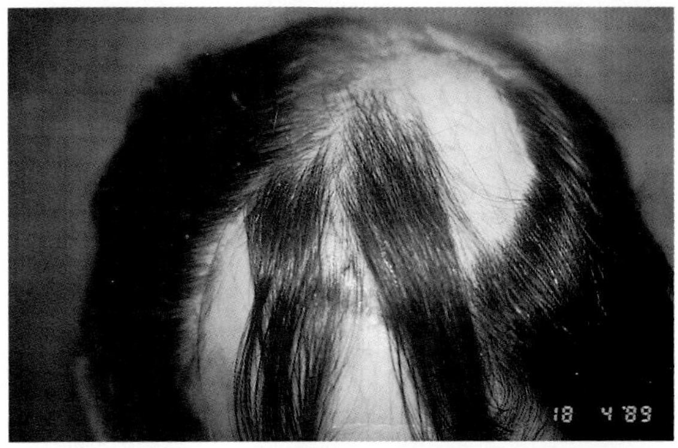

d

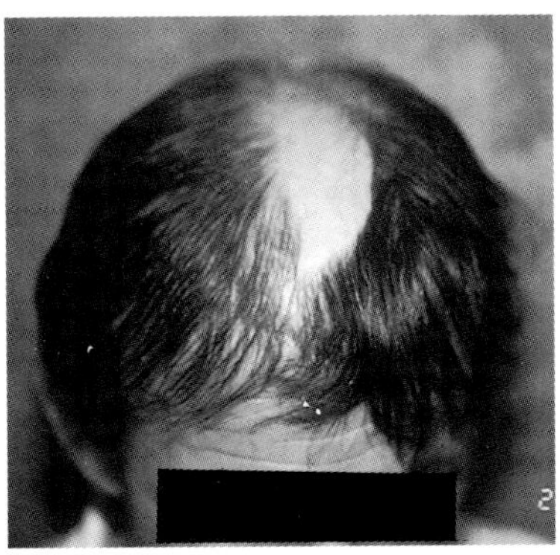
e

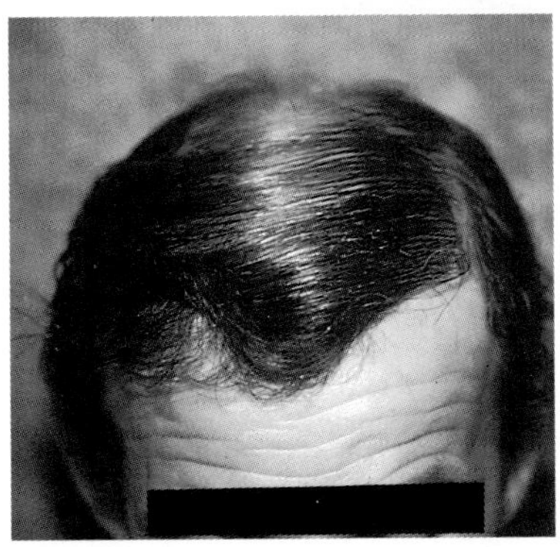

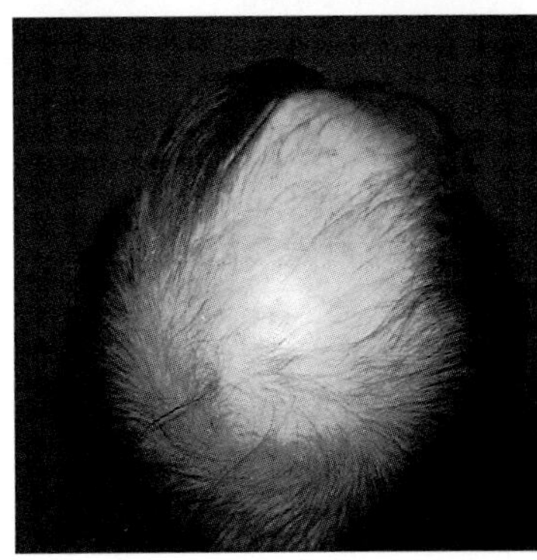
f,g

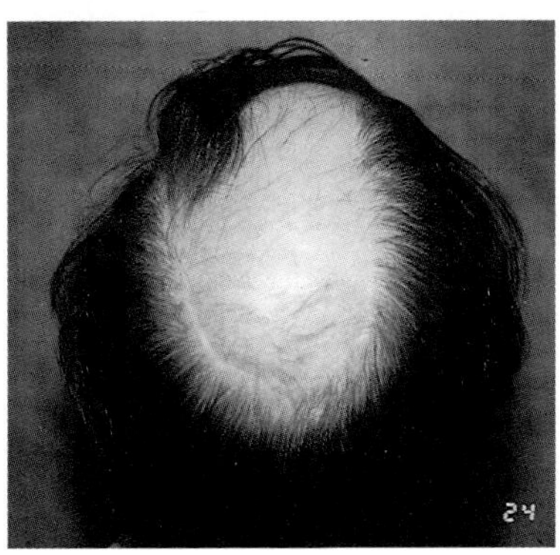
h

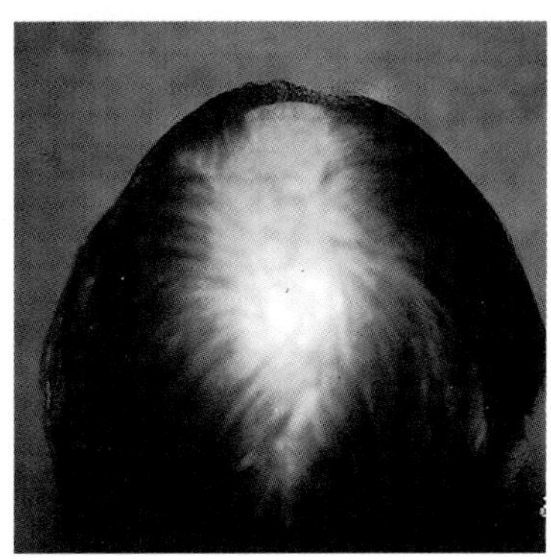
i

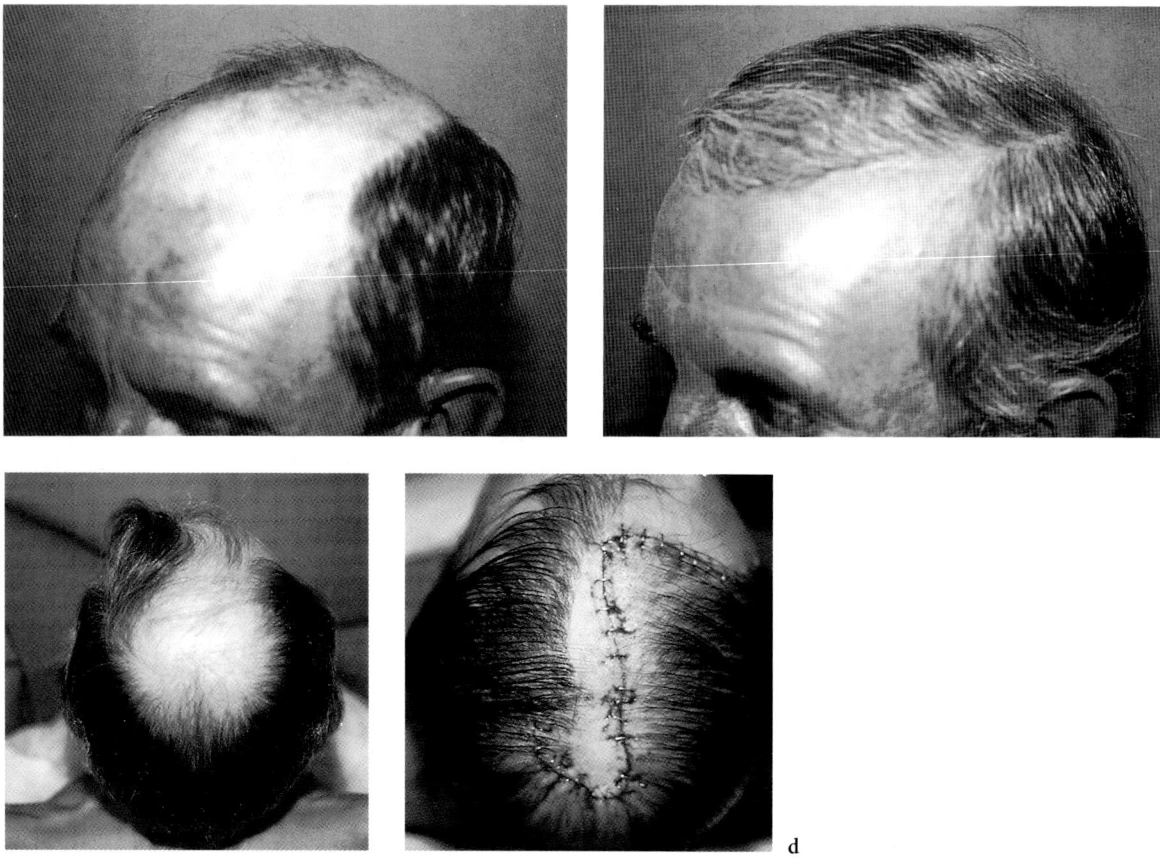

a b c d

Photo 22. **a** Baldness stage 3, C1 F4 T4, height of crown (HC)=10 cm, S=1. **b** Result after pre-auricular flap. **c** Result after pre-auricular flap (superior view). **d** Immediate result after scalp lift

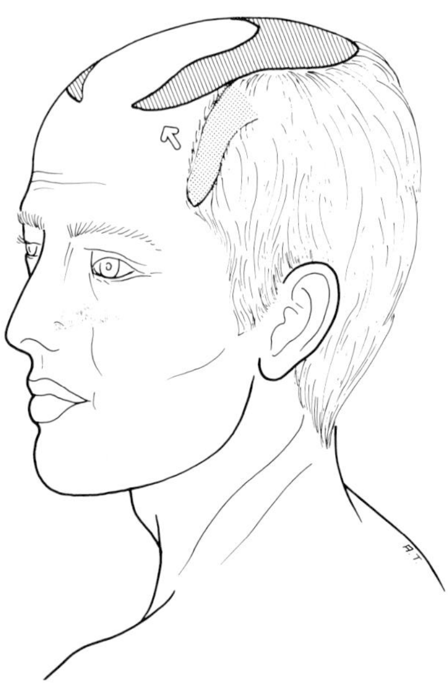

Fig. 12. Scalp lift by peripheral route combined with two vertical flaps: vertex and frontal thinning

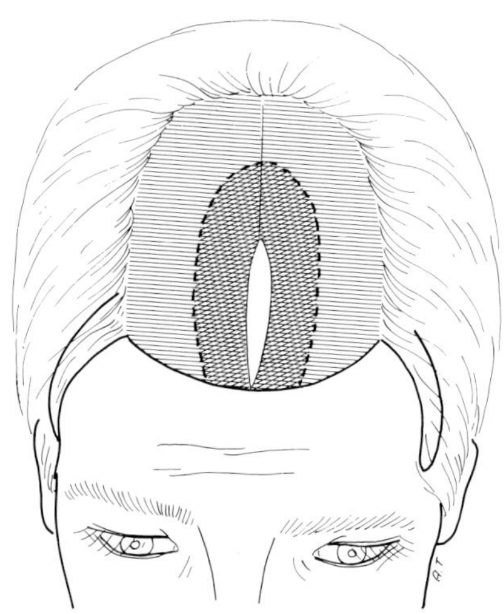

Fig. 13. Peripheral lifting: design of incisions and excisions at the two operative stages

Fig. 14. Result after two liftings by peripheral route

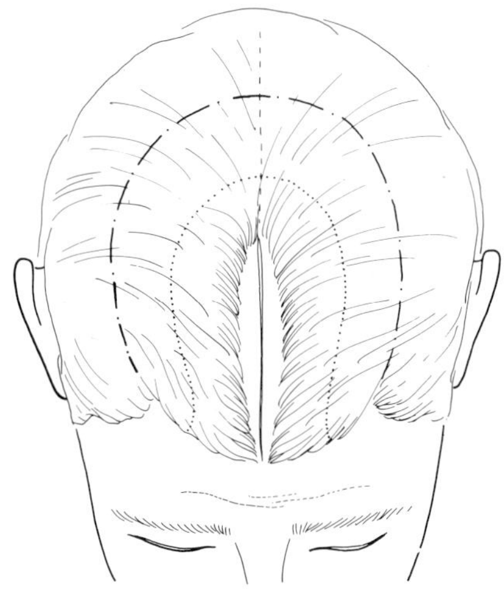

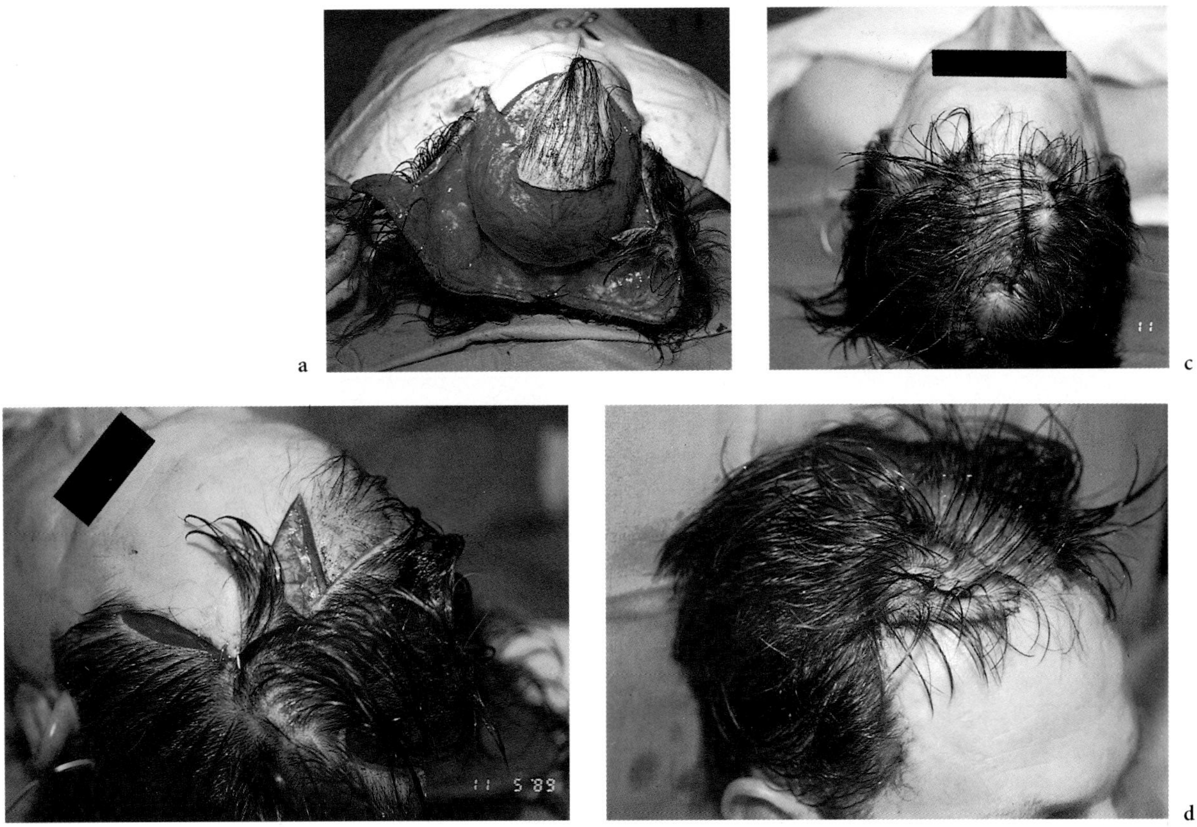

Photo 23. **a** Repeated lifting of scalp by peripheral route combined with two vertical mini-flaps: second stage. **b** First flap raised and transposed inward while a second flap takes its place next to it. **c,d** Final aspect obtained showing both flaps side by side on each side

tal reduction. Further, if S is 1, the giant reduction completely covers the residual zone, allowing complete treatment in two stages.

b) Two scalp lifts 4 months apart are an excellent alternative, especially in this type of baldness, as they often allow rapid achievement of total and symmetric coverage, avoiding the risks, minimal as they are, of a flap (Photo 29). In smokers, we have no hesitation in automatically considering this indication.

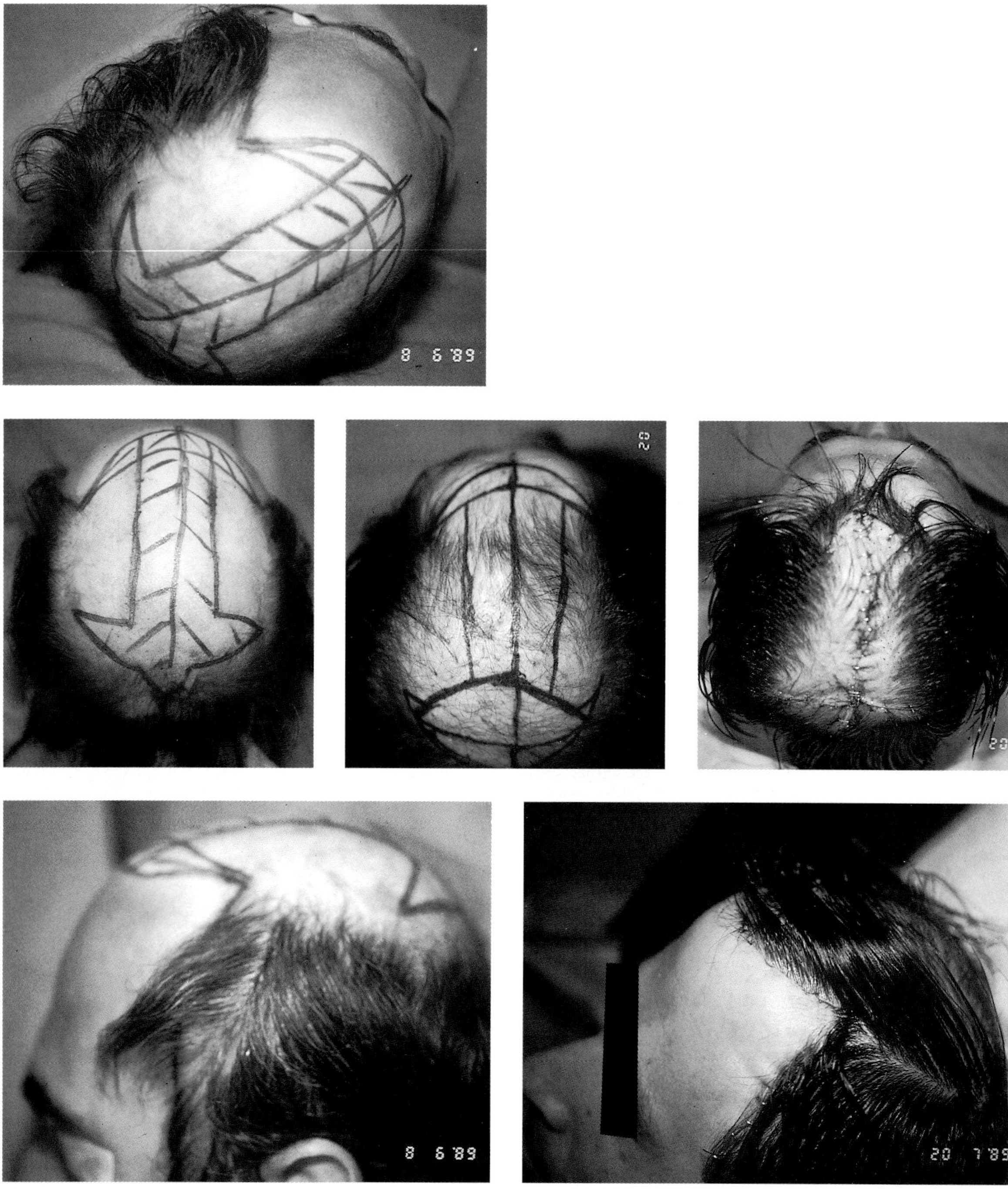

a b c,d e f

Photo 24a–c. Same patient in all three photographs: design of scalp lift and two vertical mini-flaps by sagittal route. **d–f** Same patient in all three photographs: scalp lift by sagittal route combined with two vertical mini-flaps: pre- and immediate postoperative aspect after first stage

Frontal Baldness

There are several possible cases of frontal baldness:

1. Simple recession of the fronto-temporal recession, i.e. C1 T1 F1 (F2) *t*1 (*t* 2) *f*2. We advise a uni- or bilateral mini-flap, which very rapidly provides the desired result by means of a very easy procedure and which is also of superior quality to three or four sessions of autografts (Photo 30). The objection may be raised that this technique fails

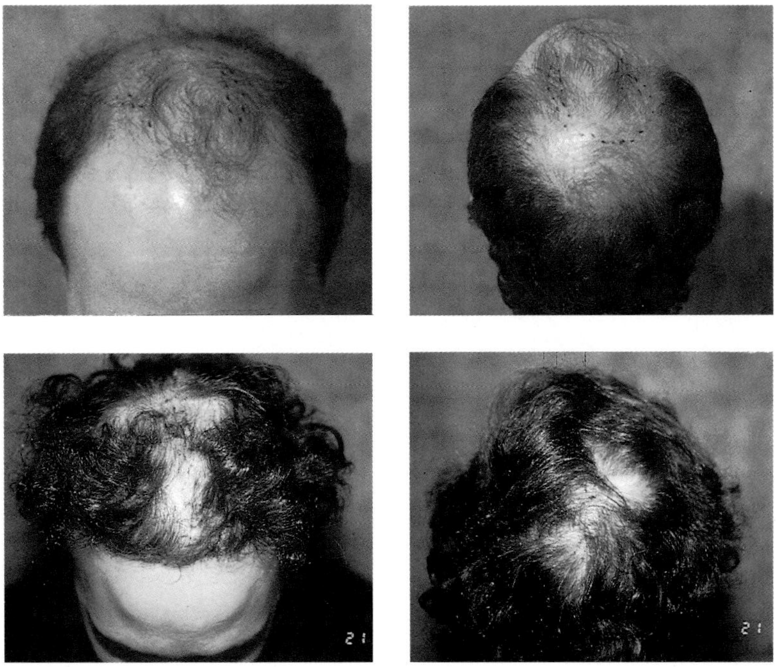

a b c d

Photo 25. a,b Baldness stage 3, C1 T4 F4, height of crown (HC)=10 cm. **c,d** Result after two scalp lifts by sagittal route, each combined with bilateral mini-flap: complete coverage of baldness

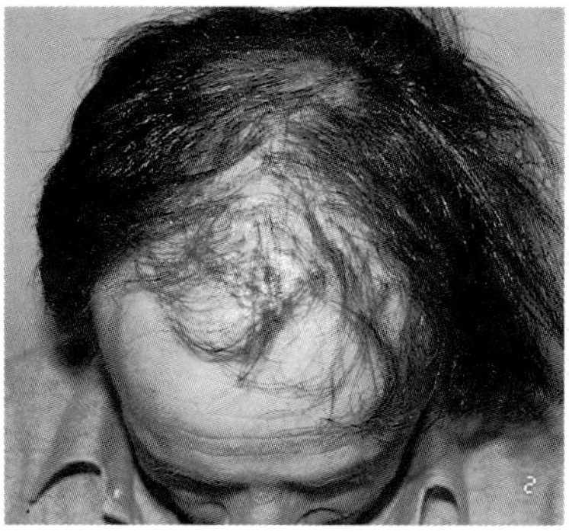

Photo 26. Upper limit of crown fuzzy, indicating median sagittal resection rather than peripheral resection

to allow for subsequent progress of the baldness. In fact, we believe that it is still possible to supplement the result obtained by autografts behind the flaps, should the alopecia extend. However, in a very young patient, or when it is certain that the baldness will seriously progress, we believe that an initial pre-auricular flap is necessary. The transplantation of two long-haired fusiform grafts may give an acceptable result in some cases. If the patient wants simple increase of density at the fronto-temporal recession, micro- or minigrafts can be transplanted in the knowledge that the solution is a temporary one (Photo 31a–f).

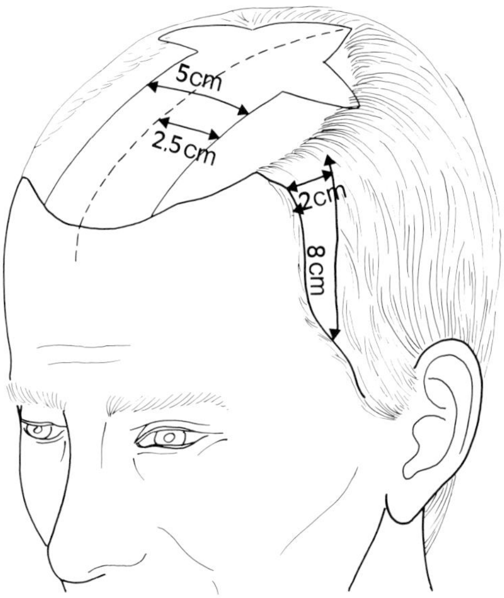

Fig. 15. Scalp lifting by sagittal route can cover half of extensive bald area

2. If the fronto-temporal recession is more marked, i.e. *f*3 G3 (Photos 32, 33), we consider performance of a pre-auricular flap mandatory. The result obtained is spectacular and calls for only one procedure. Moreover, if the baldness progresses, the flap will form the first stage of the operative sequence that we advise for major bald-

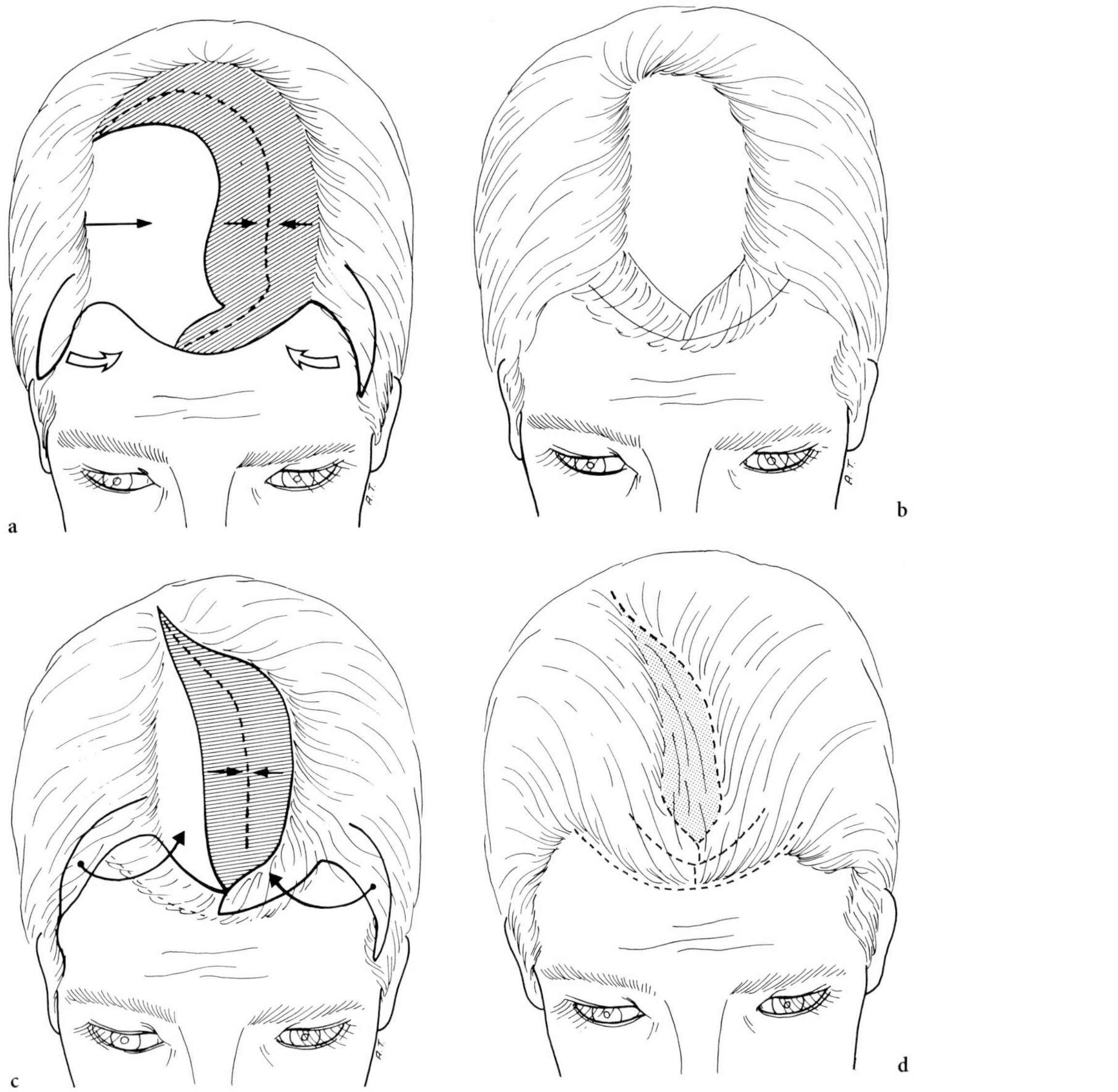

Fig. 16a–d. Scalp lifting by parasagittal incision. **a** Incisions in *thick lines*, resected zone *hatched*. **b** Result after first procedure. **c** Second stage: incision in *thick lines*, resected zone *grey*. **d** Result after second stage: a median smooth zone sometimes persists (*hatched*)

ness. As against this, several sessions of autografting risk compromising the subsequent execution of this programme. For the same reason, in this case, we advise against performance of a second vertical flap, which, by eliminating the second superficial temporal artery, would prevent the later performance of a giant reduction (Fig. 17, Photo 34).

3. Certain cases of extensive anterior baldness, i.e. C1 T4 F4. When the crown is considerable (HC >11 cm and HO>18 cm), these patients may benefit from a Dardour-type pre-auricular flap combined with a Passot flap placed side by side and then a secondary reduction of the residual bald zone between the two flaps (Photo 35).
4. Isolated anterior baldness, i.e. C1 T1 F4 (Norwood's stage IV). The first stage is a vertical pre- or retro-auricular flap. A second vertical flap would have the disadvantage of leaving a median smooth zone which could only be filled by two or three autograft sessions. We therefore think it preferable in such cases to do the grafting first, so that a second graft becomes unnecessary (Fig. 17). The second possibility consists of making a vast rotation flap allowing advancement of the vertex and intended to partially fill the residual smooth frontal zone (Fig. 18).

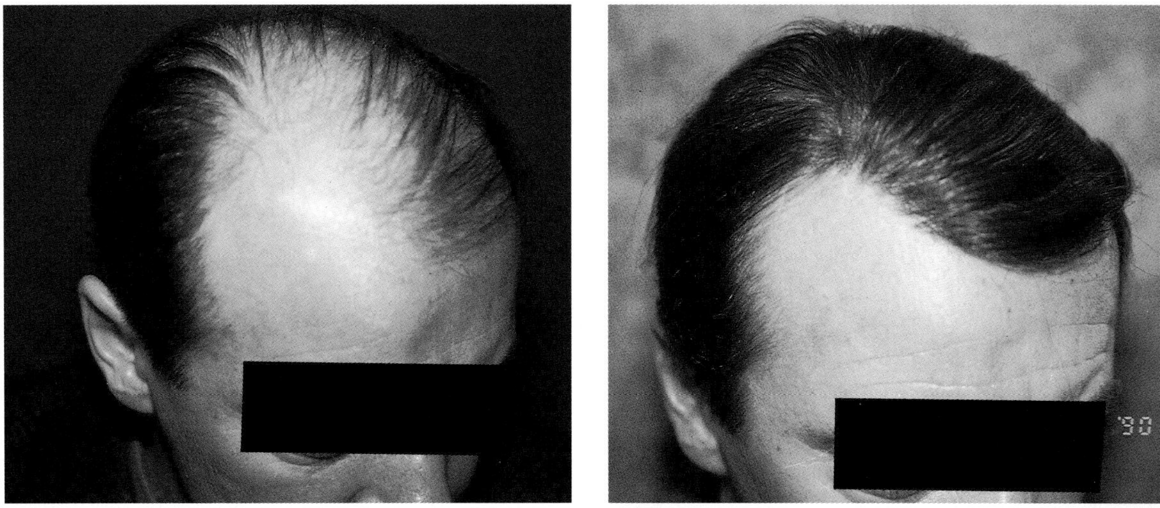

27a 27b

Photo 27a,b. Retro-auricular flap in a patient where *t* is 3

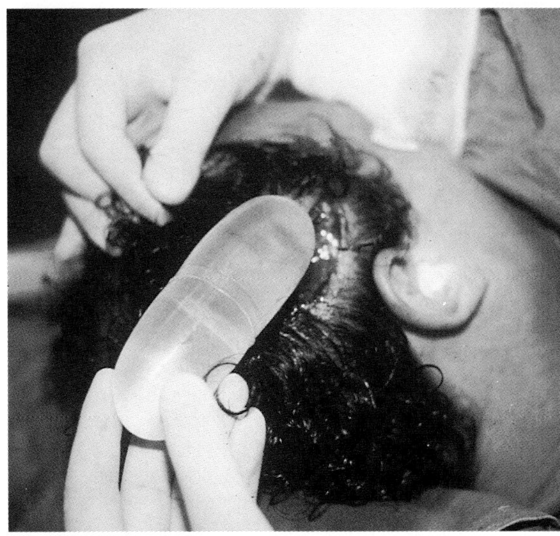

28

Photo 28. Removal of small expander which allows performance of a pre-auricular flap

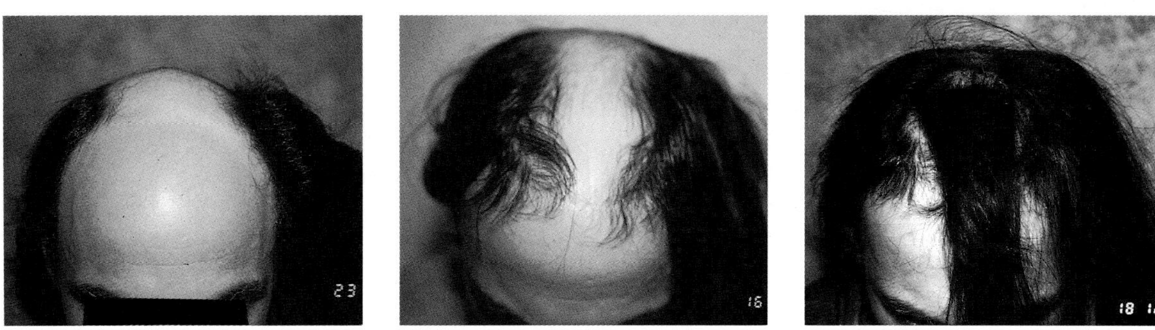

a b,c

Photo 29a–c.

Posterior Baldness

The indications in posterior baldness are more difficult to define in some cases.

1. In cases of isolated vertical baldness, i.e. C1 F1 T4, the operative indications are often difficult to establish:
   - Treatment by cylindrical autografts involves three or four operative sessions and renders any other subsequent technique impossible if the baldness deteriorates.
   - Repeated vertical reduction gives good results in moderate vertical baldness if the scalp is supple. Its peformance prevents that of a subse-

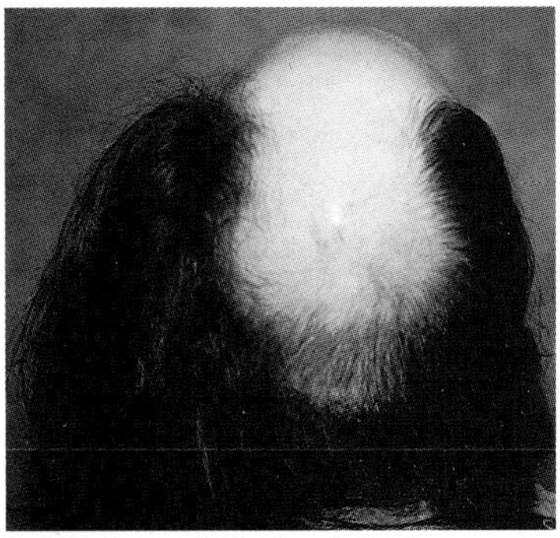
d

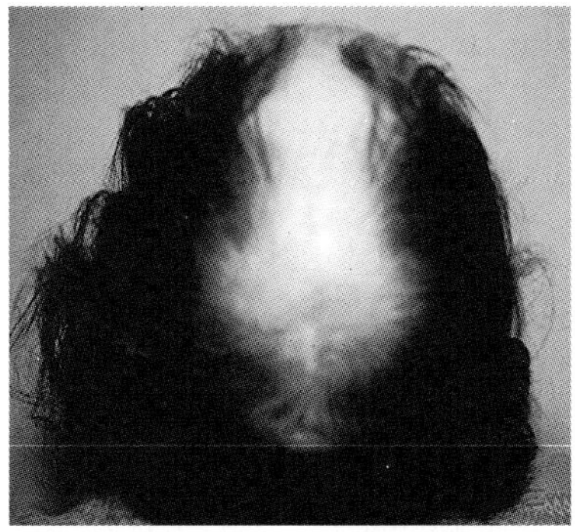

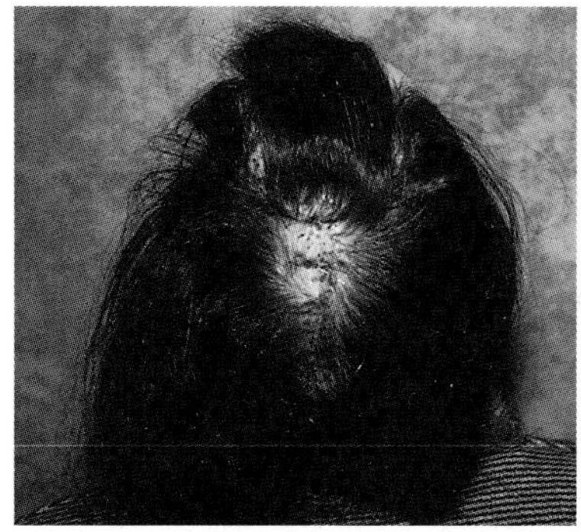
e,f

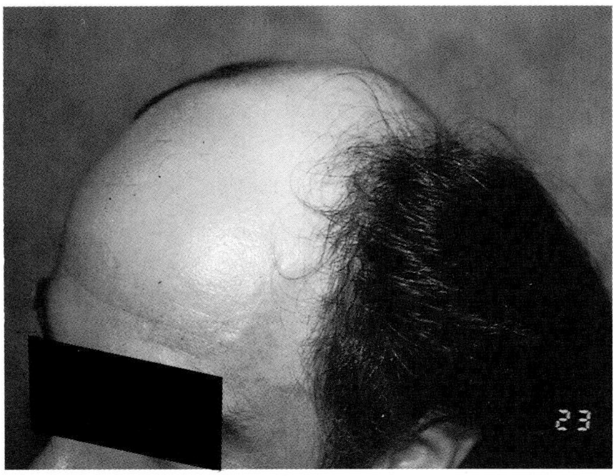
g

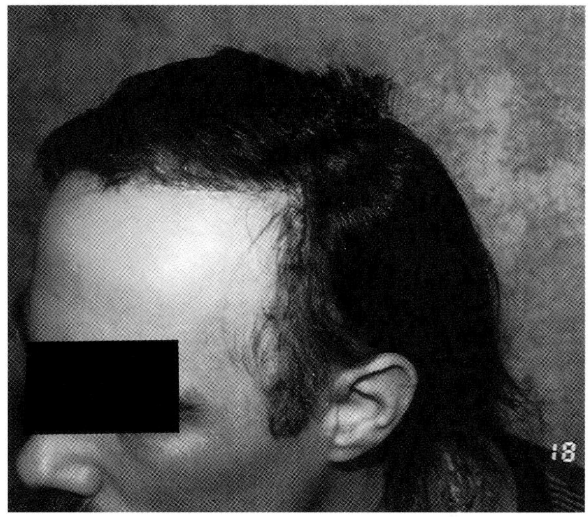
h

Photo 29a–h. Treatment of major baldness by two scalp lifts combined with two vertical flaps by parasagittal route. **a** Preoperative aspect, anterior view. **b** Aspect after scalp lift combined with two mini-flaps by parasagittal route, anterior view. **c** Aspect after two scalp lifts, anterior view. **d** Preoperative aspect, superior view. **e** Postoperatively, superior view. **f** After two scalp lifts, superior view. **g** Preoperative aspect, three-quarters view. **h** Aspect after two scalp lifts, three-quarters view

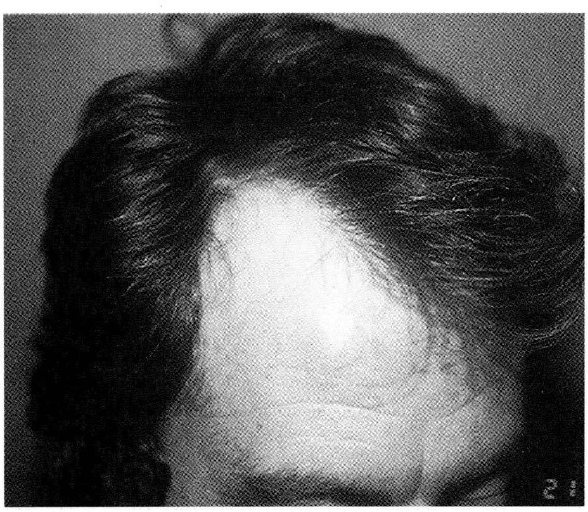
a

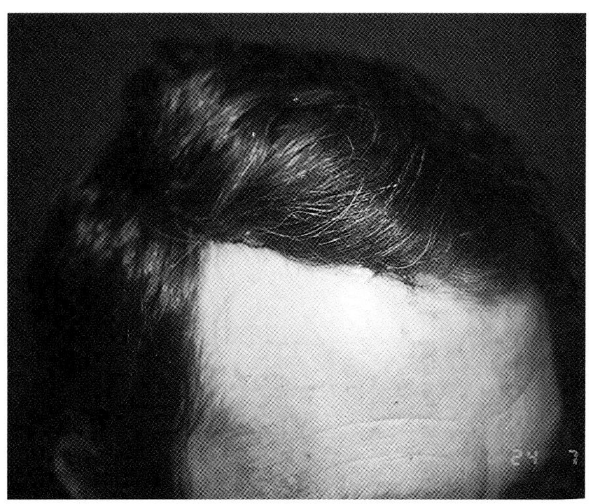
b

Photo 30. **a** Minor frontal recession *f*(2). **b** Correction by vertical mini-flap in one stage

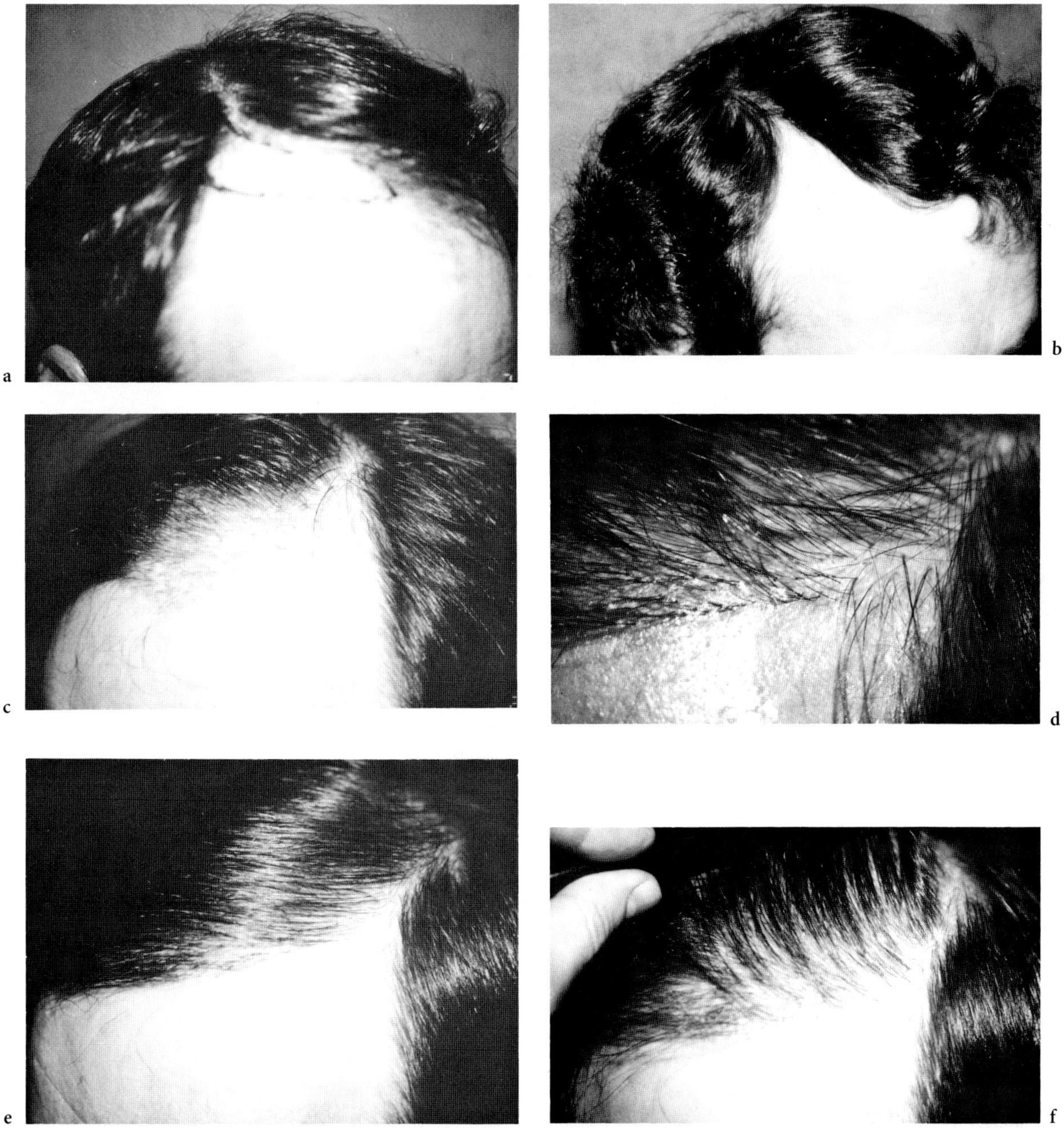

Photo 31. **a** Early stages of baldness, recession from the frontal line. **b** Result after treatment using one vertical, preauricular flap. **c** Treatment of the opposite side using micrografts; result after the first treatment session. **d** Result after the second treatment session. **e** Result after three treatment sessions using micrografts. Hair combed to form a side-parting. **f** Hair combed to show the hair density obtained

quent vertical flap but is compatible with lifting of the scalp. The design is adaptable to the shape of the vertex.

- Performance of a flap is always difficult in this region as, during its placement, one often arrives at a sharp demarcation between the flap and the frontal region (Photo 36) or obvious differences of density with adjacent zones (Photo 37).
- Lastly, when S is ½, we perform repeated vertical reductions; if S is ¾, we prefer mini- and micrografts.

2. For the quite common type of baldness rated C1 T3 F2 *f*2, where HO is 15 cm and HT is 6 cm

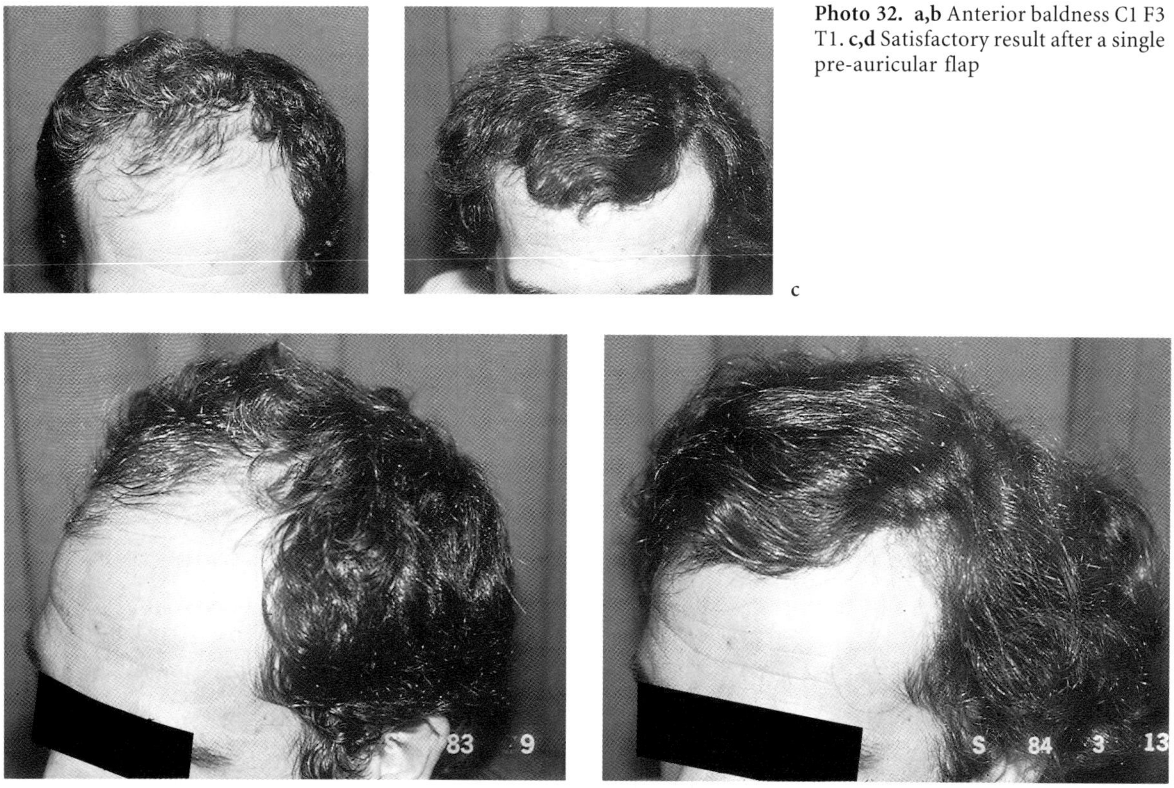

a c b d

Photo 32. a,b Anterior baldness C1 F3 T1. **c,d** Satisfactory result after a single pre-auricular flap

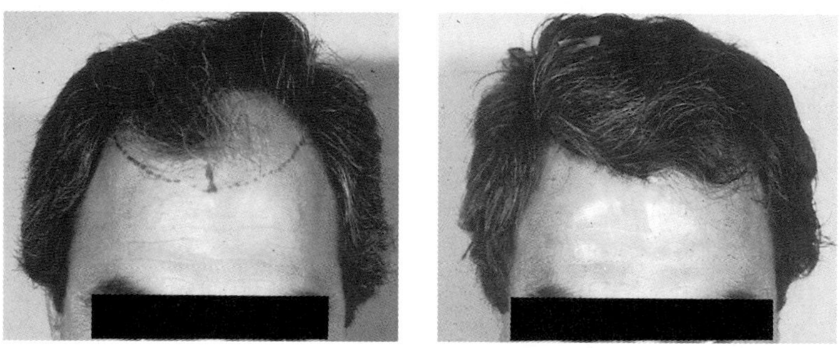

a b

Photo 33. a Frontal baldness. **b** Immediate result after Dardour-type pre-auricular flap

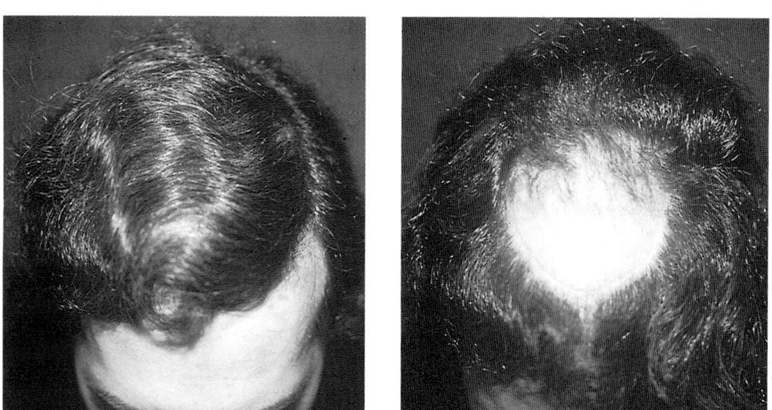

a b

Photo 34a,b. Two pre-auricular flaps may appear satisfactory for coverage of frontal baldness; actually, they leave a central triangle very difficult to cover secondarily except by autografts and sacrifice of both temporal arteries

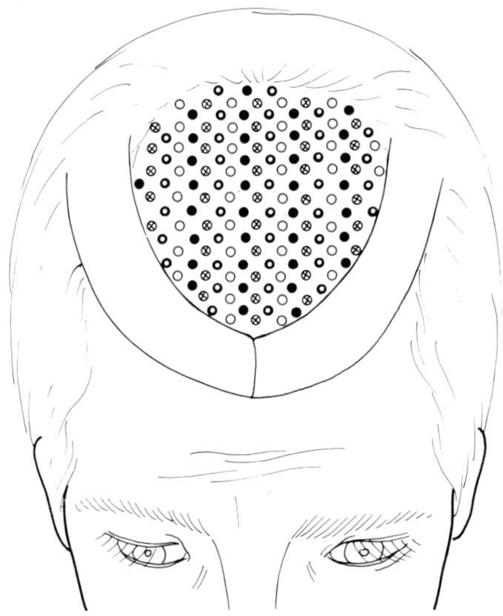

Fig. 17. Placement of two vertical flaps leaves a smooth median triangle which cannot be covered by grafts

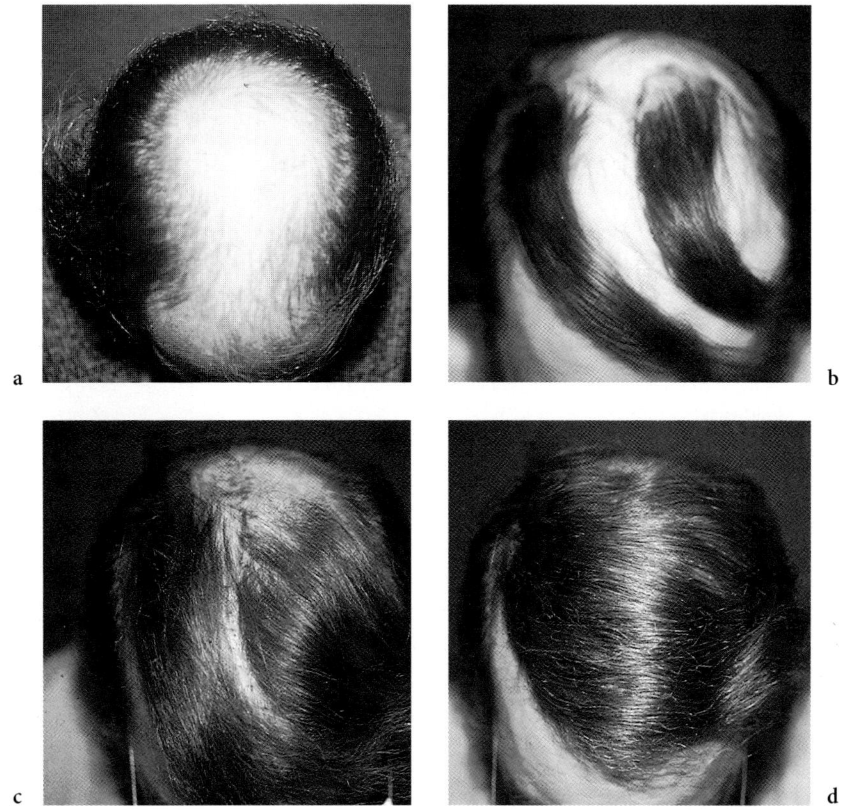

Photo 35. a Baldness stage 3. **b** Result after two vertical pre-auricular flaps in parallel. **c,d** Aspect after excision of intermediate bald zone

(patient with a vertex of around 6 cm in the antero-posterior direction, a very slightly thinned frontal region and fronto-temporal areas a little receded), we suggest an original procedure: giant reduction or lifting of the scalp by the peripheral route combined with one or two vertical flaps at the same time (Photo 38). The gain in reduction allows advancement of the temporal line at the same time as ascending the vertex. A vertical flap with a postero-superior pedicle can then be fashioned on one or both sides situated at the most anterior part of the biparieto-occipital flap.

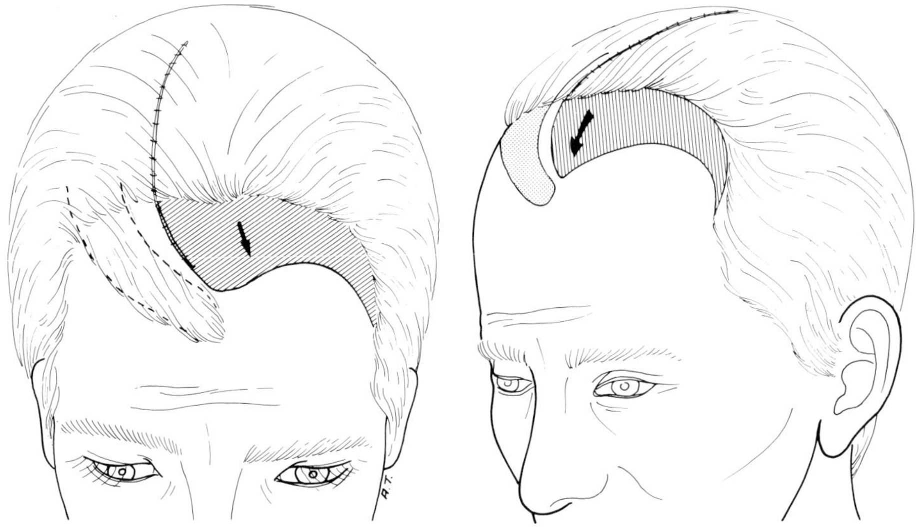

Fig. 18a,b. Pre-auricular flap and rotation flap

This flap, which may be 5–7 cm long and 2 cm wide, is transposed forward to recreate a frontal line.

If the flap reaches the mid-line, it is impossible to shape another flap on the opposite side as their junction at the mid-line would demarcate a posterior oval zone at the vertex deprived of any peripheral vascular supply. However, it is possible to construct two small flaps which, when tilted forward, leave an anterior and median skin bridge of 4 cm, which allows vascularisation of the vertex.

3. In the case of baldness type C1 T2 F2 G1, there is simple decrease in density in the frontal or temporal zones; it is usually best to do nothing as no technique will give satisfactory results. However, the placement of micrografts may sometimes be considered to slightly densify a region. In all cases the result obtained by flaps or reductions can be improved by limited sessions of autografts or micrografts, as required, particularly to improve the appearance of an anterior scar or to fill in a small residual smooth zone.

Conclusion

Certain rules may be deduced from these indications:

1. When F is 3 or 4 and/or *t* is 2 or 3, at least a vertical flap is necessary: pre- or retro-auricular flap (if *t*=3) or in some cases a mini-flap (*f*=2), alone or combined with scalp lifting.

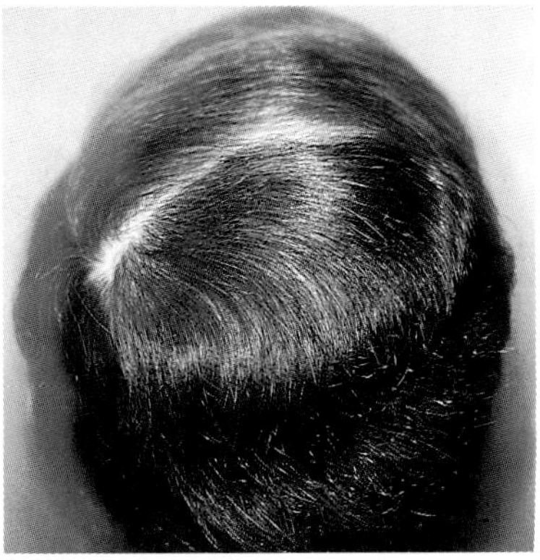

Photo 36. The vertical flap often raises the problem of its demarcation with the frontal zone

2. When T is 3 or 4, several vertical reductions may be indicated. If these need to be combined with a flap, they can be performed chronologically after the flap(s), or simultaneously in the context of a scalp lifting.
3. We consider grafts as the technique of choice to improve the result.
4. Lifting of the scalp is finding ever-increasing indications.

For the reader's information, we compare these indications with those of other authors (Unger) using Norwood's classification:

- Types I and II: 150–175 grafts, i.e. four sessions. We prefer two mini-flaps, i.e. two operative sessions.
- Type III: 175–225 grafts, i.e. four procedures. We prefer one or two pre-auricular flaps.

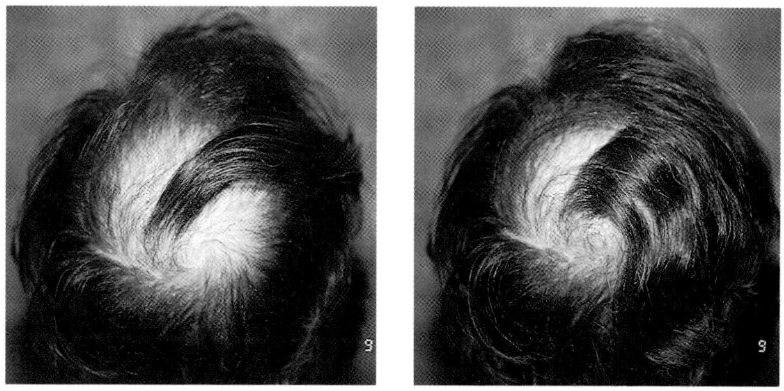

Photo 37a,b. The vertical flap covers the bald zone when the hair is dressed, but often raises problems of different density from the adjacent anterior zone

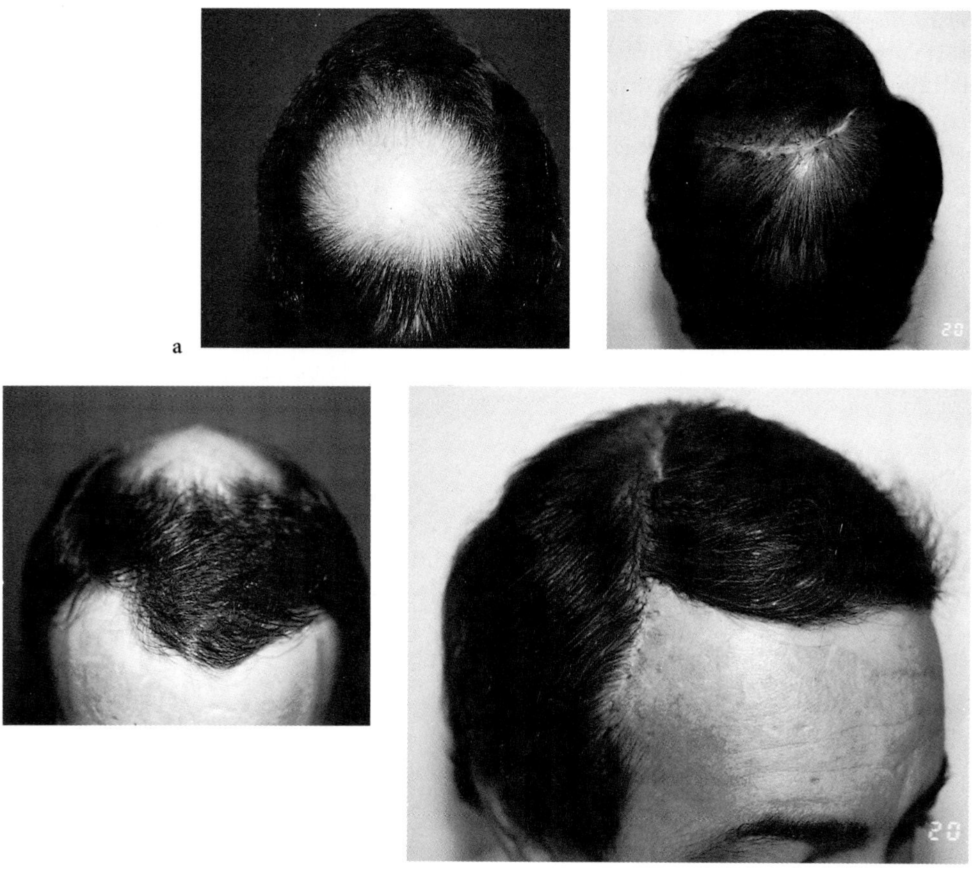

Photo 38. a,b Baldness T4 F2 (wide vertex and fronto-temporal recession by 1–2 cm). **c,d** One-stage treatment by scalp lift combined with right vertical pre-auricular flap (personal technique)

- Type IV: 300–400 grafts at the back and 200 grafts or two reductions at the front (six to eight operations). We prefer a pre- or retro-auricular flap followed by scalp lifting combined with a vertical mini-flap (two operative sessions) or two scalp liftings with a 4-month interval.
- Type V: two or three reductions followed by 300–400 grafts, i.e. six or eight sessions. We prefer a pre-auricular flap followed by one or two scalp liftings, sometimes supplemented by a sagittal reduction, i.e. two or three procedures.

- Type VI: 800 grafts or four reductions followed by 500 grafts. We prefer a pre- or retro-auricular flap followed by two giant reductions and possibly supplemented by two grafting sessions. The first flap can also be replaced by a scalp lifting.

Variation in Operative Indications Related to Certain Factors

Age

Although our statistics do not supply any proof of a higher incidence of necrosis in elderly patients, we usually prefer not to construct flaps in subjects over 60 years, though this limit is naturally variable in terms of physiological age. In a very young subject with commencing early baldness, we consider that an initial large flap is indicated rather than a mini-flap, since this flap will be only the first stage of the treatment of advancing baldness.

Heavy Smokers

Smoking more than 60 cigarettes a day is in our view a contraindication to the use of flaps, even if performed in three stages, the incidence of necrosis appearing greater in such cases.

Scalp Elasticity

Scalp elasticity (S) may modify the operative indications; in general, very poor elasticity (S=4) may indicate a preference for autografts rather than reductions of doubtful efficacy. Similarly, it may call for the use of an expander before construction of a flap.

Hair Colour

Hair colour may modify certain indications. In subjects with light skin and very light or greying blond, white or chestnut hair, autografts give good results, always provided they are thick enough, as their covering power is less than that of dark hair. In contrast, subjects with brown hair, particularly against a light skin, are very poor indications for autografts, as the "doll's hair" aspect here is very difficult to conceal. It is here that micrografts are particularly valuable.

Crinkly Hair

Crinkly hair has excellent covering power and several sessions of autografts often give a spectacular result.

Thinned Crown

In the case of a thinned crown (C=2), the donor zone is a poor one and, in our opinion, a contraindication to any form of surgery, as is often also the case in the alopecia of elderly subjects and women.

Variation in Indications Related to Patient and Surgeon

Variation Related to the Patient

Some patients routinely decline a technique, usually a flap, either because they believe that it is too "surgical" or more often because a non-specialist colleague or even a magazine has claimed that the method is dangerous. Once the surgeon has given his patient the fullest information, he must either accept the patient's choice or decline to operate.

Some choices must be suited to the patient's activities. If he is in frequent contact with the public, he will be reluctant to accept the use of an expander and similarly autografting on a completely bald frontal region, which will produce a considerable cosmetic defect for about a year. A patient who is not available for follow-up after operation is unsuitable for a flap or skin expansion.

Variation Related to the Surgeon

Some surgeons do not know how to construct flaps, while others do not have the patience to perform autografting properly. Obviously, such considerations will, consciously or unconsciously, influence the surgeon in his choice. It is normal to prefer to advise those techniques with which one is most familiar, provided of course that they lead to equivalent results. However, we believe that a surgeon should not completely refuse a technique on any grounds whatever.

Special Cases

Some patients who have had a Juri flap often consult us for cosmetic improvement of their result, complaining particularly of hair growth backward, a defect for which nothing can be done. However, they also very often complain of insufficiently hollowed areas of fronto-temporal recession and the aspect on the side of the flap of major frontal creases, sometimes even ptosis of the eyelid, due to an excess of skin supplied by rotation of the flap (Photo 39).

To correct these defects, we have developed a technique for replacement of the pedicle of the flap at the site where it was raised. This replacement is always rendered very difficult by secondary skin contracture and by the zones excised at the original procedure. This is why we recommend the following technique (Fig. 19):

- Repetition of the anterior frontal incision on the side of the pedicle from near the mid-line as far as the anterior temporal line over about 2 cm (line AB).
- Stripping the forehead and performance of a unilateral frontal lift.
- Stripping the scalp backward as far as possible.
- This creates a flap BCD, which corresponds to the origin of the Juri flap but is wider by 2–2.5 cm and is rotated backward into its original position at BC'D.
- Backward reopening of the entire incision of the donor zone to the origin of the flap, then incision of the origin of the posterior margin of the flap over 5–6 cm.
- Replacement of the upper scalp with separation of the margins, yielding a triangular flap with the apex forward (D), which is normally placed at the base of the fronto-temporal recession at the junction of the frontal and anterior temporal lines. The dog-ear can be ignored or dealt with by a small triangular resection at the posterior apex.
- The flap fashioned at the start of the procedure is placed in the loss of substance created (BC'D), thus replacing the hair in the right direction (Photo 40).

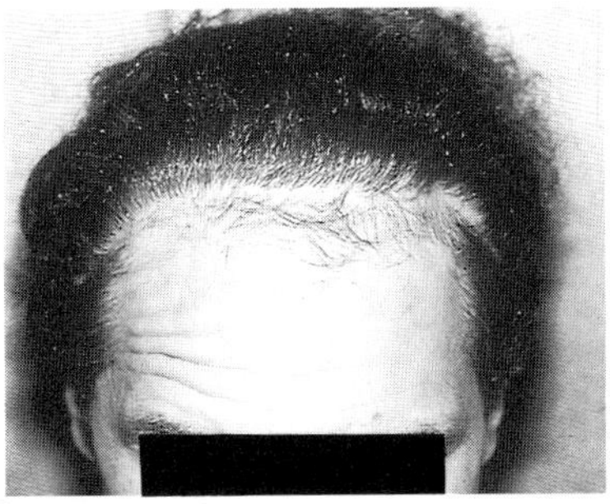

a

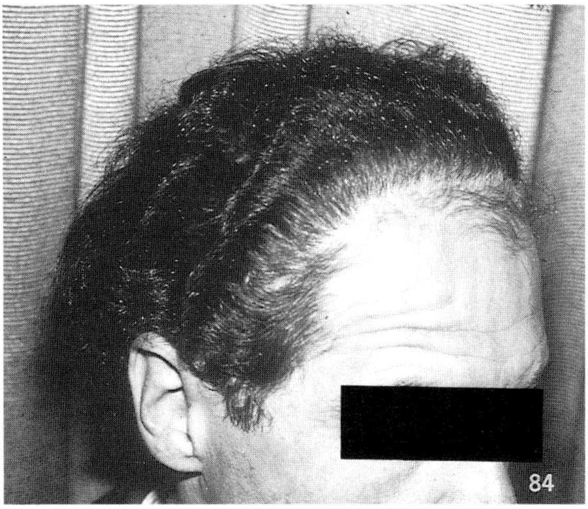

b

Photo 39a,b. Juri flap with classical defects: hair growth backward, absence of fronto-temporal recession and side-parting

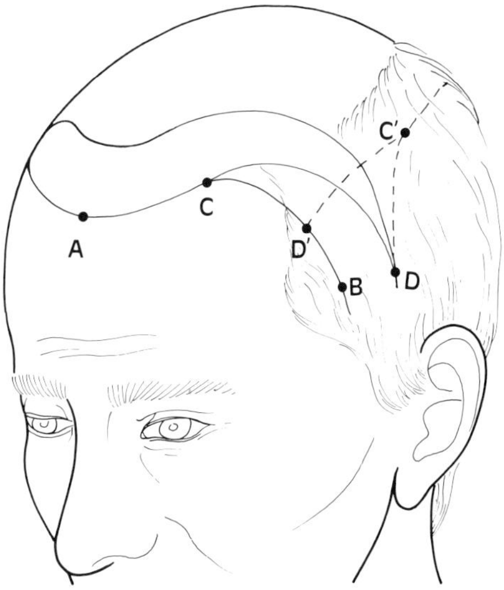

Fig. 19. Principle of correction of defects of Juri flap

Frontal Lifting in Bald Men

Scalp lifting in men essentially raises the problem of choice of incisions in both the pre-auricular and temporal regions. This problem is particularly acute in frontal lifting for bald men, and no solution has been put forward to our knowledge. In the normal subject two choices are possible: a posterior bi-coronal incision and a marginal incision, which can be extended laterally into the temporal region, marginally or within the hair-bearing zone (Fig. 20). The marginal incision raises the problem of secondary recession at the frontal line, which will unmask the scar. The posterior incision causes recession of the frontal line, which is always embarrassing in men as it deepens the fronto-temporal recession. In the bald subject, the scar of frontal lifting is always obvious and therefore unacceptable. For this reason, we propose simultaneous correction of the baldness by two vertical pre-auricular flaps as already described.

Description of Technique

The flap is begun 4 or 5 cm behind the temporal hair line and is concave towards the front; its first part is vertical and the second transverse, and it ends above the ear. This is the Dardour type of pre-auricular flap, as previously described. It is 15–16 cm long and 3.5 cm wide at its origin and 2.5 cm at its extremity. So designed, the temporal incision allows raising of the flap intended to correct the baldness and to perform frontal lifting (Fig. 21, Photo 41). If facial lifting is required, the incision descends in front of the ear. If cervical lifting is unnecessary, we halt the incision at the level of the ear lobe.

We then perform the frontal lifting by an incision at the level of the theoretic marginal line (Fig. 22). For greater convenience, the exact position of this frontal marginal line is marked on the underlying periosteum, as it is more difficult to determine after stripping of the frontal region and vertex. The frontal lifting is made in the classical manner, and the excess skin is resected using the bony landmarks as stated. Before suturing the frontal line, we raise the lateral flaps. This zone is actually the skin resected in a classical frontal lifting. To obtain a wider flap we perform very major stripping of the parietal scalp behind the flap. In this way both flaps can be 3.5 cm wide and suture of the donor zone can be made without tension.

The two flaps are then put into place in the frontal region, always using the same bony landmarks.

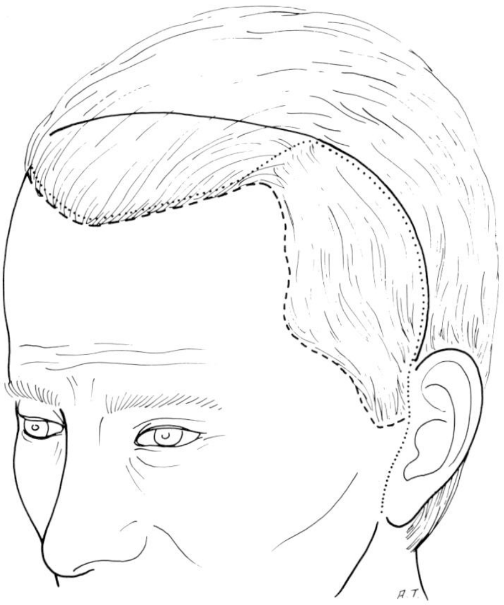

Fig. 20. Possible incisions for frontal lifting

a 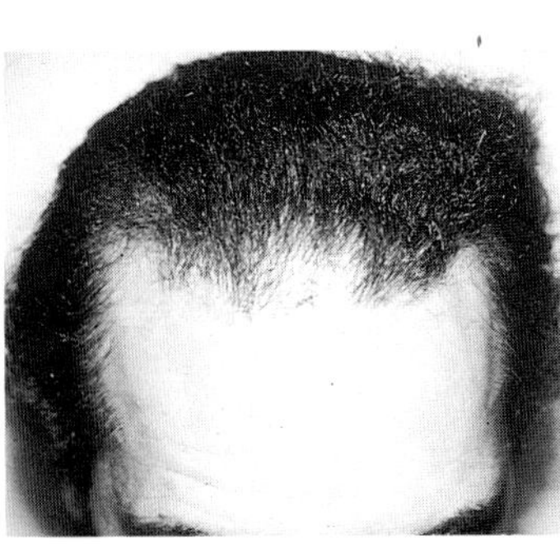 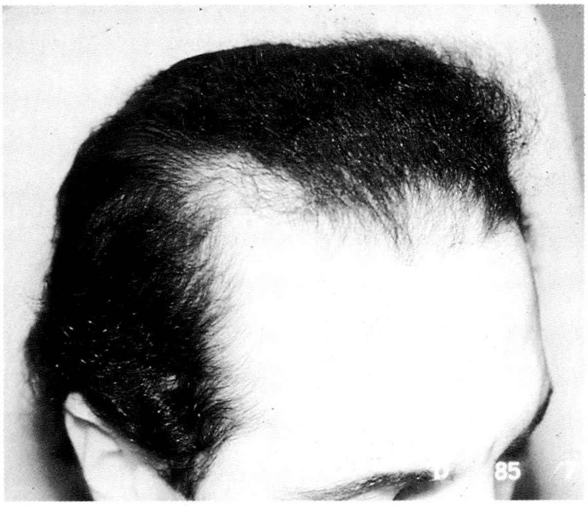 b

Photo 40a,b. Correction by our technique of reposition of initial segment of flap

This technique provides deep fronto-temporal recession with a natural appearance and hair which grows forward in the physiological manner. Thanks to this technique, it may be stated that correction of the baldness is at least as important as lifting as regards the rejuvenating effects obtained. Moreover, the scar of the frontal lifting is then completely invisible (Photo 42).

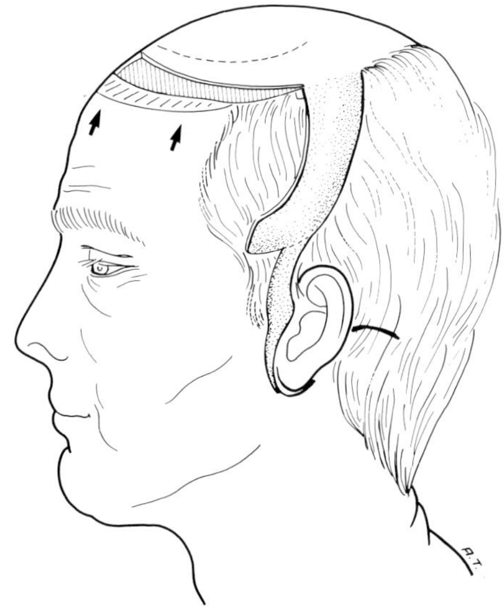

Fig. 21. Lifting combined with flap

Lifting for Frontal Thinning in Men (Photo 43)

When frontal lifting is required for slight thinning, the risks of two classical marginal and posterior incisions have been noted: one risk being unmasked as baldness progresses, the other moves back a frontal line that is already too posterior. In this case we advise an anterior marginal incision combined with two vertical mini-flaps, which we now perform to correct simple fronto-temporal recession in commencing baldness.

The line of incision is located at the anterior limit of the frontal and temporal lines. The two vertical mini-flaps with superior pedicles are then designed to begin at the anterior temporal line. They are 2 cm wide and 10 cm long. One must foresee the excision of an anterior frontal scalp zone, which is the thinned zone that will receive the two flaps after their transposition. After having made the fronto-temporal incision, this line is located on the periosteum as before. The frontal skin is stripped as far as the eyelids to allow frontal lifting with excision as required of 1–2 cm of excess skin. The two vertical flaps are then raised and the temporal scalp is stripped backward for 6–7 cm to allow closure without tension, thus avoiding receding of the temporal line (*t*).

The flaps are then transposed forward and sutured to the frontal line, after excision of a zone of

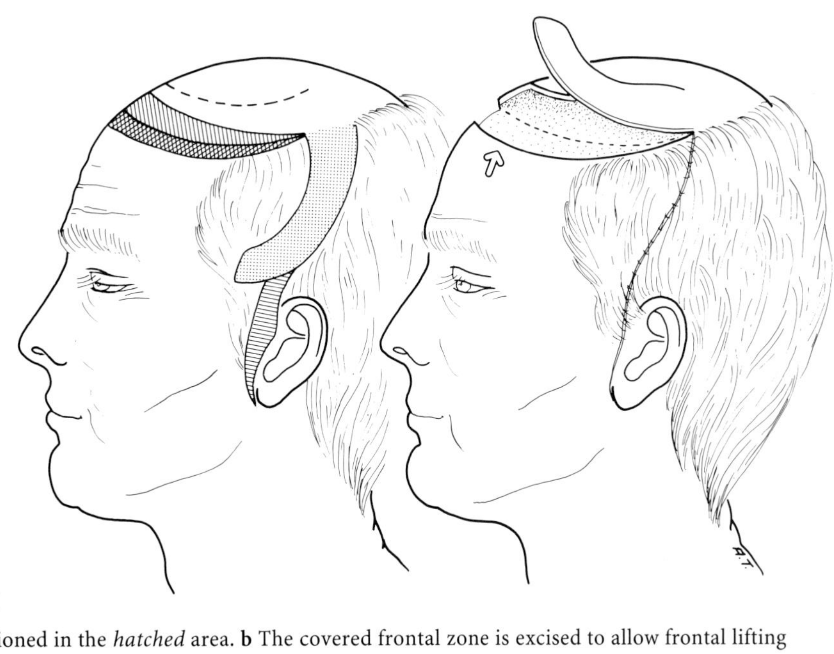

a b

Fig. 22. a The flap in *grey* is positioned in the *hatched* area. **b** The covered frontal zone is excised to allow frontal lifting a 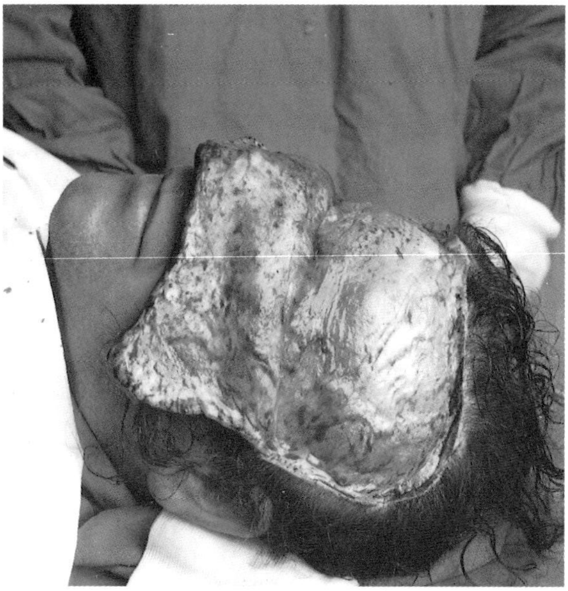

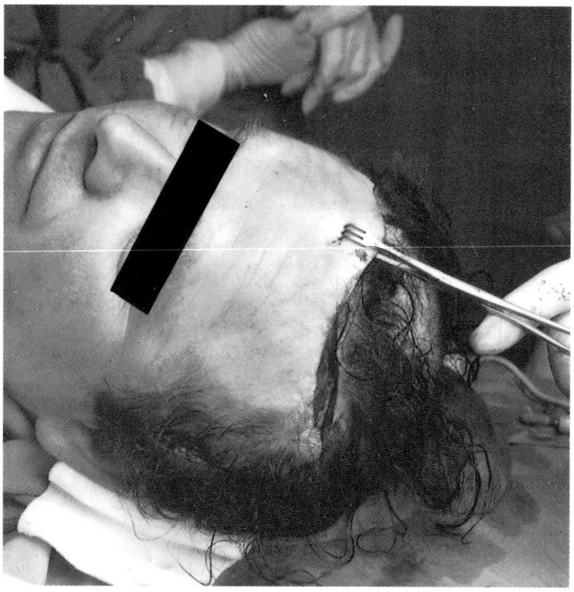 b

c 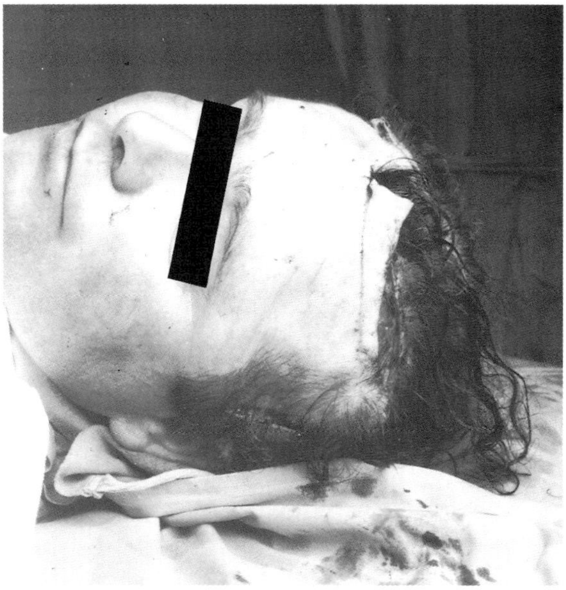

Photo 41. **a,b** Frontal lifting is done before the flap. The temporal incision corresponds to the former flap incision. **c** Resected frontal zone

frontal scalp 1–1.5 cm wide. This gives a guarantee for the future, as these grafted hairs never fall out.

In cases of advanced baldness, it is possible to combine this procedure with scalp lifting by a sagittal route, which permits simultaneous removal of an antero-posterior sagittal strip of scalp of about 5 cm. In this case a second intervention is arranged 4 months later; this allows repeated excision of 5 cm of the smooth area, i.e. in general of the residual smooth zone, and coverage of the frontal region by two other vertical flaps transposed in place of the former flaps, which are themselves transferred medial to the above.

Correction of Grafted Fronto-temporal Recession by Frontal Lifting

It is common to see frontal recession treated with poor cosmetic results by cylindrical autografts. The doll's hair aspect may be due to an insufficient number of grafts, to a poor indication (light skin with dark hair) or too vertical an implantation of the grafts.

Correction may be made in these cases by the addition of properly positioned grafts very oblique towards the front, fusiform grafts or micrografts, but in some cases the patient asks for simple excision of these grafts.

In cases with bad implantation which completely obscures the fronto-temporal recession, such excision of the grafts is obligatory. In such cases, we perform a frontal lifting, which allows excision of the frontal skin zone carrying the grafts in one stage, and then redesign the fronto-temporal recession as required (Photo 44). The technique of the frontal lifting is classical. However, if it is unnecessary to lift the eyelids the stripping stops there, making lifting below this zone ineffective. Sometimes, when the area of the grafted zone is too large, two similar procedures at some months' interval are required to excise it completely. This technique of frontal lifting seems preferable to that of excision of the grafts one

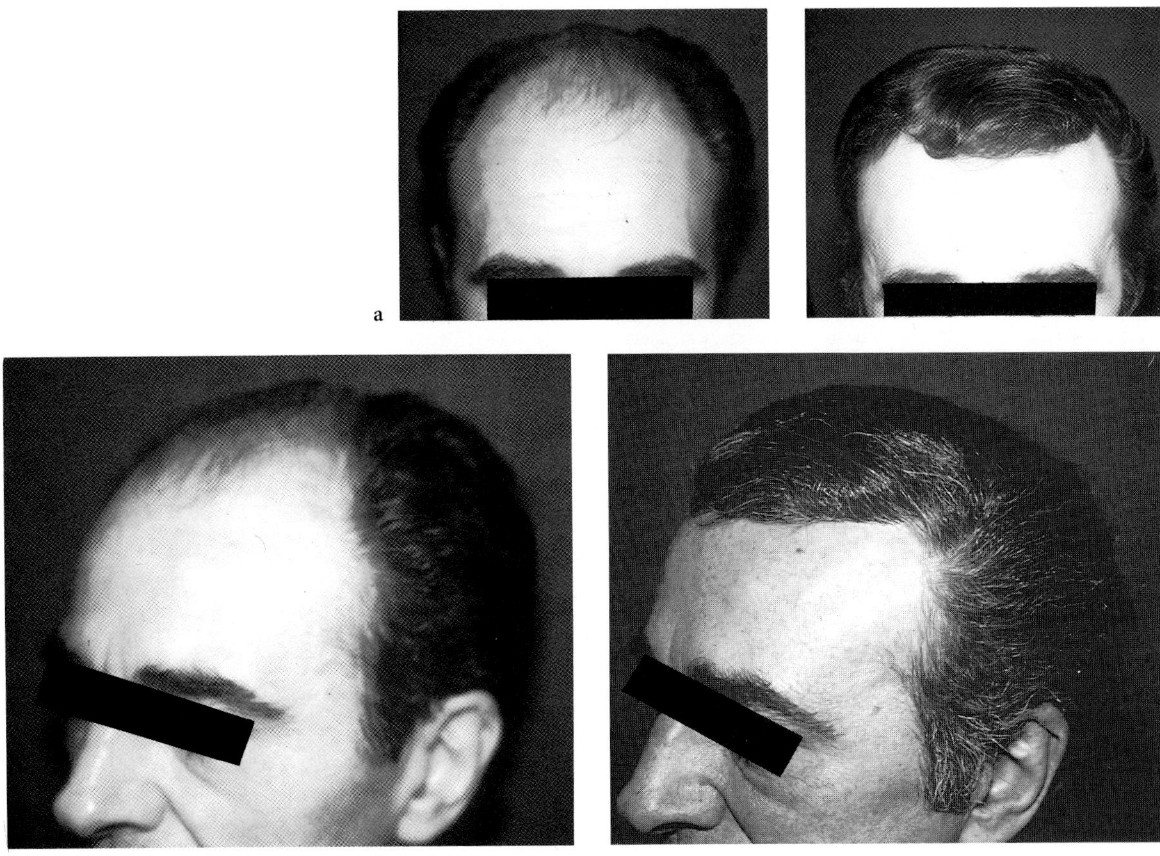

a c b d

Photo 42a–d. Frontal lifting combined with two pre-auricular flaps of the Dardour type. **a,b** Preoperative. **c,d** Postoperative

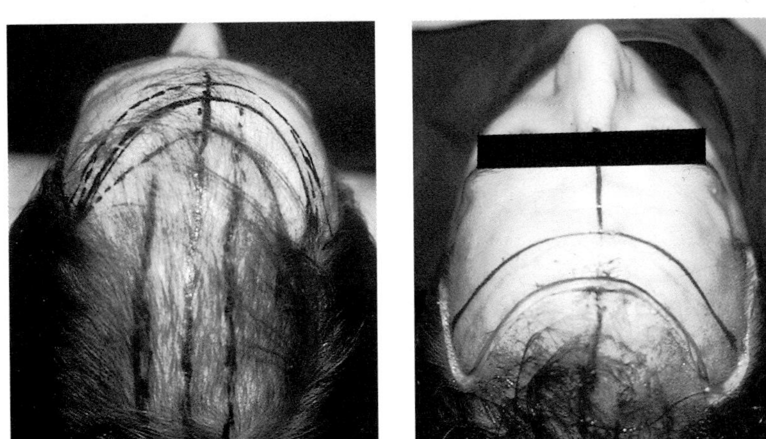

a b

Photo 43a,b

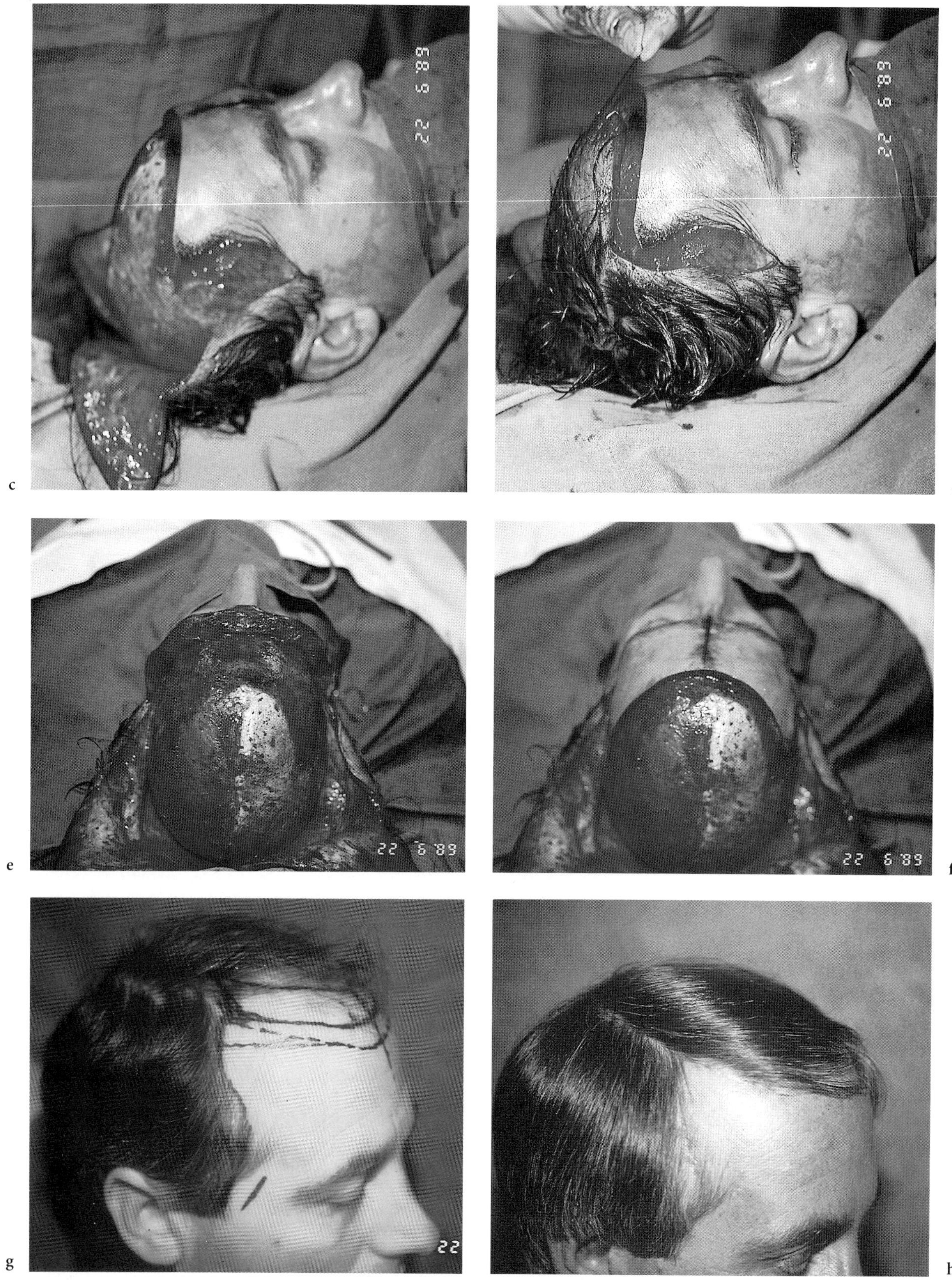

Photo 43. a,b Frontal lifting in man with onset of baldness: design of excised zones. **c,d** Incision and stripping of scalp with fashioning of two vertical temporal mini-flaps. **e,f** Stripping of scalp and frontal skin up to eyebrows. **g,h** Pre- and immediate postoperative aspects: obliteration of frontal creases and camouflage of anterior scar by two vertical mini-grafts

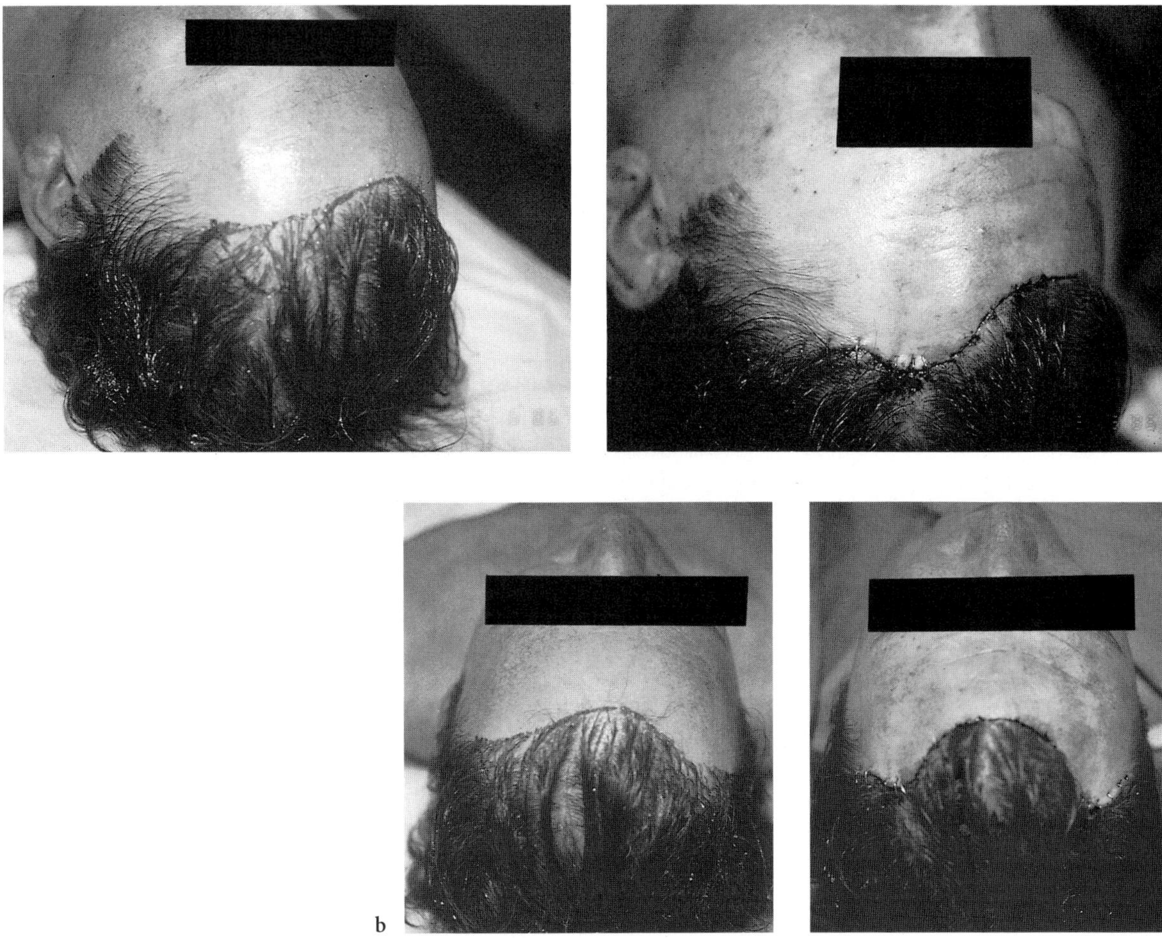

Photo 44. a,b Unaesthetic filling of fronto-temporal recession by cylindrical autografts. **c,d** Correction by excision of grafted zone combined with frontal lifting allowing recreation of harmonious anterior line

by one, which has the disadvantage of leaving an often unpleasing pattern of scars.

Flap–Grafts and Graft–Flaps

The combination of a vertical pre- or post-auricular flap followed by three or four sessions of autografts is a possible sequence in the correction of progressive baldness. It involves correction in four or five stages, but it allows uniform distribution of the hair behind the grafts with a lesser density than that of the flap. For safety reasons, the flap must precede the autografting. The flap will mask the temporary unaesthetic effect of the latter.

Some patients originally treated by autografts are sometimes unsatisfied because the number of grafts implanted is insufficient, because the technique was poorly executed, leaving partial, irregular or badly distributed regrowth, or because the indication was doubtful: subjects with stiff, dark, thick hair on a fair skin. In all these cases, the placement of a flap with a superior pedicle will allow correction of a poor result in a single procedure.

Two conditons are essential for the performance of this technique:

- The number of grafts originally performed must not be too great, and in particular they must not have been implanted close to the future pedicle of the flap, i.e. in practice on the vertex.
- It is usually preferable for safety reasons to perform a three-stage technique, i.e. with two preliminary stages of autonomisation.

Very useful results have been obtained with this technique (Photos 45–47).

Alopecia in Women

Alopecia in women is usually rated C2 F2 T2 S4. It therefore combines diffuse thinning with an al-

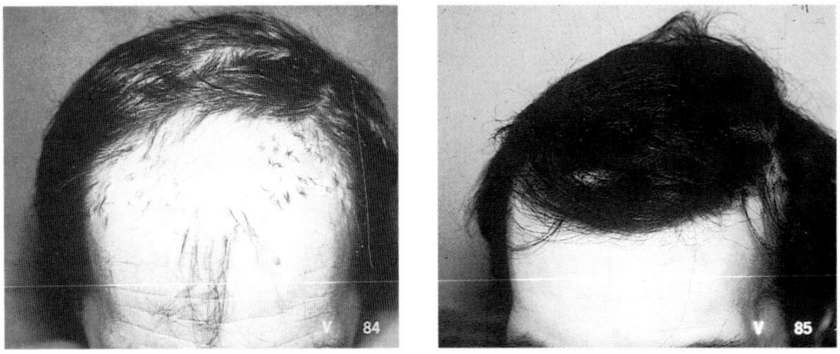

a b

Photo 45. **a** Failure of cylindrical grafts. **b** Correction by Dardour-type pre-auricular flap in one stage

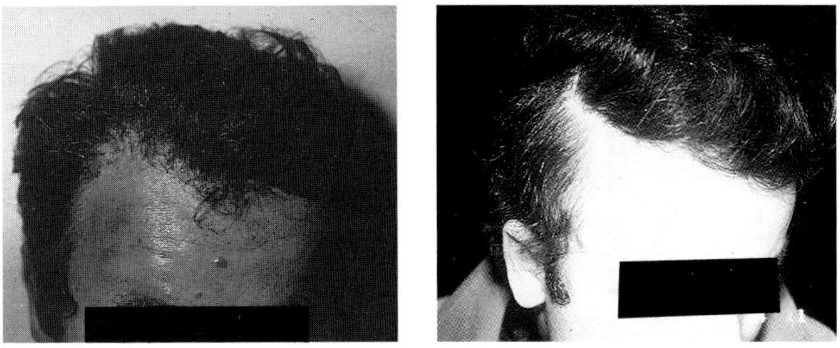

a b

Photo 46. **a** Classical doll's hair aspect after inadequate cylindrical autografts. **b** Correction by Dardour-type pre-auricular flap in one stage

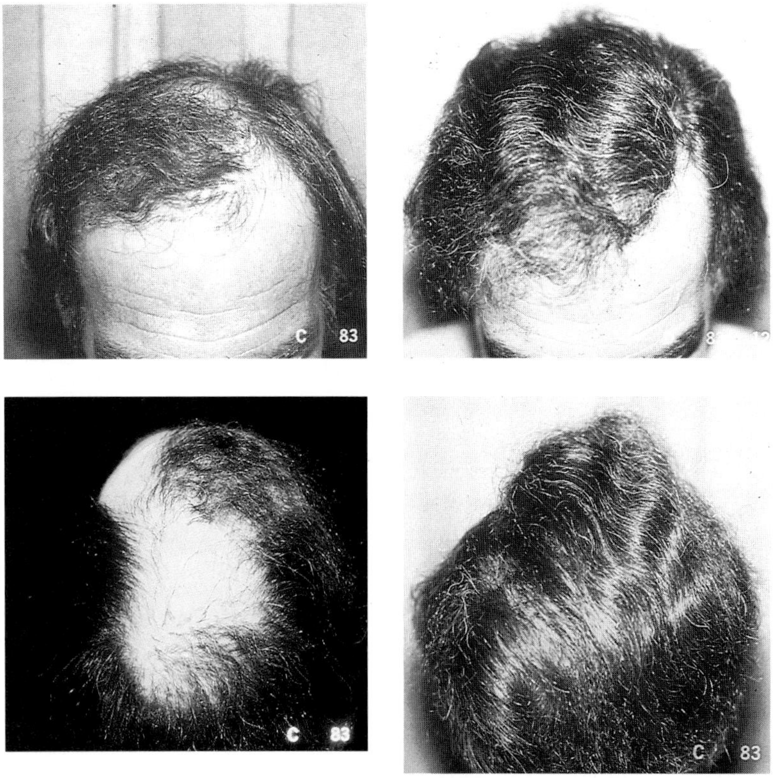

a b c d

Photo 47. **a,b** Inadequate result after implantation of 350 grafts intended to correct baldness stage 3. **c,d** Result after correction by pre-auricular flap made in three stages because of increased risk of necrosis due to scars of grafts

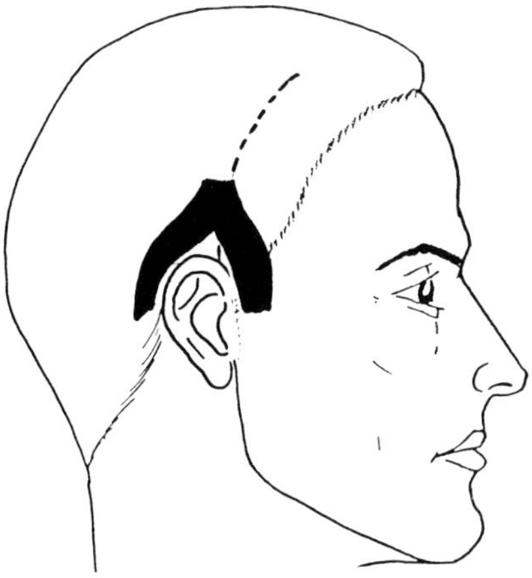

Fig. 23. Retro-auricular flap

most total absence of scalp laxity, which contraindicates any flaps or vertical reduction. The sole solution is the judicious distribution of mini- and micrografts at the vertex. If the patient chooses to dress her hair backward, the grafts are placed at the frontal region. If she dresses her hair at the side, with a parting, the grafts are distributed over this parting, over a breadth of 3–4 cm and possibly supplemented over a frontal band.

Treatment of Temporal Alopecia Secondary to Lifting

The difficult problem of temporal alopecia secondary to lifting may be solved in different ways depending on its origin. The wide temporal scar is usually due to closure under excessive tension or sometimes to an incision perpendicular to the scalp. A correct incision with the scalpel parallel to the follicles and suture in one layer by staples is sufficient. Recession of the temporal line may justify a rotation-advancement flap, which is easier and quicker to perform, when possible, than micrografting.

Sometimes the sideburn disappears completely, because it is thrust upward and backward. In these cases we use a small retro-auricular flap. The anterior border of this flap must lie in the extension of the temporal lifting scar (Fig. 23).

Conclusion

The great variety of types of baldness and the multiplicity of techniques make the operative indications very difficult to establish. Systematic refusal of a technique handicaps the surgeon and is harmful to the patient. Before undertaking treatment, the surgeon should always have drawn up a strict plan in order to deal with the possibilities of each technique.

References

1. Bouhanna P, Nataf J (1976) À propos des transplantations de cuir chevelu. Critiques et propositions. Rev Chir Esthet 7(2): 17–23
2. Bouhanna P (1989) Greffes à cheveux longs immédiats. Nouv Dermatol 8(4): 418–420
3. Bouhanna P (1990) Les lambeaux de cuir chevelu à charnière haute. Ann Chir Plast Esthet 35(5): 397–404
4. Bouhanna P (1993) Newer techniques in hair replacement. In: Roenigk RK, Roenigk-Martin H (eds) New trends in dermatologic surgery. Dunitz, New York, pp 527–553
5. Dardour JC (1989) Traitement moderne de la calvitie. J Head Neck Pathol 4: 123–130
6. Dardour JC (1983) Treatment of male baldness with a one stage flap rotation. In: Transactions of the VIII Congress of Plast Surgery, Montreal, June 26–July 1, pp 680–681
7. Dardour JC (1989) Les réductions de tonsure. Principes et innovation: le lifting du scalp. Ann Chir Plast Esthet 34(3): 234–242
8. Dardour JC (1991) Treatment of male pattern baldness and post-operative temporal baldness in men. Clin Plast Surg 8(4): 775–790
9. Mahe E, Camblin J (1974) La ligne frontale dans le traitement de l'alopécie idiopathique masculine. Ann Chir Plast Esthet 19(1): 61–68
10. Mayer TG, Fleming RW (1985) Aesthetics and styling in hair replacement surgery. Facial Plast Surg 2(3): 235–244
11. Norwood OT, Shiell RC (1984) Hair transplant surgery, 2nd edn. Thomas, Springfield
12. Unger WP, Nordström R (1988) Hair transplantation. Dekker, New York

Conclusion

Great progress has been made in the surgery of male baldness in recent years. The technique of grafting has developed toward miniaturisation, going as far as micrografts, which have abolished the "doll's hair" aspect so prejudicial to such treatment. The techniques of flaps have become more reliable, leading to more cosmetically successful results. The techniques of classical reduction and sometimes of lifting the scalp allow rapid treatment of major baldness.

All these procedures, far from excluding each another, should be combined in the same patient or be performed as supplements to yield the best result. The importance of the operative indications must be stressed.

In women, on the other hand, only the transplantation of judiciously distributed minigrafts is compatible with the diffuse nature of alopecia.